PSYCHIATRIC NURSING

Nursing Reading Series

A BOOK OF READINGS

PSYCHIATRIC NURSING

Developing Psychiatric Nursing Skills

Volume One

Second Edition

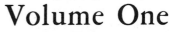

Dorothy Mereness
Dean, School of Nursing
University of Pennsylvania

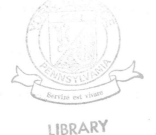

WM. C. BROWN COMPANY PUBLISHERS
Dubuque, Iowa

NURSING SERIES

Consulting Editor

ANNA KUBA

Copyright © 1966, 1971 by
Wm. C. Brown Company Publishers

ISBN 0–697–05513–2

Library of Congress Catalog Card Number: 76-142229

Fourth Printing, 1975

Printed in the United States of America

preface

In the hope of making available to students of professional nursing a convenient collection of articles about psychiatric nursing, two volumes of readings have been compiled—*Developing Psychiatric Nursing Skills* and *Understanding the Nurse's Role in Psychiatric Patient Care*. These volumes comprise many of the most helpful articles which have appeared in nursing literature within the past fifteen years. As far as the editor is able to determine, no other publication has attempted to present a similar compilation.

Teachers agree that one of the best ways to assist students to gain a broad professional view of the role and function of the nurse in relation to the prevention of mental illness and the care of mentally ill patients is to encourage wide reading in appropriate professional literature.

It is especially meaningful to students of nursing to have the opportunity to experience through reading the understandings and professional practices which skilled psychiatric nurses have developed and described. Although some excellent articles by representatives of other professional disciplines have been included, the editor has attempted to emphasize the work of nurses in compiling this material, which is presented in two convenient volumes. With the expenditure of the minimum amount of time and effort on the part of students, these volumes make it possible for them to enlarge their understanding of both the psychological skills involved in the practice of psychiatric nursing and the nurse's role in psychiatric patient care.

Volume One, entitled DEVELOPING PSYCHIATRIC NURSING SKILLS, is divided into five sections with material on self-understanding, communicating with patients, nurse-patient relationships, therapeutic

v

approaches to patient problems, and information about the therapeutic community.

Volume Two, entitled UNDERSTANDING THE NURSE'S ROLE IN PSYCHIATRIC PATIENT CARE, includes five sections which present material on understanding unusual behavioral manifestations, the aged patient, the alcoholic patient, the nurse's role in psychiatric therapies, and community aspects of psychiatric nursing.

Experienced psychiatric nursing practitioners will welcome these two volumes as a handy compilation of material with which they are already familiar, but to which they may return repeatedly as they seek to deepen insights and perceptions.

In addition to the course in Psychiatric Nursing, teachers in schools of nursing will find these volumes useful as a readily available supplement for concepts being taught in courses such as Fundamentals of Nursing, Care of Patients with Long-Term Illnesses, and Medical-Surgical Nursing.

Those who are familiar with psychiatric nursing literature may discover that a few of the most helpful articles which have been published in the past are not included. Unfortunately, some highly-prized material was not made available to the editor because of the policies established by the publication in which the articles originally appeared.

It is anticipated that READINGS IN PSYCHIATRIC NURSING Volumes One and Two will prove to be an indispensable supplement to any of the currently popular basic texts in psychiatric nursing.

Dorothy Mereness, Editor

introduction

As the psychiatric hospital grows more complex and as a variety of specialists are introduced to meet demonstrated patient needs in an ever-increasing number of special areas, new aspects of therapeutic nursing responsibilities will develop while at the same time some old and familiar roles will continue. It is a serious oversimplification to suggest that there is only *one* role for the nurse in a psychiatric situation. Instead it seems reasonable to believe that there will continue to be a need for nurses to fill many roles with which they are familiar and comfortable. At the same time, new roles will evolve and those with which nurses are just beginning to become acquainted will develop and expand. These new and evolving roles will require much of the same skill, understanding, and professional sophistication possessed by other well prepared professional workers in psychiatric situations.

It thus seems logical to believe that for some time to come psychiatric situations will provide an opportunity for many nurses to make a contribution in their chosen field if they are sincerely interested in understanding human behavior and willing to work hard at developing new attitudes and refining old skills. In addition, it seems likely that there will be unique opportunities for nurses with special educational preparation to develop a high degree of skill in providing interpersonal therapeutic experiences for patients.

Many nurses employed in psychiatric settings must rely upon the traditional roles with which they are familiar. Functioning within one of these roles the nurse may complement the work of the psychiatrist in the classical sense of the nurse-doctor unit, at the same time working toward developing and transforming the role in order to bring into reality the concept of a psychiatric nurse-psychiatrist team. In addition to traditional symbolic values, the nurse adds skills and knowledge not usually available to the psychologist and social worker. These involve recognizing and understanding physical aspects of mental illness including reactions to drugs and their side effects, such as hypotension and dizziness.

One important aspect of the traditional role of the nurse is as the dispenser of medications. Many nurses reject this function and feel that it is not worthy of the attention of a well-prepared psychiatric nurse. They suggest that any intelligent, accurate person can dispense drugs to psychiatric patients and point to the fact that many nonprofessional workers assume this responsibility when a nurse is not available. Drug treatment, however, is an absolute and unqualified necessity for many mentally ill patients. Some patients could never return to their homes if one of the psychopharmocological agents were not available to them. A few patients would not be able to function at even a minimal level in the hospital community if such drugs were withheld.

The dispenser of medications has an opportunity to have more frequent contacts with many patients than do other members of the staff. She has the opportunity to talk with the individual and to draw conclusions concerning his physical and emotional response to the medication and the hospital environment. If this data about patient response to treatment is gathered with insight and understanding it can be invaluable to the physician, the social worker or other professional colleagues involved with the patient and his family. If the nurse is imaginative and alert to the cues the patient presents, it is possible for her as the dispenser of medications to develop the nurse's role into a dynamic and meaningful part of the work of the psychiatric team. On the other hand, it is possible to dispense medications in an unfruitful, routine, and dull way which will contribute little to the welfare of patients or to the therapeutic work of the hospital. How the role is developed depends upon the nurse: her intellectual curiosity, her ability to learn, and her interest in and concern about the welfare of other human beings.

A second significant nursing role is that of the creator of a therapeutic environment. In many situations where a therapeutic environment is being developed, a nurse is in immediate charge of each ward and attempts to establish surroundings which reflect to the patient a consistent, rational, and safe place in which to live and learn. Maximum opportunity is provided for interpersonal interaction with both staff and other patients in situations in which skills of successful living can be learned or relearned and practiced. High expectations for socially acceptable patient behavior are held by the staff. Honest feedback for antisocial acts is provided for patients. The hospital environment is developed as much like a normal home environment as possible, with patients being encouraged to function in as many areas as practicable. Assistance is provided with only those aspects of living in which the patient is clearly inadequate.

The ingredients of a therapeutic environment are defined somewhat differently in different centers. Most people agree, however, that a therapeutic milieu provides a consistent, rational, and safe environment which is as homelike as possible where the patient is encouraged to function as independently as feasible. Role models and healthy group relationships, developed around planned activities, are included as an aspect of most situations where a therapeutic environment is being developed. The nurse is a vital factor in planning, developing, and participating in the therapeutic environment.

Other key and essential roles which the nurse in the psychiatric setting is uniquely equipped to develop include coordinating the activities in which the patient is involved; serving as the center for gathering and recording information about patients which must be communicated to the treatment team; giving physical care to those patients who require it; and initiating and directing resocialization activities with patients who need to remain on the treatment unit.

The nurse can no longer feel secure in the knowledge that if she will but follow the orders the doctor has written the patient will recover. If meaningful therapeutic decisions are to be made, the nurse must communicate effectively to the treatment team. Time spent attemping to ease the patient's adjustment to the hospital is no longer thought to be the nurse's major contribution to the care of the patient. Rather, time and effort should be directed toward strengthening the social abilities of the patient and emphasizing and re-emphasizing his role as a member of the hospital community.

If it is true, as many authorities believe, that verbal exchange between the emotionally ill individual and a healthy person is the therapeutic tool which helps correct faulty perceptions and pathological communications, the nurse who functions in a psychiatric setting has a unique therapeutic opportunity in this area. It is encouraging to observe that more and more emphasis is being placed by nurses in psychiatric settings upon the development of therapeutic relationships with patients, upon seeing them frequently and regularly, and upon working with them consistently until something positive has been achieved. Thus one of the potential therapeutic roles which the psychiatric nurse can develop even more than she has done to date is the therapeutic verbal relationship in which she helps the patient get his mind on his problem, focus on the problem, and move toward resolving it.

Since group therapy has come to be recognized as an important part of the treatment for many emotionally ill patients it seems reasonable to expect that all prepared psychiatric nurses will be pressed into service to provide this important experience. There is reason to believe that many nurses, when properly supervised, are capable of developing the skills needed to fill the role of group leader and to participate as therapist or co-therapist in group psychotherapy. Actually, when opportunities have been made available to nurses to develop group skills under proper supervision, many have become skillful psychotherapists.

When the nurse accepts responsibility for providing group psychotherapy she is confronted with the need to work in collaboration with other members of the treatment team. Although sharing information and jointly identifying treatment goals have long been one aspect of the nurse's role, accepting a peer relationship on the treatment team requires much more professional skill than many nurses have been able to achieve. With an interdisciplinary team approach, the problems of identifying role and function, of resolving the problems of overlapping, and of communication within the team become an absolute necessity. Learning the skills of collaboration, competition, and compromise is an arduous task for the disciplines involved.

A new role for the psychiatric nurse is being visualized. In this newly developing role it is anticipated that the nurse will move with ease and therapeutic skill from the hospital to the home and back to the hospital. Thus the same nurse will be able to work with the patient while he is in the hospital or at home. This role will require a great deal more knowledge and versatility than nurses have needed in the past. Concepts related to psychiatric patient care are changing so rapidly that nursing must not ignore them. As currently visualized the new mental health centers which are being developed in each state will have an impact upon the present organization of every institution now designed to care for psychiatric patients.

It is thought that large numbers of patients in state and government institutions may be able to return to their home communities within the not too distant future and be treated by the staff of the community mental health center. Many hospitals currently functioning may become the focus for such a center. The setting and the focus of these centers will present new challenges to the nurse who comes without specific preparation in psychiatric nursing. Like some of the other roles which have been discussed, the abilities which the nurse brings to the setting can be developed, supplemented, and improved by learning from other more skillful members of the clinic team. Psychiatry is on the threshold of a new era in the care of psychiatric patients and in therapeutic opportunities for all professional workers. Psychiatric nurses must prepare themselves to share in this new era.

The evolving role of the psychiatric nurse who works with patients in their homes requires that she learn more about families and more about communities, and develop skills in working in both areas. Many new and thrilling opportunities are becoming available to psychiatric nurses as well as to members of other professional disciplines who traditionally work with mentally ill patients. These challenges call for better educational preparation in order to make it possible for the nurse to accept the role of the professional peer in rendering mental health services. The key to the situation in psychiatric nursing is more and better preparation for the task ahead.

contents

Section 5

Providing a Therapeutic Community

Developing
Self-Understanding

1

The Importance of
Understanding Yourself

Norman Q. Brill*

*The nurse, like everyone else, has her share of human frailties.
If she understands them, however, she will be better able to
understand those of others.*

The popular concept of the nurse has, in part, developed from the
idealized picture of Florence Nightingale—the devoted, self-sacrificing, and
generous person, who caters to the ill with no thought of herself.

How far this concept is from reality is obvious at first glance. Nurses—
like any other professional group—represent a cross section of humanity. Some
nurses are personally ambitious; some are irritable, cross, or frustrated. A
nurse may be interested in caring for just one sex or one age group; she
may like caring for groups of patients, or prefer caring for just one patient.
While one nurse wants to be in a position of authority and give orders—to
organize and direct—another may look upon her career simply as a stepping
stone to marriage. Other nurses are personally dedicated to their life's work,
and happy in their role as helpers of the sick.

The word *nurse* refers to a member of a profession—to an individual who
has completed a certain course of training, and not to a kind of person. This
fact is frequently forgotten not only by patients and doctors, but also by
the nurses themselves.

The traditional public concept of the nurse is the bedside nurse. Yet this
concept is no more correct than the one that describes a doctor as a bearded
gentleman sitting up all night in some lonely farm house watching over a sick
child. Just as a doctor may be the head of a public health department, a re-

*From *American Journal of Nursing*, Vol. 57, No. 10 (October, 1957).
Dr. Brill is chairman of the Department of Psychiatry, School of Medicine,
University of California at Los Angeles.

search worker, or a general practitioner in the country, so a nurse may be a private duty nurse, a general duty nurse, a head nurse, a supervisor, a teacher, a public health worker, a nurse in a doctor's office, an industrial nurse, or administrator.

Nurses vary in their liking to be with other people, their interest in other people's troubles, their degree of patience, ability to sympathize, intelligence, tact, poise, ability to deal with difficult or disturbed people, and in their ability to accept supervision, regulation, subordination, and guidance. Some nurses are interested in why persons (including themselves) behave the way they do, and others are not. While some nurses understand that the state of a person's health has a definite connection with his feelings, others think only in terms of what is physically wrong—to them, treating a patient is something tangible like putting on a dressing or giving a medication.

Modern, "scientific" medicine at times also tends to lose sight of the patient as a person. Instead, he becomes an inflamed appendix, a herniated disc, a diseased kidney, or a cirrhotic liver, and treatment consists of the specifically agreed upon operation or medication for the disease. However, we do know that a knife can't operate and antibiotics can't treat a kidney. Treatment is given by a person to a person, and the personal attributes and attitudes of the one giving it play a very important role in its effectiveness.

Patients do get well, however, despite their doctors' and nurses' personality defects, and all patients do not have to be treated with "kid gloves" or approached as though they were fragile pieces of china. They get well even when treated by surgeons whom they secretly call "butchers," and cared for by nurses they call "battle-axes." Some patients who are sufficiently ridden with guilt may even respect a rude, dictatorial approach. But each patient is responsive to the personalities of those who are caring for him. The recovery of patients who are extremely responsive may depend more on *how* something is done than on *what* is done. Thus, the nurse who is alert to these differences in her patients' responses, who is flexible in her approach, will be more successful than the one whose rigid personality happens only by chance to meet the needs of a patient.

One of the best ways to achieve this flexibility is through self-understanding. The person who doesn't understand himself cannot understand others. In hospitals and clinics where emphasis is placed on treating the patient and not just his disease, the nurse must observe the patient's mood and attitude, and be as alert to what he says and does as she is to the color of his lips and the quality of his pulse.

The patient who has no desire to get well will often reveal this to the nurse before he does so to the doctor. Some patients are reluctant to tell their doctors about symptoms they fear are neurotic, but they will often tell the nurse about them. Domestic discord and anxieties that retard recovery are frequently confided to the nurse because the patient feels that the doctor is not interested in such things. Every nurse would call a doctor's attention to bleeding, yet many would hesitate to report signs of depression—some nurses wouldn't even recognize them!

There are many excellent nurses who, without self-understanding, are intuitive and do just the right thing; but there are others who because of lack of understanding have to be taken off duty—occasionally even discharged.

I can recall one nurse, assigned to a ward for mildly disturbed psychiatric patients in an Army hospital, who never once set foot inside the gate between her office and the ward—she was too frightened. Imagine the effect *this* had on the patients!

An important role of a nurse is assisting patients to accept the reality of their situations, and helping them to "stand up to it." The nurse who can't face reality herself is unable to help her patients do so. People tend to be impatient with, and intolerant of, undesirable characteristics in others which they themselves have; this is a way of denying the presence of these characteristics in themselves. For that reason nurses are sometimes irritated with, and antagonistic toward, patients who won't "face up to reality"— whether it concerns taking medication or staying in bed.

Frequently a nurse about whom the patient complains may be giving him far better care than the nurse whom he glamorizes; his "ideal" nurse may identify herself with him and be so "understanding" that she reinforces his unrealistic attitudes. An immature patient whose unreasonable expectations cannot be fulfilled by anyone is neither helped by the nurse who reacts to his criticism, nor by one who needs to be adored and leaves the patient psychologically helpless by smothering him with attention.

If a nurse has never learned to endure slights or rejections she may overprotect her patient, yet unconsciously resent the burden she has undertaken. A nurse who has felt the need to completely control her feelings may react with anger, fear, sexual feeling, envy, or anxiety, without knowing why; the one who prides herself on her extreme orderliness, cleanliness, and perfectionism may be intolerant of a patient who is incontinent, sloppy, or unsystematic, and equate these symptoms or characteristics with badness—as she did in herself in early life.

Women patients who dramatize or exaggerate the severity of their suffering will get no sympathy from the nurse who does not realize that her particular emotional allergy toward their complaints stems back to envy and resentment of a younger sister. A nurse may get abnormally irritated with male patients who tease her if she has still not resolved her problem of competing with a brother.

The nurse who never got over the need to please her mother and do her mother's bidding is relatively ineffective in dealing with an older woman patient or an autocratic supervisor; the one who unconsciously competed with her mother for her father's affection and never got over resenting her mother as a rival resents having to cater to a patient who is a mother figure to her. If a nurse inwardly wishes she had a mother who never frustrated her or denied her anything, she may "knock herself out" treating her patient as she herself wants to be treated—she may then become disappointed and turn bitter and cynical if the patient doesn't react with all the gratitude she herself would feel if she were in the patient's place. A childless nurse may become overly attached to child patients. She may find fault with the child's parents and compete with them for the child's affection—she may even unconsciously attempt to prolong the child's illness and hospital stay.

A nurse who has resented her sex from early life may be resentful of male physicians; she may envy and hate them, and unwittingly attempt to sabotage their work with patients.

These examples cannot be attributed to just ignorance. They reflect personality defects in action—defects which are purposeful and which are defended with vigor when they are pointed out.

Patients in treatment occasionally complain that psychiatrists seem to be interested only in the bad or undesirable traits of their patients and not in their good points. Similarly, if I seem to imply that all nurses are maladjusted, I wish to assure you that they are not. I am merely dwelling on the pathological traits because they are the cause of trouble.

The well-adjusted nurse can be herself without being afraid of harming her co-workers and patients. She does not feel that she has to live up to some unrealistic and nonexistent concept of perfection—no one nurse will be able to please everyone and every human being should expect some unjust criticism and disapproval. Each nurse is an individual with different characteristics because differences exist in infants when they are born. Then, every individual is molded, modified, and transformed by childhood experiences in the process of growing up, and attitudes are absorbed from parents, friends, and teachers. In later life, secret feelings and childhood dreams influence many of our decisions and objectives.

However, when life experiences and individual yearnings are dealt with in emotionally unhealthy ways, and result in an inflexible and distorted personality, there is need for concern. You have all seen persons who do not learn from experience, do not act their age, constantly blame others for their difficulties, or who never give the *real* reasons for doing things. You have seen those who vent their anger on some innocent person, and those who "live in the clouds." These are examples of mechanisms that we all use in varying combinations to keep ourselves from seeing us as we really are, and to help us maintain our exaggerated notions of our own importance and goodness.

I have not discussed such qualities as tact, tidiness, sympathy, gentleness, cheerfulness, charity, and understanding which a nurse should have, but have dwelled on the unfortunate traits that are occasionally displayed by some nurses. I have tried to show how each undesirable trait affects the nurse's job, and to emphasize that a nurse is a person who may have emotional blind spots that can impair her performance.

2

Mental Health
A Point of View

Dana L. Farnsworth*

Mental health means much more than the absence of mental illness. If we could learn to think of mental health in this way, I believe we would make more rapid progress than at present in the communities in which we work.

People with a positive idea about mental health work toward the elimination of causes—not just the cure—of mental illness. The positive concept is not something with which the great majority of people, including the majority of physicians, are in sympathy.

The field of mental health is getting so large that we can only hope to get a few working ideas, even after a life-time of study in this field. We will assume that mental health is a state in which we can work effectively and move toward the realization of our goals. Mental health defies accurate description, just as do love, mercy, justice, good, and evil.

I also think of the mental health movement as embracing a point of view toward human beings in which we take into consideration all the multitudinous factors that combine to make a person what he is. It is a departure from the idea that people are good or bad, desirable or undesirable, or otherwise sharply divided into distinct categories. Instead they are resultants of a vast number of influences—some physical and some psychological. To help an individual we must keep his own particular experiences in mind. We cannot treat patients or any other people fairly by treating them exactly alike.

---

*From American Journal of Nursing, Vol. 60, No. 5 (May, 1960).

Dr. Farnsworth is professor of hygiene at Harvard University, a member of the faculty of the Harvard School of Public Health, and director of the University Health Services. He is a Diplomate of the American Board of Psychiatry and a Fellow of the American Psychiatric Association.

Several mental health principles are central to this point of view:

Mental health education should instill in people a deep respect for human beings, regardless of origin, race, present status, or behavior at the moment. This is a simple statement, but it has more significance than any of the principles that follow.

People like to be treated as individuals and not as members of an amorphous group. They don't like to be pushed around.

Feelings and sentiments of people are real and must be dealt with as such, regardless of whether we agree with them or not.

Human behavior has causes—both rational and irrational—and can be understood if enough facts are known. That too is a statement which nurses would take for granted, but it is not understood or accepted by the great majority of people in our country.

Effective communication at all levels is fundamental to good human relations.

The development of desirable values in a given community can be achieved only when those same values are supported by example and by precept on the part of the opinion-makers or the prestige people.

The particular activities in the community which are of immediate interest to anyone concerned with mental health include marital counseling, family casework, pastoral counseling, clinics for the treatment of alcoholism, courts—especially those dealing with juvenile offenders—and public health programs.

Mental health workers are also concerned with attitudes of people toward those who suffer from physical disabilities, the effects of displacing people for housing or highway projects, attitudes toward police and other agents of the government, segregation and other unfair forms of discrimination, absenteeism in industry, and even the nuclear arms race.

These are only a few, but perhaps the most obvious, of the areas which are most closely concerned with mental health. This concept is as big as life itself. It is *not* a substitute for religion. It is *not* something with which people can solve the world's problems. It is *not* a panacea. It is simply a point of view which, if adopted on a wide scale, could certainly help to relieve some of our burdens.

MORE THAN KINDNESS

There are some other general principles that underlie this point of view. One of them is that love is generally a stronger influence toward the unification of personality than hate.

A second principle is that we should work toward greater significance for each individual as our population increases. For example, unless we take special care along these lines we will come to feel that the 36,000 people killed in automobile accidents really don't matter a great deal. Another concept, which is hardly a principle—yet should be emphasized over and over—is that the transmission of values from the older to the younger generation is a matter which we must study intensively.

We have assumed that, in our vast array of educational institutions, telling youngsters what they should do is enough. But we tell them what they should do, then we ourselves do something that falls short of that ideal. They follow the ideals that we act upon, not the ones that we say we honor.

These concepts seem to be nothing more than plain common sense, or kindness made explicit, but they are far more subtle. We need a way of organizing our thinking in this field in such a way that new ideas can be added to our present knowledge, assimilated, organized, utilized, and made a part of our working concepts.

PERSONALITY IN THE MAKING

We have never been entirely able to evolve a system of understanding or integrating personality effectively until the past decade when Erik Erikson came up with a system of concepts of child development so reasonable, logical, and coherent, that they formed the basis for much of the report from the 1950 White House Conference on Childhood and Youth. His system is incorporated in the book, *Personality in the Making* (1).

This book has not been properly appreciated by those of us in education, medicine, nursing, and all the allied fields.

The system is coherent and inclusive, but it isn't a new system of psychology in which a person has to be labeled as a Freudian, a Jungian, or an Adlerian.

Erikson is not a physician. He started life as an artist, has done a great deal of work in anthropology and some in psychology. He went in for psychoanalysis and is one of the few lay analysts in the American Psychoanalytical Association.

The basic idea back of his system is that we have certain key conflicts of different degrees. These stages are not limited to the ages which Erikson ascribes to them, but they are at their highest significance during that period.

SENSE OF TRUST. Erikson assumes that the most important task for the baby in the first 15 months of life is to develop a sense of optimism, a kind of confidence in the world around him—and the world around him is made up largely of his parents, his brothers and sisters, and a few friends. He should develop a confident expectation that somehow or other things ultimately will turn out all right.

If the child can develop a sense of trust during the first year-and-one-quarter of his life, the groundwork is set for his developing other attitudes later on that are necessary for his maturity.

This does not mean that every child must be so trusting that he takes up with anyone who comes along, or that he trusts a sharp knife or a hot flame. It means that the balance between trust and mistrust is developed in such a way that he knows in general whom to trust and what to trust, and that this mood is predominant over the undesirable one of trusting no one except his towel or his teddy bear.

During this period parents and those who are concerned with young children should be aware of the child's basic need to have a preponderance of pleasant experiences—to be dried when he is wet, cleaned when he is dirty, fed when he is hungry, have pain relieved when something hurts him, and to be loved when he is lonely.

At no stage is this more important. The idea that the child is so young that he won't remember just isn't true. The child may not observe all that goes on around him but is almost never fooled by his parents. Their attitudes shine through.

SELF-CONTROL. Beginning at about 15 months another set of needs comes into view. This is the period during which the baby is trying to develop attitudes about himself—who he is and what he is. In a very limited sense he learns that his arms and legs can come under his own control. He learns to talk.

It is during this period that he gradually puts inside himself some of the prohibitions taught by his parents, so that the built-in control starts. During this period from about 15 months up to the age of three or four the faint beginnings of conscience appear—"I ought" or "I ought not."

This is a period in which the youngster does an enormous amount of questioning and is attempting to become a separate person. We want to help him achieve self-control without the loss of self-esteem.

This is the period also in which his sense of guilt is developed. The youngster who is asked during this early period, "Why didn't you do it better?" gets feelings of guilt. If guilt feelings are too strong he cannot organize well, cannot achieve the desirable feeling of confidence. Children are apt to develop best if they are commended for what they do well.

In the period of four to five years of age we see that conscience is more fully developed, and guilt feelings become stronger. This age is characterized by a strong imagination. This is the period when youngsters have imaginary husbands or wives, imaginary playmates, and all sorts of fantasy goes on. If the proper sense of trust has been achieved and a sense of autonomy has been gained, then a sense of initiative comes more easily than if the child has had unhappy experiences earlier.

CONSOLIDATION THEN ADOLESCENCE. The age of 6 to 11 corresponds to the "latent" period in psychoanalysis, in which there is apparently a great need to learn to do things and to do them well. It is during this period that the youngster consolidates his earlier gains, develops feelings of adequacy or inferiority, depending on the sum total of stimuli which comes in his direction.

It is a period of steady, slow, calm growth. He embarrasses his parents by his frequent and inappropriate use of terms he has picked up. There is not the vigorous fantasy life about sexual things during this period as there was from three to five and as there will be in adolescence.

The next stage, from about 11 or 12 up to 16 or 18—a variable period —is the time when the youngster struggles to achieve what Erikson calls "identity." "Who am I, what am I, where am I going, and what meaning is there in life? Where do I fit in?" Children today have many more opportunities than their parents or grandparents had. But, because they have more opportunities, it is necessary to make more choices, and they cut themselves off from more things than their parents did as each choice is made.

Hence the level of anxiety of our youngsters is somewhat higher because of the multiplicity of opportunity, instead of being lessened as we might assume.

If a person is brought up in a rural area in which he knows he is going to live eight to ten miles from home, marry someone from one of the neighborhood families, go to the same church his parents attended, and do the same things, there isn't much anxiety about it because, whatever choice is made, he is not cutting himself off from much. True, he has to choose one person as compared to another, but by and large the choice is not such a limiting factor. A child brought up in an urban area may be confronted with many choices regarding schools, religion, and future mate.

The necessity to choose causes many of our youngsters to be uncertain about what they want to do, and many of them go in the opposite direction of achieving their identity. They may even lose their identity completely or have what is called "role diffusion." They may even develop a negative identity, making a temporary career out of hating anything that is conventional, proper, good, or what their parents want. We see this in its nearly obscene form in the so-called "beatnicks."

How we treat a youngster who has just begun to violate some of the social restrictions which are necessary for the community to function is very important. If we treat him as if he were a criminal he is more likely to become one than if he is treated in a more kindly fashion. People tend to play roles which they think society assigns them; so there is no more important period in the life of a youngster than the first time he violates the social codes and gets caught.

I emphasize the latter, because there are very few people who do not violate the social codes when they are growing up. The fact that parents or some understanding person is there when a young person makes a mistake helps him to learn something that is beneficial. Or, even more common, the young person makes a mistake, but no one else knows of it. He knows that his parents would not tolerate that kind of behavior. He knows that the church and the law do not, and his anxiety is so great about getting caught that he does his own reforming.

The next stage that Erikson portrays in the development of a mature person is that of intimacy. The development of intimacy depends in part on knowledge of self. It is hardly possible to become intimate with another person until one has a pretty good notion of what one's self is like. The term "intimacy" here refers to the capacity to have a warm and trusting relationship with another person. It does not mean sexual relations, but it includes them. Intimacy is the word that most nearly expresses the quality of a good home— the capacity to trust, to give, to receive, to share relationships, feelings, sentiments, aspirations, and the like.

The capacity to develop intimate relations with others is furthered most advantageously if the other stages are well mastered as the young person goes along—a sense of trust, of autonomy, of initiative, of industry, and of identity. If a person cannot develop intimate relationships with others, he tends to withdraw in various ways.

A person who has developed the capacity for intimacy can usually withstand bereavement, suffering, and the like, and come back and be a sweet and agreeable person, no matter how old he is. Someone has said the older we get, the more like ourselves we become.

DEVELOPING CREATIVENESS. If these first six stages have been successfully managed, if development has been more or less on an even keel, then the seventh of Erikson's stages—that of developing a sense of creativeness, a parental sense, a sense of generativity, a feeling that one has something at stake so far as the welfare of mankind is concerned—is readily developed. This we see in its most clear-cut form when people become parents. What we so often see is that they turn away from their self-centered attitudes and think of the welfare of their children. Not all people do so by any manner of means.

It seems to me that one of the basic difficulties with our present generation of late adolescents is that their parents by and large have too much of this element of self-absorption. There has not been enough of the creative sense for the whole community. I suppose that has always seemed so to the people who are confronted with the problem of adolescents.

The development of a preponderance of the parental sense, as compared to self-absorption, is most vital to developing good family life.

INTEGRITY, NOT DESPAIR. Then a final developmental stage, which has been neglected, interests me particularly. It is the development of integrity as compared and contrasted to a sense of despair or discouragement. Integrity, as Erikson uses it, means the state of mind in which one accepts himself as he is. He does not feel that he wants to live his life over again. He has had experiences that to him seem vital and significant.

He values the common attributes we think necessary to hold society together—justice, valor, courage, ideals he has obtained from some source.

The intriguing thing, from my point of view, is that the development of a sense of integrity can be achieved in a given community only when large numbers of people exhibit that same quality. If the great majority of people do not have integrity, we cannot expect very many of the youngsters to develop it. We see the problem in its most acute form in the crowded urban centers of any country in which people feel "left out." They have a strong competitive urge. In Cambridge—to use an example—we find that the areas with many social problems have a low incidence of home ownership. The population is quite transient. There are many broken families. Church attendance is low. The incidence of juvenile delinquency is quite high.

But there are some exceptions. There are some sections in Cambridge in which there is a strong family structure reinforced by religious teachings, where these same undesirable conditions prevail. Yet, youngsters grow up with integrity and fairly desirable attributes.

So we don't have to say we must give up our struggle to develop a good society simply because we are in an urban society. It is just as possible to become a responsible person when there are a larger number of people around as when there are a few.

I have gone into some detail on Erikson's scheme, because I very much hope that nurses will be stimulated to study it carefully. The best beginning can be found in the books, *Personality in the Making, A Healthy Personality,* and *Childhood and Society* (2, 3, 4). There will be some duplication in these books, but this will do no harm.

DISTORTIONS OF NORMAL LIFE

What are some of the distortions of normal living which produce emotional or social conflicts? Isolation is one of them. Rejection is another. Unfair discrimination is always prevalent. We live in a society which is highly materialistic, and competitive attitudes frequently get out of hand.

Inadequate knowledge is another condition that produces distortion of normal living. All kinds of improper attitudes are manifested in our own communities. They show up in the form of working ineffectively, relative failure, a person not doing as well as he might. These attitudes cause crippling anxiety, so that the person feels beset by some deep inner distress. This, of course, results in relative failure, in a feeling that the environment is hostile.

11

We see these indices in the form of divorces, neurosis, character disorders, drug addiction, alcoholism, hate groups, and frank mental illness.

TOWARD MENTAL HEALTH

It does seem to me that if we take the point of view that a person is the product of all that he has met, and if we work in the community to relieve people who are made unhappy by some custom or behavior of others, we will get further than if we try to formalize a type of activity which we call promotion of mental health.

If nurses devote their energies to understanding people, to relieving them of distress or promoting through their own attitudes those points of view which will be most likely to dissolve crises, to promote techniques of love as compared to those of hatred; if they work to ease the burden of people who are having marital difficulties, or who have committed some indiscretion which gets them into trouble with the law; if they take an understanding attitude toward the person who drinks too much; if they try to understand people in terms of the system that I have outlined, then we can say that they are working toward better mental health.

I don't think that we should develop a separate group of mental health specialists. I think that is going at it in the wrong way. I think that we as nurses, as teachers, as doctors, as lawyers, and as ministers should think in terms of promoting the mental health of our communities without becoming full-time specialists in this field.

In the schools I should like to see some of the teachers become mental health resource persons. In the nursing profession I should like to see some good nurses become quite skilled in how to interpret mental health principles to others, but not to cease being good nurses as they do this.

I have spent all my professional life furthering mental health, I hope. But I do not consider myself a specialist in mental health. My field is medicine and psychiatry. Mental health is not something that we can leave to specialists. It is something that all of us can try to promote.

If we can only become aware of the issues of immediate concern to optimum mental health and make our neighbors aware of them, appropriate solutions can be found. All too often people have not even been aware of the factors which encourage or inhibit the development of well-integrated, stable personalities. As professional people we can utilize mental health concepts with great profit to our patients as well as to ourselves and to society.

REFERENCES

1. Midcentury White House Conference on Children and Youth. *Personality in the Making; The Fact-Finding of the Conference,* ed. by Helen Leland Witmer and Ruth Kotinsky. New York, Harper and Brothers, 1952.
2. *Ibid.*
3. Conference on Problems of Infancy and Childhood. *Symposium on the Healthy Personality; Transactions of Special Meetings of the Conference, June 8-9 and July 3-4, 1950,* ed. by Milton J. E. Senn. New York, Josiah Macy, Jr., Foundation, 1950.
4. Erikson, E. H. *Childhood and Society.* New York, W. W. Norton Co., 1950.

3

Reflections on Self

John A. Lewis*

When a nurse recognizes and has ability to use self, she offers greater assistance to the patient.

Nurses, too, are human beings. That sounds like a simple, obvious statement. But when examined against the background of the nursing profession, its history, present concerns, and the strivings of individual nurses and their organizations for self-improvement to give better care to their patients, the word "too" stands out sharply. The statement can then be seen as a complaint, a protest, that others are regarded as human beings but that some people do not act as if nurses are human beings "too."

There is some justice to the protest. The public image of a nurse still is that of someone who carries out the doctor's orders. Traditionally, the nursing profession has been labeled ancillary, more recently paramedical; ancillary, meaning a female servant or hand maiden, paramedical, alongside of the doctor.

Both labels avoid the issue that nursing, though closely allied with the medical profession, is not a part of the medical profession; that nursing is a profession in its own right with its own theories, practices, and code of ethics; that a nurse is a human being, not an instrument to carry out anyone's will; that she is free to choose and decide with due appreciation of the skills and knowledges of others; that she is a dependable and responsible person; that she has contributions to make of her own as a nurse and as a unique personality to the care of the patient.

We have learned in mental health that it is damaging to the Self of a person if he is used to blindly carry out another person's will. This principle

2

*From *American Journal of Nursing*, Vol. 60, No. 6 (June, 1960).
Dr. Lewis is psychiatric consultant for Region III of the Department of Health, Education, and Welfare in Charlottesville, Virginia.

is clearly seen in the development of children. We learn from psychoanalysis that the young child takes within himself the behavior patterns of the parent and that he, in his immaturity, acts as if he were his parent. This phenomenon can be seen in the little girl who delights in putting on Mama's shoes and prancing around saying, "Will you have another cookie, dear?" The child slowly develops a Self of his own. This Self proclaims to the world, "I am John, I know I am because I can feel it and I know I am different."

For this Self to grow and further differentiate itself from others, it must be permitted to act on its own initiative, even encouraged to act, though there may be mistakes. If the Self is afraid to try, afraid of the wrath of the parent or of others, its development is thwarted. The child must explore his world and discover how he sees the world and himself as a person. He must have an opportunity to observe how others see the world and how they see him so that he can correct his own mistakes. If the others with whom he compares his observations have distorted views about their worlds and about him, then he will find it very difficult to develop a Self that sees people and himself as they really are.

We observe frequently that when a child with a mental disturbance is seen in a child guidance clinic there is also mental pathology in other members of the family. Treatment of the child alone is seldom effective in producing a lasting remission of his symptoms. It is necessary to also treat various members of the family, especially the mother, with whom the child has the most intense and numerous interactions.

In healthy people development of the Self continues on from infancy to adulthood. There is a push that comes from within the person toward becoming a more mature person, an impulse to growth and positive mental health.

When the nurse is treated as an instrument to carry out someone's will her Self is required to forego translation in its own terms. Her Self is deprived of the opportunity to act on its own behalf and is, therefore, deprived of the opportunity to grow and to perform a creative act of nursing. One should not be surprised at an act of protest when the nurse finds her Self ignored and she is treated, not as a thinking, feeling, creating person but as an instrument or a tool to carry out acts of another Self.

NURSES' MATURITY RECOGNIZED

Many articles about the professional status of nursing have appeared in recent issues of the *American Journal of Nursing*. Nurses are examining what they do carefully and critically with the intention of preparing themselves to act more responsibly and thus to give better care to their patients. The push for professional development can be interpreted as a logical consequence of nurses awakening to higher levels of consciousness of themselves and of the creative contributions that the nurse can make to helping people get well.

The patient stands to benefit in many ways by the Self-awakening of the nurse to her real Self, and by the recognition by others that she, too, is a human being with manifold creative potentialities.

The direct and personal contact with patients is her opportunity to see her patient as one human being can see another human being. She can, in a sense, enter the world of the patient and, to some extent, see what worries him through his eyes. She does this, not completely, exactly, or even expertly, but often enough for the patient to feel that here is one person of whom he need not be afraid, who can appreciate how he feels. When the nurse does this she establishes communication with the Self of the patient. She breaks the spell of loneliness of the patient, who often can get attention for his paralysis or increased blood sugar level but not for his Self that may be starved for recognition and expression.

The nurse's awareness will be evident to the patient by her manner as she enters the room, by the attention she gives as a part of her awareness to every expression of her patient. The expressions of the patient are meaningful to the Self-awakened nurse whether verbalized or not and which, taken collectively, give the nurse an appraisal of her patient's Self, corrected or confirmed as she continues to work with him. Such a nurse is a delight and a reassurance to a person whose interactions with family and friends have been interrupted by the illness.

REGRESSION AND ILLNESS

We all know that with every illness there is a falling down of the person's level of functioning which can be called regression. Involved in the process of regression is psychological as well as physical functioning. The conception of regression expressed here is not exactly in psychoanalytical terms. In psychoanalytical theory regression means a falling back of the level of performance to certain fixed points of earlier development such as early infancy (oral or anal), or to adolescence (genital). I do not believe that regression takes place so drastically or to fixed points in every case of illness. I simply mean by regression that behavior is not up to par; it is on a lower level. The nurse needs to have a concept of regression, of her own and of her patient's. The nurse, whom we have agreed is a human being, too, will, of course, experience regression herself from time to time.

It is remarkable that at each level of functioning we see the world outside of ourselves differently and that at each level what the person sees and feels is real for him. A crude analogy that conveys the meaning is that a person on the 50th floor of a building sees the world differently than if he were on the 10th floor; his situation in the world is different. Likewise, a person who is ill sees and feels the world differently than when he is in good health; his situation, too, in the world is different.

Without thinking about it we are continually testing our perceptions of things and people—our world—so as to be able to act appropriately. A part of our world is also ourselves— so we test how other people see us and thus correct or confirm our notions about ourselves. The truth of this conception comes out in the joke about the two psychiatrists, one of whom asks the other, "How am I today?" The nurse, awakened to her own Self, with a conception of the patient's level of functioning and respect for the patient's Self, will act in ways which permit expressions by the Self of the patient, expressions that are necessary for the patient to gain an appropriate perception of his situation in the world.

Disorders of the Self manifest themselves in different kinds of mental illness, and mental illness can be thought of as a way of living—that is, a way of being in the world. The Self of the mentally ill person has its own reality, it is a construction that the Self has created to fit its own needs. How the mental patient sees and feels about the world and about himself is so different from the reality of others about him that the difference is noticed by the others. It appears that the Self of the mental patient expresses both regression and distortion of functioning, and the mental symptoms as we see them are the patient's attempt to remake his world as he sees and feels it.

One of the symptoms frequently seen is anxiety and the nurse needs a conception of anxiety as it is related to her functioning and her patient's. Anxiety is a state of the person that occurs when the Self feels threatened. The kinds of threats that produce anxiety vary widely with different people. For some it may be a threat of loss of job, or loss of a loved one, or loss of approval from a significant person, depending on the particular sensitivities to threats of the person. Usually the source is not recognized by the person experiencing anxiety; we say that often the source is unconscious—that is, not in conscious awareness. Anxiety is experienced as a state of tension, tightness is felt in the muscles and in the body generally. There is a feeling of apprehension, that something dreaded is about to happen.

Anxiety, if unrecognized in the patient, can cause the nurse to become anxious too. The cause of anxiety in the nurse might be apprehension about what the patient might do or that the nurse might feel she is going to fail in working with the patient. There are many sources of anxiety. Because the nurse is a human being, too, she also has sensitivities to threats that may produce anxiety. In any case, if the nurse develops anxiety, then regression in her performance is likely to take place with consequent changes in how she sees her world which includes the patient. Her perception of the patient then becomes distorted which in turn causes the nurse to misinterpret the communications of the patient.

If the nurse can reduce the patient's anxiety by making him more comfortable, by communicating to the patient her awareness of and respect for the Self of the patient, it is possible for the reduction of the patient's anxiety to permit the patient's level of functioning to be elevated—that is, for the process of regression to be reversed. With the reversal of regression the mental symptoms begin to subside. Much of the good result public health nurses are having when they visit in the homes of patients with mental illness is due to the reassuring presence of the nurse which causes a reduction of anxieties in the patient and in other members of the family which also affects the patient.

Deficiencies in the education of nurses in mental health are being overcome so that nurses can receive as much satisfaction in their work with the mentally ill as with the physically ill. Nurses are not going to become psychiatrists. It is reasonable to expect, however, that nurses will gain greater knowledge about their Selves and, in so doing, be able to understand more about their patients.

As the nurse grows in knowledge of her Self and as others begin to see her as a human being, too, a real person, with abilities to use her Self and her skills that are unique to her as a person and as a nurse, she will be better able to help her patients achieve higher levels of functioning and living.

4

Look at Yourself

Catherine Ring*

A frank account of a student's reactions while caring for an attractive young man who was emotionally ill.

"There he is," I said to myself as I walked into the day room that very first day. I was referring to Fred, slouching by himself on the couch, peering from beneath drawn eyebrows. I knew he must be Fred, because he fit the description which I had received from my head nurse, except for one thing— how bitter his eyes were! I was soon to learn just how bitter, and just how little I was really prepared for him.

My first reaction to him was one of wonder and perhaps even pleasure. He was a tall, extremely good looking boy about my own age. He was dressed in a crew neck sweater, chinos, and had a crew cut. He looked so normal. How could he be sick? A mentally ill person looks—well—looks ill, I thought. I know my preconceived idea of a mentally ill patient was a little unrealistic, for I pictured patients running around, making strange faces, talking to themselves, and being destructive. I realized that this wasn't true in all cases, but inwardly I really expected this to be the case.

"Look closely," I said to myself. "Look again at his eyes. No eyes should be so bitter, glaring at everything and everyone around them. Watch his hands; they are moving constantly, jerking to his face, rubbing his eye, poking himself all over." Why? Why is he this way? Why do these things happen to young people? All these questions deluged my mind, and with

*From *American Journal of Nursing*, Vol. 60, No. 8 (August, 1960).

Miss Ring is a senior at the University of Vermont School of Nursing in Burlington. She wrote this article in her junior year during her psychiatric nursing affiliation at the Boston University School of Nursing and the Massachusetts Mental Health Center.

a sigh, a smile, and a secret crossing of my fingers I went to him and said, "Hello, Fred."

I told him that I was to be his nurse, and that I would be working along with him for the next 10 weeks. Expecting a somewhat sociable reply, my confidence was shattered when he said, "Oh no, not another one." I asked him if he had worked with a student nurse before, and what he thought about it. He shrugged his shoulders and informed me that he didn't see the sense in it and proceeded to jump up and dart away. "What did I do?" I wondered. I had the feeling that everyone had seen this episode, and I wished I were miles away. I was embarrassed almost to the point of tears.

The rest of the afternoon Fred was in and out of the day room. He avoided me completely. When he saw me coming toward him, he would go away. Throughout that first week I saw him talking with other student nurses. I realized that I was becoming resentful of them, and became infuriated when the other students talked with him. I could not express my feelings to them, but became tense and quiet when around them. I was alone. I was unused to loneliness, and the jealousy that I felt toward my best friends frightened me.

The little contact I did have with Fred during that first week was extremely unpleasant for me and probably for him also. His whole outlook on life was so bitter. I am quite sensitive, too sensitive, perhaps, and I took his sarcasm as a direct attack on me. Our conversations went something like this:

"Good morning, Fred."

"Oh, hello, hello, hello." He would either get a false smile on his face (at least I thought it was false) or else a look of sheer boredom.

"How is everything," I might say.

"Oh, fine, fine," and again that smile. I didn't seem to be able to reach him at all. One day I asked him about his hopes and future plans. "I think I shall be Emperor of Iran, or King of Tunisia." I was taken aback so that all I could do was to look at him. He was making a fool of me, and how I hated him for it! I was oversensitive and began to do some serious thinking about "why." The conclusions I came to were that there was something about him that was attractive to me, and I wanted his approval very much, and was sure I could get it. I was not used to being rejected. My life had been so full of love, protection, understanding, and security that I hardly knew what rejection meant. I experienced the feeling of being completely rejected for perhaps the first time in my life, and was hurt, confused, angry, and utterly dejected.

When I had figured this out, I began to really look at Fred. I began seeing him as a challenge to be met, still thinking of my own selfish satisfaction. I wanted his approval to mend a hurt pride, so I played along with Fred's sarcasm, giving him a taste of his own medicine. I laughed at his sadistic jokes and mannerisms, met wisecrack with wisecrack. Fred responded to this, but just how did he respond? Was I really helping him? Just what was I doing, anyway?

For the first time I began to think of Fred as a patient who was ill and needed help. This was not another man to be conquered; he was a sick boy to be helped. As I gave more thought to this I began again to talk to my classmates and share my ideas with them. All of us decided to change our approach to Fred. It gave me a feeling of security to have their support. I was no longer alone. I would no longer accept his sarcasm, no longer play along with him in his make-believe world. It was doing him no good at all; it was even hurting him and the wall he had built around himself was being strengthened. He was safe within this wall—safe in his sarcasm; people wouldn't get too close to him and he didn't have to become close to anybody. I shared these ideas with the doctor who went along wholeheartedly with the idea.

This was the real turning point in our relationship. The day I changed my approach to Fred, he changed his approach to me. When he said something of which I disapproved, I let him know of my disapproval. When he talked of conquering worlds, I told him to stop being foolish and to talk about something that was within reach. I was used to "going along with people in a sympathetic understanding"; this blunt facing of reality—actually showing anger at a patient when I felt it—was a little difficult. I didn't want to hurt him, but I was angry enough with him not to care if I did hurt him a little. I felt this was going to be for his good anyway.

Fred sensed what was going on, I felt sure, and began to realize he was not going to push me away so easily. I wasn't sure whether he would bolt away again, but when he asked me to go to the coffee shop with him during the second week, I was amazed. This was the first time he had ever made any kind of approach to me, and I was thrilled. However, in order not to frighten him I accepted his invitation with a smile—as though he had asked me many times before. I was nervous about going, not knowing what to expect next. Fred walked quite a distance from me, which also irritated me until I realized why he was doing this. Now that he had committed himself by asking me to the coffee shop, he was not going to commit himself further by walking with me.

We talked small talk for awhile, and I was pleased at his lack of sarcasm. I began to feel sympathetic toward him. He told me that he felt that he could tell his real problem only to his doctor, and wouldn't talk about it to anyone else. I respected this, although I think I resented it also. I never let him know that I knew about his problems, feeling that when and if he ever wanted to talk about them with me, he would.

Twice while we were talking he got up and darted away, only to come back again after a minute or two. When the conversation got too close to his problem he would dart away; however, he always came back. Examples of subjects that triggered his quick departures were in talking of his stepmother, his feelings about work and responsibilty, and about me.

As time went on, I began to think about my feelings when he would bolt away from me in the middle of a conversation. At first I hated it when he did this; "What would the patients think? They must think I said something terrible to him to frighten him so." I came to realize that this was Fred's way of protecting himself. I realized that it was no reflection upon me, and didn't care what the others thought. I knew why Fred did this, and that was what mattered.

Now when Fred leaves I start talking with other patients, and when Fred comes back I greet him and begin again where we left off. The other patients sense that I understand this trait of his, and treat it casually along with me.

Actually, I have the feeling that they understood him all the time, but were embarrassed because I was.

I began to look forward to seeing Fred each day, and wondered at this. I could remember how I hated him at first. But did I ever really hate him? I hated being made a fool of and I hated being rejected, but I didn't hate him. I realized that I had always liked him, and this is one reason why I was so hurt and disappointed in his behavior.

One day at the end of the first month Fred appeared quite restless. I was talking with another patient and could not go to him right way. Before I knew it it was lunchtime. As I was returning from lunch, I heard someone call me. It was the first time Fred had called me by name, and I knew then that I had been accepted. Not only had I been accepted, but he accepted the responsibility of a relationship with another person besides his doctor. I was glad that I was that person.

He fell into step beside me, and we walked to the day hospital together. For the first time I felt at ease with him, and I am sure he sensed this, because he stayed with me and talked for about an hour.

Things progressed very well; Fred now greeted me enthusiastically each day; he suggested our doing things together—we played pool and shuffleboard and frequently went to the coffee shop to talk. He was entering more in the group. He was talking with other patients more easily. I watched him grow in self-confidence, and felt myself growing with him. In having this solid relationship behind me, I felt more at ease with other patients.

The first real crisis in our relationship occurred at the end of the second month. I had a new patient who happened to be another fairly young, attractive man. I spent a good part of the day with him, and when I did go to Fred I found him to be quiet but restless. Unfortunately I had class at the university that day, so I couldn't discuss it with Fred then.

The next afternoon I could not find Fred. I suspected that he might be at occupational therapy, so I went to the department. There he was, slouched down in a chair staring into space. He looked utterly despondent, and guilt boiled up inside me. I sat beside him, and received a sarcastic "hello" much the same as on our first meeting. For some reason, I could not bring myself to .discuss my new patient. I knew it had to be discussed, but at that moment I was afraid. Perhaps I thought he may bolt away again, something he rarely did now, but something for which I had thought I had conditioned myself. Perhaps it was simply an old trait of mine coming out again—my tendency to stay away from issues that may be unpleasant. Perhaps I simply could not bear to be rejected again after such a fine relationship. At any rate, I did not bring up the issue. Soon Fred did bolt up, and before I had a chance to tell him that I had class in five minutes, he said, "Wait here," and was gone. I waited as long as I could, and finally decided to look for him. As I stepped into the elevator, Fred was stepping out and in his hands were two cups of coffee. The elevator door closed, and I didn't see Fred until the next day.

I worried about this incident all evening. I was sure Fred had gotten me coffee, and I felt extremely guilty about it. I felt that I had let him down by not being there to accept his kind offer. However, I also knew that I must let him know that he had not "lost me" to this other patient, and that he did not need to buy back my friendship. The next day I told him I was "sorry

I had had to leave, and if that extra cup of coffee had been for me, 'thank you.' " I also told him that I had a new patient who needed some of the time I usually set aside for him, and wondered how he felt about it all. He looked at me and said, "Aha, you feel guilty about it, don't you? You were really worried about it." He didn't know how right he was.

His sensitivity to my feelings bothered me at first, or rather frightened me a bit, because some of my feelings I did not want him to sense or know. But, I found out that I could not hide anything from him. Our relationship grew stronger along with my relationships with my friends and co-workers. I spent time with Fred when my other patient was around to show him that our relationship had not changed. Throughout all, the helpful guidance of my supervisor in that situation, was appreciated by, not only us, but Fred too, I think. My psychiatric nursing experience was nearing an end. It was really more of a crisis for me than for him. I began mentioning my departure every once in awhile from the very beginning of our relationship, but Fred ignored it. Two weeks before the date I began discussing it at length with him. I told him I was very pleased in his progress and that he had helped me a great deal in my own growth and maturity. He seemed amazed at this, so I explained how my friendship with him and my understanding of him had indeed helped me in understanding myself, because some of his problems were my own. When I asked how he felt about my leaving, he put on his "indifferent" act. However, he knew I could see through him nearly as well as he could see through me, so he finally said he didn't want me to go.

For my own selfish satisfaction I had hoped he would say this, because I didn't want to leave him. I was a little resentful of whomever would take my place, but hoped it would be someone who would establish a happy, growing, and learning relationship, as Fred and I had. I was very thankful I had the chance to work with Fred, and thankful also that I did not give up as I almost did at first. I felt that he would be more accepting of a new student nurse than he was of me, because he is more accepting of people in general, and more ready for closer relationships.

Fred will never know how much he taught me, in tolerance, in frankness, in self-understanding, in sensitivity to others, in self-confidence, and confidence in others. His initial rejection of me taught me to understand what rejection is, what it feels like, how to deal with it. His later acceptance of me helped me to know real satisfaction, and working with him taught me to appreciate satisfaction in small victories.

5

Understanding Ourselves

Leonard F. Stevens*

Understanding one's own behavior is basic to understanding others. The nurse who is aware of her own needs, as well as those of her patient, can keep them from coming into conflict and interfering with the effectiveness of her nursing care.

All patients are entitled to good nursing care. In order to provide good care, nursing personnel have to be aware of patients' psychological needs—and they should also be aware of their own. They should understand the frustrations that develop when these needs are not satisfied and the problems that may result from attempts to satisfy them.

All of us should think about whose needs receive first consideration in our work with patients. Sometimes our own personal needs take priority and keep us from giving a patient the kind of care that he requires and that we think we are providing. Unconsciously, we may be using him to satisfy our needs. Therein lies our problem—not in the fact that we all have certain definite personal needs, but rather in the means that we may use to satisfy them.

We must recognize that the demands arising from our basic psychological needs do affect our daily relationships. The needs of nurses do not lie dormant but actively affect their relationships with patients and also with co-workers.

Our most familiar needs—like those of other people—are related to self-preservation, security, self-esteem, and worth; but we also need to feel that our efforts are understood and recognized by those whose opinions we value.

*From *American Journal of Nursing*, Vol. 57, No. 8 (August, 1957).

Mr. Stevens (McLean, Waverly, Mass.; B.S., M.S., Boston University) is chief of the nursing service at the Veterans Administration Hospital, Jefferson Barracks, Missouri.

We want people to conform, and to react as we expect them to. We have a picture of how nurses should be treated and we are unhappy when we are not treated in that way. We have our "entitlements"—those considerations and rights we believe are due us. It seems natural to meet one's own needs first rather than to give first consideration to the needs of other people. It is possible that even as we consciously attempt to meet our patients' needs, we may be giving priority to our own interests without being aware of it.

All persons are growing, changing, living organisms, trying to adapt to the world and the situations they encounter here. This adjustment process is sometimes described as "homeostasis."[1] Homeostasis is a tendency toward balance; whenever there is a disturbance, activity occurs in order to bring back a balance. This activity accounts for human behavior and, in the case of illness, for patients' symptomatology. This partially explains, too, the reaction of nursing personnel to patients.

All nursing personnel are bound to react to people and to situations and not all of these reactions will be positive or constructive ones. The degree and type of reactions that occur will vary considerably, depending on the individual's previous experiences and his adaptability. We should understand that a patient may cause us to react in a negative manner and that this may be difficult for us to deal with. These reactions can occur because of one or more of the following situations:

1. The patient does not conform to our expectations of a patient.
2. We do not conform to the patient's expectations of a nurse.
3. The patient prevents us from conforming to our expectations of a nurse.
4. We prevent the patient from conforming to his expectations of a patient.

In discussing plans for patients' care, nursing personnel are often heard to make such comments as these: "He is a good patient" or "He is a difficult patient." Why do we think in terms of "good" and "difficult" patients? What are the criteria for classifying patients as "good" or "difficult"? Apparently we have definite ideas of what a patient ought to be like, how he should behave, how he should respond to a nurse. When a patient does not fit our concept, we may become baffled, frustrated, and perhaps angry. We are unhappy and "off balance."

What can we do in such a situation? *We must accept the patient as he is and begin our planning at this point.* Our problem is how to handle our own reactions and how to deal with the negative feelings that are aroused in us.

HANDLING NEGATIVE REACTIONS

This is a challenging problem but we must resolve it in the situation in which it exists, if at all possible. Our first step should be to recognize that negative reactions will occur and that they can even be used as assets if we can sublimate by pouring the energy they generate into constructive activities.

---

[1]This term is usually associated with physiological factors; in this article, the author applies it also to psychological factors. For a discussion of homeostasis, see Walter B. Cannon's *The Wisdom of the Body,* published by W. W. Norton in 1939.

Most important, we should try to understand our reactions and why they are occurring. It may be well to discuss our reactions with others who are likely to understand and in whom we have confidence.

The ways in which we react to others, the intensity of our reactions, the amount of resistance or blocking which occurs in situations that trouble us are all highly personal. The amount of frustration a person feels depends on his tolerance and on the acuteness of the problem facing him. Everyone meets a certain amount of frustration in daily living but, if it is not so intense as to be overpowering, it serves as a stimulus to problem solving.

But there can also be negative reactions to frustration. Some of the common ones are *fear*, either of a physical object or of being inadequate to cope with a problem; *preoccupation* with the problem to the extent of being unable to organize, plan effectively, or exert constructive effort; *flight*—with the individual running away, leaving his position, changing his assignment, or having physical symptoms which keep him away from the problem situation; *projection* of blame onto others or the situation; *rationalization* to save face in explaining a failure; *depression* or *worry*, or both, in any degree.

The degree to which we manifest these negative reactions determines how much they interfere in planning or giving effective nursing care. The patient often reflects our reactions and if we see in his attitude any suggestion that we are inadequate or lack skill, we may become angry or "off balance" again, contributing to a circle of reactions which preclude our building the kind of relationship in which we can give good care.

WHAT IS GOOD NURSING?

Good nursing is equated with meeting the patient's needs and is present when a patient derives physical and emotional comfort as a consequence of his care. More difficult to answer is the question, often asked, "What makes a good nurse?" In giving their answers to this question, patients have described the good nurse as "one who treats me as a human being," "one who inspires friendly confidence," "one who implies that she wants to help," "one who understands herself and is humbly aware of others," "one who gives a feeling of security," "one who is sensitive to the patients' needs."

These patients have said nothing about technical skill, but perhaps this is because they assume all nurses have it in abundance. The usual listing of characteristics that make for a good nurse includes orderliness and the ability to organize, establish routines, have a place for everything, and have things done on time. Such activities are good to the extent that they help to meet the patient's needs. They are harmful when they interfere with his care and perhaps are only providing satisfactions for the nurse. Moreover, some nurses use them excessively to avoid direct contacts with patients. When this situation occurs, obviously the nurse is meeting her own needs.

If she is to give therapeutic nursing care, the nurse must develop an acute sensitivity to her patient's needs—an awareness of him as a complex human being. Her observations, as she appraises his needs, should be based on a vivid appreciation of his motivations and an understanding of the tensions reflected in his behavior. Only the nurse who has some understanding of her own behavior and her own motivations will be able to do this.

IMPROVING SELF-UNDERSTANDING

Very few people ever achieve complete self-understanding. But most persons are capable of improving their understanding of themselves and becoming aware of some of the motivations which cause them to act as they do. And nurses certainly should make a sincere effort.

How does one go about achieving greater understanding of oneself? There is no pat formula but certain approaches can be helpful.

The first step, of course, is to accept the fact that self-understanding is necessary and basic to understanding others. There must be realization that knowledge about one's motivations is essential in achieving psychological and social harmony. Goals must be defined, understood, and accepted, and then the premise accepted that ways and means to reach them can be found.

Here are some of the activities which can help the nurse who is struggling to achieve self-awareness. She should:

1. Develop an awareness of her own inappropriate reactions that are repeated. This will help her not only to free herself from such reactions, but also to become more aware of all reactions.

2. Study the factors involved in basic personality formation and the common adjustment devices that are used. She should learn to recognize destructive devices as well as more constructive ones, such as sublimation.

3. Attempt to learn from all interpersonal relationships. Any situations in which she reacted in a way she considered negative should be reviewed and discussed. Discussion of positive reactions may also prove to be helpful.

4. Learn from all supervisory and administrative counseling or guidance contacts. These discussions can be positive forces to help her increase her insight and understandings. With guidance, she can evaluate her personality traits but she should not attempt a "self-inventory" alone.

5. Attend and take an active part in discussions, seminars, and workshops designed to increase general understanding of self and of others.

6. Participate in professionally guided group therapy sessions.

7. Take part in guided readings and discussions of selected books and articles related to the general areas of personality development, interpersonal relationships, mental hygiene, and emotional maturity.

8. Participate in individual or group conferences with other professional personnel—psychiatrists, psychologists, social workers, nurses, and others.

9. Learn as much as possible about good mental hygiene practice in daily living. Develop a philosophy of life that is outgoing and compatible with the social milieu. If possible, set aside some time for a little introspection or a "quiet period" for thought.

10. Work and grow a little each day, so that the goal, "Know thyself," comes over a little closer.

BIBLIOGRAPHY

Anderson, Camilla. *Emotional Hygiene, the Art of Understanding.* 4th ed. Philadelphia, J. B. Lippincott Co., 1948.

Bischoff, M. W. and Connolly, M. G. New skills are needed. *Am. J. Nursing* 51:576-578, Sept. 1951.

Black, Kathleen. Appraising the psychiatric patient's nursing needs. *Am. J. Nursing* 52:718-721, June 1952.

Cannon, W. B. *Wisdom of the Body.* New York, W. W. Norton and Co., Inc., 1939.

Kalkman, Marion E. *Introduction to Psychiatric Nursing.* New York, McGraw-Hill Book Co., Inc., 1950.

Karnosh, Louis J. *Psychiatry for Nurses.* 4th ed. St. Louis, C. V. Mosby Co., 1953.

Leino, Amelia. Planning patient-centered care. *Am. J. Nursing* 52:324-325, Mar. 1952.

Matheny, Ruth V. *Psychiatric Nursing.* St. Louis, C. V. Mosby Co., 1953.

Mueller, Theresa. *Nature and Direction of Psychiatric Nursing.* Philadelphia, J. B. Lippincott Co., 1950.

Saul, Leon. *Emotional Maturity.* Philadelphia, J. B. Lippincott, 1947.

Symonds, Percival. *Dynamics of Human Adjustment.* New York, Appleton-Century-Crofts, Inc., 1946.

[The statements and conclusions presented in this article are the author's own and do not necessarily reflect the opinions or policy of the Veterans Administration.]

6

As You Enter
Psychiatric Nursing

Werner Tuteur*

*When the Illinois Department of Public Welfare opened its af-
filiate program in psychiatric nursing at Elgin State Hospital
in September 1954, Dr. Tuteur extended to the entering students
their first introduction to this new experience. His counsel seems
useful not only for students and their instructors, but also for
all graduate nurses who are about to embark on a first experience in psychiatric nursing.*

The requirement of psychiatric training for student nurses was added
rather late in the development of nurse education. Formal psychiatry itself
has been a late development and has had difficulty in keeping pace with the
sometimes very rapid progress made in other medical specialties. There are
no miracle drugs in psychiatry. There are no operations which may bring
about a magical cure. Time has always been a great factor in this field, and
human nature, which is inclined to be impatient, was alienated by the mentally ill, who would not respond to treatment and get well.

The stigma that mental illness always bore, and continues to bear, did
its part to prevent progress in this field. Clouds of superstition, fear, and
hate shrouded mental illness during the Middle Ages. The mentally ill
during that time were considered to be "possessed of the Devil." Only 200
years ago a mental patient was publicly burned to death. At that time general
medicine and surgery had already made much progress.

The French Revolution in 1789, the great symbol of human liberation
and free thinking to many historians, has been considered to mark the true

*From *American Journal of Nursing*, Vol. 56, No. 1 (January, 1956).
Dr. Tuteur is clinical director at Elgin (Illinois) State Hospital and clinical
associate at Loyola University's Stritch School of Medicine.

end of the Middle Ages. In 1793 Philippe Pinel freed the mentally ill at the Bicetre in Paris of the chains with which they had been bound in dismal dungeons.

Psychiatry has come a long way since then, but it remains shadowed by many undesirable deficiencies. Of the nine million people in this country who suffer from some form of an emotional illness, one million are confined to mental hospitals.[1] But only about 15,000 of the more than 350,000 registered nurses in this country are actually engaged in caring for them. Although $41,000,000 are spent annually in this country in care and research for all types of illnesses, only $6,000,000 are set aside for mental illness These figures may make you wonder—does psychiatry remain a clouded mystery; does the care of these patients represent a thankless task to the present-day registered nurse? Could it possibly be that the rewards are too insignificant? That is a misleading concept which we shall try to dispel. There are rewards, and they are great.

As you enter this new experience you will be confronted with human beings who, only 200 years ago, were considered criminals and outcasts, and your task will be far from easy. There will be an unavoidable impact on your first meeting the patient and on the patient's first meeting you. There will be embarrassment, uneasiness, self-consciousness on your part and on the patient's. The mental hospital situation is new for both the patient and you.

At times the demands that mental patients make on you will seem unreasonable, if not impossible to cope with. At other times your feeling of pity may be aroused to such a degree that you will feel wholly incompetent or incapable of meeting a certain patient's needs. At still other times you may become so alienated that you feel these patients do not deserve your care. You may at times even compare a patient's behavior with that of another person of your acquaintance or your family, and you will find that the patient reminds you very much of a person whom you have known to be inadequate and unpleasant as long as you can remember.

Any one of these attitudes is unwholesome, and they will further complicate your already difficult task. To feel comfortable in the presence of a mental patient, one must drop all that prejudice which still hangs heavily over mental illness. One must possess the mental freedom to assess the patient as an ill person who is in need of help.

This help, by its very nature, must be intense. It will involve your entire person. It may involve far more sacrifice on your part than you have made in caring for the other patients with whom you have associated so far—those suffering from illnesses that fall within other medical specialties. The latter come to a general hospital, usually for a well-circumscribed illness, for a certain length of time. They leave cured or considerably improved, leaving you with a sense of accomplishment—and your feeling is thoroughly justified, because you were an important link in the team which brought about this improvement.

You will, likewise, be a very important link when you attend those who are emotionally deranged. You will notice from the beginning that a

---

[1]Appel, K. E. The present challenge of psychiatry. (Presidential address) *Am. J. Psychiat.* 111:1-12, July 1954.

hospital taking care of mental patients will cater to much greater and more various needs of the patients than a general hospital does, and you will soon compare the general hospital from which you came with this institution. One may say that a general hospital oftentimes serves as a convenience for the attending physician. He sends his patient, leaves his orders, and knows that they will be carried out painstakingly, to the ultimate benefit of his patient. The operating room will be carefully prepared, and the patient's after care is assured.

For us these are merely skeleton functions. Besides attending to the patient's illness, we must carry out many other functions necessary for his mere existence.

The length of the patient's stay in a mental institution is usually uncertain. In many instances it will involve months, if not years. The patient, during this prolonged period, will need clothing, supervision of personal appearance, entertainment and recreation, to mention only a few. Most of our patients are not capable of taking care of their own affairs, and so considerable administrative work falls to the social service department and the record librarian. Many patients cannot be left to themselves, for various reasons. Visits by relatives will have to be planned; so will patients' visits to their homes, which we strongly encourage. Their personal property and valuables will have to be carefully checked and kept, yet they must be available when they are wanted, if it is feasible to let the patient have them.

You spend more time with patients' relatives and have much more intensive dealings with them than you do in a general hospital. Members of the patient's family are having just as new and strange an experience as you are today as you enter this institution. Not only will the relative need an explanation of the patient's symptoms but, after leaving the interview with the physician, he will be in much need of reassurance and warmth. Your professional training has already brought you into contact with persons who have a great need of both. Your contacts with the mentally ill patient's relatives will bring you a great sense of satisfaction and accomplishment during your stay with us. And they will help both to bring you into contact with the patient and to grasp the nature of mental illness.

But there will be many other sources of satisfaction. The vast majority of mental patients, those suffering from schizophrenia, develop this mental illness as a result of the severe rejection they experienced during early life. In becoming acquainted with our patients' histories, you will soon discover that every human being has a fundamental need of being accepted, appreciated, and loved. If these needs are not properly satisfied, especially during childhood and puberty, the person is apt not to withstand the strain and stress of everyday life, and will, through mental illness, return again to an age level at which he feels he can induce and even force his environment to take care of him. Thus, you will see patients who will have to be fed, and have their other personal needs attended to.

While the possibility is great that you will feel estranged from a young man in good physical health who needs such attention, your opportunities to help him again to reach a higher and more adult level of behavior are practically unlimited. Always remember that these unfortunate ones failed in their relationships to others; let them, and help them, relate to you. Let them gain the confidence and trust in others that they so utterly lack. Having gained confidence in you, they will learn to trust others.

Remember that mental patients are extremely sensitive. It was this sensitivity which played a major part in the development of their illness. It will take considerable self-control on your part, sometimes self-control of almost inhuman proportions, to display constantly a reassuring and friendly attitude. If you fail, the disappointment you may experience may be great but, if you succeed, there are no bounds to the rewards.

There is one type of patient with whom both the challenge and the awards are especially great. Since Biblical days and before, we have given special honor and respect to the aged. In the days before man had writing and printing as a means of communication, the elderly necessarily had an important role in the household and the family. They transmitted knowledge and maintained tradition. This has changed as our civilization has developed. The elderly no longer fulfill this purpose, and at times it seems to be difficult for the young to remember and to understand that elderly persons have a right to exist, even if they have, as the cruel expression goes, "outlived their usefulness." A person remains "useful" much longer than is commonly thought, and usually elderly people appear to become "useless" only because they have been forced into idleness.

Modern living has done its share to expel the elderly from the homes they had firmly established—they thought—with their grown-up children. Physical and mild mental handicaps in the elderly bring them to us to be taken care of, frequently against their wishes. The first gesture of appreciation, the first words of thanks from an elderly patient, helplessly confined to his chair, will amply reward you for your efforts and will give meaning to the time you will spend and to the work you will do.

You will find many patients who have come here because of a physical illness. With them you will make use of all the knowledge you have acquired and the sympathy you have been practicing during your experience in general hospitals.

There are many other types of patients you will meet and who will require your services. The individual who is addicted to alcohol is merely another person who failed to find the approval and esteem of his environment he so avidly craved. Alcohol, for him, is the escape that the schizophrenic finds by returning to his immature level of thinking and behavior. The alcoholic patient needs the same respect we give to others, lest he become convinced that he is completely outcast, unacceptable to our society. This would only provoke him to further indulgence.

You will see pregnant women for whom the thought of giving life is unbearable and who already feel intolerably threatened by their own future offspring—and you will meet women in late middle age for whom being no longer capable of giving life is disaster.

All these people have one thing in common. They are in great need of care, recognition, and approval. You will witness and assist with our physical and organic treatment methods. You will see improvement resulting from them, but you will also see their inadequacies and their fallacies. You will soon see that they cannot possibly replace the one factor that is so indispensable for harmonious living: self-respect. This can come only from other human beings, never from a machine or any kind of mechanical device.

With your patients you will experience a feeling of togetherness through which you will learn to share with the suffering patient, enabling him to carry on, enabling you to become a better human being.

There is so much communication without words. You will learn to communicate by manner and attitude, by facial expression, by gesture and tone of voice. These are great assets, not merely for one who cares for the mentally ill, but for one who communicates and lives with people in general. Love and understanding attention will always remain indispensable requisites for any human relationship. Remember the importance of tolerance, recognition of other people's point of view and, above all, your interest in others.

While you are here you will meet with an army of other employees. Some of them might not have the technical and academic knowledge of illness you have acquired during your previous training, but these people will lend you a helping hand in your difficult task. They have known mental illness for years. They know mental patients. They have proven themselves. If you extend your hand to them, you will harvest additional rewards.

Once you leave us, you can readily apply to any patient in your care the principles you have observed here. You will have learned that nursing is more than the administration of medicine, or the diligent preparation of an operating room, or routine procedures in general. One of the reasons why you spend a period of time with the mentally ill is to give you an understanding of the human needs of others and the catastrophe which ensues if they are not fulfilled or are fulfilled inadequately.

You have seen small moles and other harmless looking lesions grow into cancer. Really, the difference between physical and mental illness is not great. You will see here the final stage of a criminally neglected sore, a sore involving the whole person, not just one part, a sore which went unnoticed for some time, then was neglected, possibly even ridiculed. But this neglected and ridiculed sore took formidable revenge on the patient and all others in his environment.

Thus, as you start your work with the patient, steel yourself against the early disappointments. These are unavoidable. Prepare yourselves for the most difficult part of your education and, most of all, apply yourselves as persons tending to those who never reached maturity, those who have returned to immaturity, or those whose advancing age has taken them beyond it.

Section 2

Communicating with Patients

7

The Skills of Communication

Anne J. Davis*

These cannot be learned from a blueprint or a procedure sheet. Like all other skills in nursing, communication skills must be derived from the basic principles and concepts that determine the relationship of one person to another.

We hear a great deal today in nursing about the importance of establishing therapeutic relationships with patients. If we are to teach students to do this, however, we must do more than simply present them with a "blueprint" for relating. The skills needed for effective relationships with others—like all skills in nursing—need to be based on concepts and principles derived from a body of clinical knowledge and research. A theoretical frame of reference is necessary if there is to be any systematic method of viewing and evaluating behavior and of relating to patients.

Consequently, at the University of California School of Nursing in San Francisco, we have for the past several years utilized Jurgen Ruesch's theory of communication as the framework for teaching psychiatric nursing skills. This particular frame of reference was chosen for several reasons.

First, it seemed wise to give those students who often view the psychiatric setting as somewhat strange and frightening some principles which they could use immediately in relating to mentally ill patients. Second, we believed this approach would lead to the students' developing improved skills in com-

*From *American Journal of Nursing*, Vol. 63, No. 1 (January, 1963).

Miss Davis (B.S., Emory University School of Nursing; M.S., Boston University) was instructor in psychiatric nursing at the University of California in San Francisco at the time she wrote this paper. Since February 1962 she has been traveling in the Middle East and is now living in Israel, doing some sociological research and some teaching, dividing her time between Tel Aviv and a rural Kibbutz.

municating not only with patients, but also with families and fellow workers. And, finally, we conceived of these skills as pertaining to the care of all patients, not only of those with mental illness.

We know today that the so-called normal person is not radically different from the mentally ill person; it's mainly a matter of where the breaking point occurs. This knowledge has blurred previous distinctions between normal and abnormal, neurotic and psychotic. Therefore, professional people in many disciplines have been searching for a universal factor operative in the healthy and ill alike, and this has led to an intensive study of human communication.

Focusing on the process of communication makes possible a consideration of normal and abnormal behavior on the same continuum, deviant communication being viewed as simply ordinary communication distorted, due to a variety of reasons. Furthermore, according to Ruesch's theory, an individual's psychotherapeutic skills depend primarily upon his ability to communicate: to observe, interpret, express, or act. Therefore, the basic concepts of communication as outlined by Ruesch, seemed appropriate to present to students in an initial effort to help them develop therapeutic relationships with patients.[1]

WHAT IS COMMUNICATION?

According to Ruesch, communication embraces all the modes of behavior that one individual employs, consciously or unconsciously, to affect another: not only the spoken and written word, but also gestures, body movements, somatic signals, and symbolism in the arts. Nonverbal communication, as a matter of fact, is considered to be a more reliable expression of true feelings than verbal, because the individual has less conscious control over his nonverbal behavior.

Communication functions to mediate information across boundary lines of the human or group organization, and calls for three necessary operations: perception, evaluation, and transmission.

Perception is the reception of incoming signals which circulate either inside or outside a human organism. *Evaluation* involves summary and analysis of information provided, through retention of past experiences, and leads to prediction and decision-making. *Transmission* is expression of information by verbal expression, gestures, movements, and social actions. These three basic operations should be looked upon as a unit.

The developmental sequence through which individuals learn use of language and hence of communication is, briefly, as follows. During the process of maturation, a child uses three types of language: somatic, action, and verbal. In early life, somatic language is the means of communication. For example, the infant shows distress by his increased rate of breathing and reddened skin color. As he grows and gains more control over his body, he adds action language; thus, when he wants something, he may crawl or walk toward it. When he learns to speak, verbal language supplements his other languages. Now he

---

[1]No attempt is made here to outline Ruesch's theory of communication in full. Only a few of his basic concepts, as interpreted and condensed by the author, are included.

can communicate in all three ways when he runs into the house, fists clenched, face red, and says, "Paul and I have been fighting." As an adult he will be able, ideally, to use any one of these levels or a combination of them, according to what he perceives and evaluates as appropriate in a situation.

The individual, however, does not learn these three languages in a vacuum—the presence of other persons is crucial to such acquisition. Equally important, how others act toward the child impedes or enhances his language mastery. If, when the child is just learning a language level, his new statements are consistently not acknowledged so that he receives no gratification from his communication, he will find it difficult to master this level and to proceed to the next level. Or, if the parents acknowledge one language level to the exclusion of another—if they respond to action language, for instance, rather than verbal—the child will tend to use the level that is acknowledged, whether it is appropriate or not, because of the gratification he experiences.

Either situation, consistently occurring, results in a failure to master the language, and the individual's continued participation in such inhibiting networks results in impaired communicative ability. Thus, within Ruesch's framework, disturbances in communication become psychopathology.

From this theoretical view we can therefore assume that successful participation in communication systems which involve other people is necessary if the individual is to function effectively in society. Failure in communication is experienced as frustration. If this frustration is intense or extended, the person's thinking, feeling, and reacting become progressively more disorganized and inappropriate.

Prolonged frustration diminishes the person's ability to establish and maintain social relations. In contrast, the pleasure that individuals derive from well-functioning communication prompts them to seek human relations. Gratifying communication is, therefore, the keynote of mental health.

CRITERIA FOR SUCCESSFUL COMMUNICATION

The presence of four characteristics, Ruesch maintains, determines whether communication is successful or not: feedback, appropriateness of reply, efficiency, and flexibility.

Feedback circuits provide an opportunity for a receiver to relay back to the sender of a message the effects that the sender's statement has had. In one way or another, the receiver's reaction is relayed back to the sender and serves to clarify, extend, or alter the sender's original idea. Feedback, therefore, refers to the process of correction through incorporation of information about effects achieved.

Appopriateness means that the reply fits the circumstances, is relevant, and is matched to the initial statement. If the communication is appropriate, individuals do not feel overloaded with too much stimulation, or underloaded with too little.

Communication is efficient when the language used is simple, and when instructions are clear, agreed upon, and understood by those involved. Messages are timed so that the listener has enough time to perceive and evaluate them.

Flexibility means that there is neither exaggerated control nor exaggerated permissiveness. Messages are not redundant and information is not lost.

Communication is successful, Ruesch states, when the individual experiences the feeling of being understood, and this feeling derives from and is dependent on the presence of these formal characteristics. The absence or malfunction of one or more of these characteristics, on the other hand, leads to disturbed communication and, usually, disturbed relations with others.

When feedback circuits fail, there is interference with the free flow of messages. Messages either do not get through or they are damaged. It is impossible under these circumstances to receive appropriate replies, hence correction through feedback does not occur. Or, if the content of a message elicits fear, anxiety, shame, or guilt, the individual will feel threatened and his reactions are likely to disrupt the communication process.

Inappropriateness of reply results when the content of a situation is misconstrued or when an individual cannot make clear to others in what capacity he is acting or in what frame of reference he is speaking. He produces messages that do not fit the circumstances, are irrelevant, and are not matched to the initial statement.

The capacity to handle signals in transit characterizes every communication network. When the load is too heavy, the machine breaks down; when the load is too small, the machinery may deteriorate for lack of use. Every person has limits in terms of his tolerance for stimulation. Overstimulation may lead to disorganization and breakdown, whereas lack of sufficient stimulation, particularly in the form of emotional deprivation, can result in an individual's losing much of his communicative skill and frequently showing signs of apathy. Both overload and underload lead to inappropriateness of reply.

Inefficient communication manifests itself in the use of clumsy language or circumstantiality, producing either redundancy or a loss of information. If the information is conflicting or unrealistic, or if the information contains verbally stated goals which differ from the implied purpose, then communication becomes inefficient. Inefficiency also occurs when the statements of two persons are separated by too short or too long a time interval.

When there is exaggerated control or exaggerated permissiveness, then the communication lacks *flexibility*. In overcontrol, every message is checked and counterchecked; every action is prescribed. In exaggerated permissiveness, everyone can say and do anything he wishes, rules are disregarded, and chaos exists. In overcontrol and undercontrol, information is inefficiently disseminated.

THE IMPORTANCE OF ACKNOWLEDGMENT

The most important force one person can exert on another is to acknowledge the other's intent. Rarely, however, is such intent explicitly formulated. Out of a multitude of both verbal and nonverbal impressions, the therapist must sift out the relevant signals.

If, after attentive listening and observation, the therapist is unable to decipher the patient's message, he has to acknowledge this difficulty. Sometimes it may be possible to verbalize that part of the patient's message that is clear. Thus, *acknowledgment*, with progressive delineation of the part that has been understood, acts as an incentive toward further clarification.

Ruesch contends that the patient learns acknowledgment by being acknowledged. By acknowledging a facial gesture of the patient, or an abortive attempt to say something, the therapist teaches the patient to react. By focusing upon the patient's intention, by acknowledging his wish to communicate, by replying to the content of his message, the therapist strengthens the patient's desire to communicate and also increases his pleasure. Acknowledgment, thus, is the principal tool by which the therapist promotes communication within the therapeutic situation and motivates the patient to seek further improvement.

Devious acknowledgment, however, or a tangential response, can lead to a breakdown in communication. Here the receiver recognizes the sender's intention to communicate but disregards the content of the statement. For instance, Johnny, age five, runs in to his mother, shouting with glee, "See, I found a snail!" His mother replies in a cold, unpleasant voice, "Go and wash your dirty hands!" Johnny then experiences confusion and disappointment. His mother has recognized his intention to communicate—but not that statement which was most important to him.

If a reply does not fit the sender's statement in terms of language, content, and emotional concomitants, then the sender will experience a varying degree of tension. Another type of devious and frustrating reply is the quantitatively inappropriate response—too much or too little—or an acknowledgment that is poorly timed.

The dynamics of psychotherapy, Ruesch believes, derive from the patient's experience of pleasure when a message has been appropriately acknowledged. Successful communication is gratifying; it brings a feeling of inclusion and security and leads to constructive action. Disturbed communication is frustrating; it brings a feeling of loneliness and despair, and it leads to destructive action. The therapist's task, therefore, is to convert disturbed communication into successful communication and thus to improve the patient's relation to self and to others.

APPLICATION IN NURSING PRACTICE

Utilization of Ruesch's theory in the clinical practice of psychiatric nursing means that the nurse herself must learn how to communicate successfully as she helps correct the patient's disturbed communication. Of major importance in this process is her understanding of the criteria for successful communication—feedback, appropriatenes, efficiency, and flexibility. These, therefore, receive initial emphasis in our classroom discussions.

The presence of efficient feedback circuits is perhaps the foremost criterion of successful communication since it leads to correction of information, and correction is basic to all forms of learning including adaptive, healthy behavior and successful communication.

To maintain feedback circuits the nurse must often repeat the patient's verbal statement, as if to say, "This is what I heard; is that what you meant?" At other times she may need to transmit this message: "I hear you but I do not understand what you are saying. Would you tell me again?" Or, "I see what you are doing but I do not know what you are experiencing." This sort of communication helps the patient to begin to know when he is and is not being understood by the nurse. If the nurse continues to feed back to the patient the effects his messages have had, she gives him a better chance to learn successful communication because he has participated in this relationship.

Naturally, there will be occasions when the patient does not understand the nurse. If the latter has some doubt about whether the patient has understood her, then she, as the sender, needs to ask the patient, the receiver, if he understood her message. This gives the patient an opportunity to say that he has or has not understood or what part of the message was unclear.

Sometimes, too, the patient is unable to feed back verbally the impact the nurse's statement has had on him and may manifest only a nonverbal response. To help the student to become aware of responses like these, we encourage her initially to observe such gross behavior as whether the patient stayed or left the interaction, or whether he looked at the nurse or turned his back on her. Later the class considers more minute elements of the patient's nonverbal communication—that is, facial expression, position and movement of the hands and feet, and posture.

In the beginning of their practice, students are much more aware of the patient's verbal than of his nonverbal communication. Then, as discussion in class and conference begins to focus on the patient's nonverbal cues, students start to take these into account. They still need guidance, though, because at this point they may take one nonverbal cue out of context and jump to a conclusion without "checking it out" to ascertain the reality factors.

For example, a nurse may conclude that the usually depressed and slowed down patient now walking very rapidly up and down the hall is anxious, and this interpretation will influence her nursing intervention. Mr. Jones may indeed be anxious, but it is also possible that he is frightened or angry, or may want to go to the bathroom but it is locked. The nurse must therefore learn to approach Mr. Jones for more data as to the real explanation for the situation.

Nonverbal communication expresses a variety of emotions or needs, depending on who is communicating with whom, when, in what context, and what the individual's communication pattern is. The nurse must consider these factors in interacting with patients. By so doing, she no longer views the patient's behavior as if it occurred in a vacuum but as a response to the people who make up his environment.

Thus, when the patient's behavior changes as in the illustration just given, the nurse can acknowledge this changed behavior. When she does not know the patient very well, she uses simple acknowledgment, stating what she sees the patient doing, for what she hears him saying. For instance, noting the usually inactive patient now pacing the hall rapidly, the nurse could simply say, "Mr. Jones, I noticed you walking up and down in the hall. Is something bothering you?"

This type of simple acknowledgment is a tool that allows the nurse to state what she has seen or heard but does not understand. She can thus open circuits for the patient to express verbally that which he is experiencing. Further, she can approach the patient without a premature and false conclusion and also avoid such a question as, "Mr. Jones, why are you walking in the hall?"

Mr. Jones may not be fully aware of the why of his behavior and would find such a question difficult to answer. The underlying message in simple acknowledgment, however, merely says, "I see you there; I see you are doing something or saying something different from the usual. I do not yet understand but I will try to understand. Talk with me about it."

As the nurse spends more time with Mr. Jones, she will become aware of his pattern of communication and therefore will begin to understand what his behavior means. Eventually, for instance, she learns that just before Mr. Jones has a special kind of treatment he walks up and down in the hall. They have talked about this before and Mr. Jones has expressed how frightened he is. So, at these particular times, Mr. Jones' pacing means he is frightened. With this much information, the nurse can now acknowledge Mr. Jones with understanding. She can go over, walk up and down with him, and say, "You are upset about going to your treatment this morning. I will go with you and stay with you until it's over."

Acknowledgment with understanding may also be accomplished nonverbally. For example, on being told that a relative cannot come for a planned visit, a patient expresses her feelings of anger and disappointment by crying. Since the nurse sees this response as an appropriate expression of feeling within this situation, she may choose to acknowledge this nonverbally by simply staying with the patient until she feels better. By not avoiding the patient or trying to stop her crying, the nurse's message is, "You are hurt and angry and you are getting rid of these feelings in a healthy way."

The art of acknowledgment involves knowing what, how, and when to acknowledge. Like any other tool, acknowledgment, indiscriminately used, loses some of its effectiveness as an instrument of feedback.

APPROPRIATENESS, EFFICIENCY, AND FLEXIBILITY. We discuss the concept of appropriateness with our students from two approaches: first, the matter of overload and underload, and, second, the matching of verbal and nonverbal messages. If the nurse does most of the talking in an interaction with a withdrawn patient, then she is probably overloading this patient. On the other hand, underloading may occur if a nurse fails to respond when a patient repeats an action or verbal statement which previously has not been evident in his communication pattern.

The second aspect of appropriateness, matching verbal and nonverbal messages, involves helping the patient learn to make his actions, thoughts, and feelings coincide. To do this he needs to interact with another person who does this successfully because he, like many patients, may have experienced receiving two different messages simultaneously and may have learned to mistrust words. Such patients have to experience many times a situation wherein actions and words can and do give one message before they can learn to make their own actions, thoughts, and feelings coincide.

Efficiency—the third criterion of successful communication—means that the nurse must time her messages adequately, giving the patient enough time to receive and to evaluate a message and then transmit a response. The nurse may find it difficult at first to participate in conversation when the pace is slower than usual, but with experience she learns that a period of silence can be used as an effective tool.

Use of simple language is another way the nurse learns to maintain efficient communication. For example, when talking with a patient, it is better to use the words "mad" or "angry" rather than the more technical word, "hostile." This concept applies also to communication with staff. Rather than characterizing a patient as "suspicious," it is much more informative and efficient if the nurse describes what she actually sees and hears him do and say.

Flexibility, it is explained to the student, means that she could operate on the immediate cues from the patient. It is today that is important, not yesterday or tomorrow.

For example, yesterday Mr. Smith was in fairly good spirits so he and the nurse spent a pleasant, relaxed afternoon at the zoo. Today, however, Mr. Smith is obviously in very low spirits. If the nurse is happy and gay in her approach today because of yesterday, then she is either not perceiving the cues or, having perceived them, is not able to utilize them to help the patient.

Or perhaps the nurse decides that she wants to ask another patient about his recent visit at home. When she approaches him, she finds that he is extremely upset, talking in a loud voice, throwing his arms about, and striding around the room. If she persists in asking about the visit, then she has not changed her goal in spite of the intensity of the new cues. She needs to focus on what the patient is experiencing now.

NURSE-PATIENT RELATIONSHIPS. After several classes devoted to these criteria for successful communication, we then discuss different types of psychopathology as representative of disturbances in communication according to Ruesch's interpretation. Nursing interventions appropriate for each type of disturbed communication are suggested. Special emphasis is placed on the patient's probable childhood experiences in communication, and we speculate as to what might have gone wrong at that time to lead to the present communication problem.

Then the discussion turns to the present characteristics of the patient's communicative process. For example, we may discuss the withdrawn patient, who is usually an acute observer, especially of other's actions. He neglects, however, to evaluate the effect of his behavior on others.

Theoretically, within Ruesch's framework, the patient's acuity as an observer can be explained by the dynamics of parent-child relationships. When he was a child his parents did not respond to him on an action level and thus prevented him from learning to relate to others. Because he has never received sufficient response to his actions, in later life he seldom involves others.

In addition, he may have received from his parents simultaneous messages which did not coincide. His mother may, for instance, have said, "Of course, I love you," but communicated nonverbally through wrinkling her face a feeling of disgust to the child. The child must, therefore, become an acute observer to note others' actions because the latter may not agree with their words.

Such a discussion of the patient's history, developmental problems, and present situation helps the student to formulate appropriate nursing actions directed to communicating with the patient.

Although students know the total ward situation and relate to some degree to all patients, they work closely with one patient and keep process notes on this relationship. Therefore, the instructor confers with each student individually twice a week to discuss her nurse-patient problems. We try to help the student to develop a way of thinking about and viewing nurse-patient interaction that will allow her to work out her own methods of communicating therapeutically with the patient. Thus the student and the teacher view the student-patient interaction in light of the criteria for successful communication.

STUDENT-INSTRUCTOR DYNAMICS. Simultaneously, however, as instructor and student talk of student-patient communication, they are communicating with one another. The instructor deliberately uses this communication process to teach the student better communication. How the communication process in the student-instructor situation is used depends on the student's needs, which become evident after several conferences, and the instructor's skills. Thus the student herself begins to experience the dynamics of communication as well as the sort of relationship which she must help the patient to experience—namely, a goal-directed relationship aimed at improved communication.

Sociodrama is still another tool which we employ to help make Ruesch's theory of communication more meaningful to our students. Our over-all goal, toward which all our teaching and conference techniques are directed, is to assist students to develop more successful communication—and, therefore, more constructive relationships—with patients, families, and fellow workers.

8

Improving
Nurse-Patient
Communication

Stanley H. Eldred*

Words are but a part of the process of communication. We must also be aware of what our gestures, inflections, and movements say to patients.

Everything we do, say, or present has communicative value—the words we use, the gestures associated with the words, the clothes we wear or don't wear, the cars we drive, the house we live in, the area of the community in which we live and work. These things function as signs or symbols and communicate meanings. All of these meanings are culturally determined and members of the same culture or subculture will perceive them in approximately the same way.

At the present time, there is no *one* theory of communication. The linguist, the mathematician, the psychiatrist, and the advertising man all assess communication at levels which are pertinent to their particular field of expertness. As a psychiatrist, my particular field of interest is interpersonal communication.

Interpersonal communication goes on in three different ways at the same time—language, kinesics, and vocalizations, all going on within a context. Let us consider first the language. Language is roughly defined here as that which would appear on a typescript of a tape recording of a conversation.

The *language* used in interpersonal conversations bears only a lexical similarity to the written language found in papers and books. The grammatical forms, the sequence of words, and the frequency with which individual words are used differ greatly in spoken and written language. A person who in his interpersonal contacts talks as if he were reading a paper is very apt

*From *American Journal of Nursing*, Vol. 60, No. 11 (November, 1960).
Dr. Eldred is associate in psychiatry at McLean Hospital in Belmont, Mass.

to be considered affected, overformal, maybe even obsessional. The difference between the written system and the spoken system is even more apparent when we consider the other two ways in which interpersonal communication goes on.

When we speak we use not only words but also gestures. The term gestures is really too narrow to indicate the totality of what is communicated by our total muscular system and so the term *kinesics* has been coined.[1] Kinesics means not only the obvious gestures we all learned in public speaking but the totality of body set, rhythm, and movement of a nonrhythmical nature. This is a whole system of human behavior that has only recently been subjected to systematic analysis.

Except for a few standard gestures—such as thumb to nose, or the hand signals of a surgeon at work—kinetic movements do not have meaning in their own right. In general, the whole system of kinesics serves to support and modify the meaning of the spoken word. There are no kinesics in the written system.

Just as with our language, our kinesics are radically influenced by the culture in which we live. For instance, the way we walk says something about us, particularly in relation to our sexual identity. What, for instance, is implied when you see a male over the age of three walking along with his pelvis rolling with each step, his elbows held closely to his sides, his hands held away from his thighs, and the little finger of each hand separated widely from his other fingers? In our culture you would wonder about his sexual identity. In some African tribes, however, men are expected to conform to this set of kinesics and there is no implication of homosexuality.

The slumpng forward of the head and shoulders is frequently associated with low self-esteem. Has anyone ever seen a patient in an agitated depression who did not slump forward? These are only a few of the thousands of ways we communicate with our bodies to those around us.

The third component of interpersonal communication are the *vocalizations*—those noises, pauses, and alterations in pitch and degree of loudness which are generally lumped under the heading, "tone of voice," and which qualify or support the words that are being said. It is these vocalizations that convey a sense of seriousness, or insincerity, anxiety, anger, love, surprise, or what have you. Vocalizations convey the feeling tone in what is being said. In addition, vocalizations perform the function that is performed in part by punctuation in the written language—commas, periods, question marks, exclamation points, hyphens, underlined words, and paragraphs.

It is important to remember that vocalizations are culturally determined. There exist in any given language certain vocalization patterns which are as uniform in their function as the words themselves. These are patterns of stresses and pitches and pauses that are applied to the words to convey certain implications. For example, a question in English is indicated by a rising pitch at the end of a sentence. A declarative sentence ends with a falling off

---

[1]Birdwhistell, R. L. Kinesics and communication. In *Explorations: Studies in Culture and Communication*, ed. by E. S. Carpenter. Toronto, Canada, University of Toronto, August 1954, No. 3, pp. 31-41.

of pitch in the last bit of speech. Take the sentence, "You had your pill today." This can be a statement of fact, a question, an accusation, a criticism. All members of the English-speaking group will very likely understand exactly what the speaker is implying from the vocalization pattern he uses.

The vocalization patterns of our language are actually a whole system of interpersonal communication which we learn at a very early age. For the most part, this system functions outside of our awareness and so automatically that ordinarily we do not have to pay any attention to it. By learning to pay attention to our tone of voice, however, we can be in better control of what we intend the listener to understand in what we are saying and thus we can improve our communication.

All three elements of interpersonal communication—language, kinesics, and vocalizations—take place within a particular context. Ordinarily the context is something that our fantastically efficient central nervous systems handle automatically without our having to pay attention to the infinite number of decisions being made all the time. The context of an interaction encompasses such things as what has gone on in the immediate pasts of the participants, their total life histories, the time of day and year, their sexes, their socio-economic status, the place of meeting, and almost everything else.

Let's consider one situation: nurse talking to patient and patient talking to nurse in a particular ward in a particular hospital at a particular time. The socially defined role of being a patient is part of the context. A new patient coming into any hospital in this country is unwittingly behaving or misbehaving along culturally determined patterns. He is expected to be dependent upon the nurse and to surrender a great deal of his personal freedom.

Another part of the context is that the patient gives up some of his outside connections and makes interpersonal connections within the hospital system. This, along with learning the rules of the new small culture into which he is entering, produces *stress*. Stress—psychological stress—is always part of a hospital's context.

Also part of the context is the nature of the patient's illness. Pneumonia elicits different responses from the nurse than does a broken leg incurred while driving under the influence of alcohol.

Moreover, the social context varies from one hospital to another. Thus, a small community hospital, for example, would carry different connotations for both the nurse and the patient than a roaring "blood and guts" city emergency hospital or a quiet expensive private hospital in the suburbs would. The nurse and the patient will each perforce communciate somewhat differently in each setting.

The nurse's contribution to the social context of interpersonal communication with her patients is monumentally important to understand. In our culture, she or he represents a selfless dedication to service of mankind. She represents the ministering agent who will nurse one back to health. Whether or not she perceives herself in these terms, this is part of her social context. The limitations to this role are something to be learned by both the nurse and the patient in the course of their experience with each other. The age, sex, and specialty of the nurse also have cultural implications which define and qualify the nature of the communication which is to take place between a nurse and any given patient.

44

Having considered, if all too briefly, the context of this nurse-patient relationship, let us take the two people involved and see what can be said about their language, their kinesics, and their vocalizations.

First, the patient. It seems trite to say that understanding the patient is one way of being a more effective nurse. It is possible, however, to be rather explicit about how to arrive at a better understanding of the patient's communication.

Any patient is under stress. This may be the stress of the illness from which he is suffering or the stress of his particular way of living which has produced the symptoms. In either case, the new patient is also under the stress of having had to leave the environment to which he has been accustomed (no matter how bad it was) and to adjust to the new and frequently frightening environment of the hospital. People under stress talk differently. All three aspects of a patient's communication—his language, his kinesics, and his vocalizations—are affected, whether he has appendicitis, or a broken arm, or asthma, or schizophrenia. Unless the nurse is aware of these alterations she is apt to misinterpret what the patient is saying.

COMMUNICATING UNDER STRESS

A person who is seriously ill physically is apt to talk more slowly, more softly, less precisely, and with a narrowed range of pitch. Frequently he can't talk at all. The nurse has learned to expect these things and to respond to them appropriately. These are the socially and physiologically determined vocalizations which carry implications of helplessness and a need to be dependent for certain things. The nurse usually has no trouble in responding in the appropriate way.

A patient who is not so seriously ill, however, may talk very differently in response to the stress of this new environment. Although the alterations vary from patient to patient, let us consider the patient who is afraid of being dependent and fights it by acting in a very authoritarian way. His tone of voice may be harsh, rapid, loud, and peremptory. It is almost automatic for us to respond defensively or at best negatively to this kind of communication. In so doing we may deprive the patient of the very kind of interpersonal transaction that is needed to relieve stress. This point becomes particularly poignant if we realize that such a patient may not have the foggiest notion that he is communicating in an offensive fashion.

It is important to remember that our voices do not sound the same to us as to others. The competent nurse recognizes that very frequently a patient's offensive manner of communicating is no less a symptom of illness than his elevated temperature. She is then better equipped to treat his illness and avoid being the agent of increasing discomfort.

Psychiatric nurses probably know a great deal more about vocalization patterns and kinesics than they realize. These things are learned outside of awareness and are responded to intuitively. For example, in schizophrenia, aside from the obvious disturbances in the patient's language (his words), his use of vocalizations and kinesics deviates from the normal. The so-called flattened affect of the schizophrenic consists of a narrowing down of the pitch range, disruptions of pausal phenomena, and a narrowing down of the range of degrees of loudness. This may erroneously imply the absence of feelings. In addition, when the schizophrenic patient does use discernible intonation patterns, they are apt to be used in the wrong place. When the patient is trying to ask a question, he may use the intonation pattern which is appropriate to a flat statement. He may wonder why his questions go unanswered. He may even give up asking questions.

The nurse who is aware that the mentally ill patient is apt to use intonation patterns in the wrong place is better able to understand what the patient says with his words, and she is also able to be more aware of his feelings. She doesn't expect conformity to the cultural norm. She listens for cues and partial, parenthetical bits of communication. The important life-and-death things are frequently said in the most "affectless" tone of voice. The speech of depressed patients is characterized by squeezed-down pitch and intensity ranges, alterations in tempo, and failure to drop the pitch at ends of declarative sentences.

PROFESSIONAL AWARENESS

Now, what about the second person involved in patient-nurse communication? Most of us, by the time we have reached maturity, have been taught to be very aware of what we say in words. We are careful in our professional roles not to say the wrong things. We are unfortunately not so aware of what we communicate with the other modalities—our tone of voice and our kinesics. For example, a nurse who had a heated argument with her husband on the way to work in the morning would not think of continuing her complaints to her patient. But unless she has an unusual capacity for self-observation, she is very likely to continue to communicate her anger through her tone of voice and her kinesics in her first contacts with patients. Most of us are equipped to make allowances for this sort of thing and not take it personally. A psychiatric patient is less well-equipped and is apt to wonder what he did to elicit her angry tone of voice.

I suspect that some of Stanton and Schwartz's findings about covert discord between staff members adversely affecting the patient can be understood in terms of the nurse communicating to the patient (quite outside of her awareness) her angry feelings toward the doctor and vice versa.[2]

I have touched only on angry feelings. In fact, we are apt to convey to our patients most of our feelings, whether they be moods of depression, of being at peace with ourselves, or even of being in love.

The nurse who has had the opportunity to examine what she communicates with her movements and tone of voice is in a better position to communicate that which is appropriate to her professional role. One way for her to begin studying her communication is to listen to tape recordings of her own voice. Almost universally, the first time we do this we don't recognize our own voice. And once we do, we are very apt to wish we hadn't! Listening

---

[2]Stanton, A. H. and Schwartz, M. S., *The mental hospital: a study of institutional participation in psychiatric illness and treatment.* New York, Basic Books, 1954.

to ourselves can be a humbling experience from which we can learn a great deal about how we sound to other people.

The careful analysis of tape-recorded psychotherapeutic interviews has in some training areas become a very useful training device for the psychiatrist. Perhaps some day we will be sufficiently nondefensive to permit and to develop methods of obtaining tape recordings and sound movies of the interactions on hospital wards.

9

Interviewing with a Purpose

Maurice H. Greenhill*

*Should nurses use scientific interviewing techniques to deter-
mine their patients' needs? This authority suggests adding er-
udition to intuition.*

Interviewing involves communication between two individuals. Communication, by definition, is the act of transmitting facts, feelings, and meanings
by words, gestures, or other action. Hence, communication may be verbal or
nonverbal, and both are important.

It seems reasonable to assume that communication in an interpersonal
relationship such as the nurse has with her patient must carry with it the
transmission of feeling if it is to be meaningful. It is possible, of course, for
a person to transmit facts and avoid feelings, and such transmission of facts
may be very effective in keeping the patient and the professional person away
from their feelings.

INTERVIEWING TECHNIQUES

Interviewing is a goal-directed method of communication—a medium for
interaction between two persons. Social conversations are not interviews, but
when the professional person has a goal in mind as he converses with a patient, interviewing is in progress. Effective interviewing cannot occur without
effective interaction between two persons.

*From *American Journal of Nursing,* Vol. 56, No. 10 (October, 1956).
Dr. Greenhill is professor of psychiatry and chairman of the Department of
Psychiatry at the University of Miami in Miami, Florida. He is chairman of the
Community Services Committee of the National Institute of Mental Health and a
member of the Psychiatric Nursing Subcommittee of the NIMH Training Committee.
He also serves as consultant to the Surgeons-General of the U.S. Army and the U.S.
Public Health Service.

Nine principles of interviewing provide the foundation for verbal techniques of interaction.

1. *The patient is given the initiative.* He is prompted to begin the discussion, and the interviewer is careful not to interrupt, leaving the initiative with the patient. This does not mean that the patient manages, controls, or regulates the interview himself. Contrary to the misconception that the interviewer must be extremely passive, timely interjections or prompting are required.

2. *The approach to the patient is indirect.* The interviewer begins from the periphery. For example, in discussing his wife, the patient may say, "My wife isn't feeling well." Instead of saying, "Tell me about this problem that you must have," the interviewer might respond, "She's not well," prompting him to go on. She thus uses a more indirect approach, moving from the periphery closer to the center. This method may seem to require much more time than a direct approach does. Essentially it does not. It is surprising how rapidly the patient may open up and reach the core of the problem when a peripheral approach is used.

3. *Interviewing should be as open-ended as possible.* Statements made by the interviewer should not be closed off or sound final. One method of keeping the interview open-ended is to use an incomplete form of statement. "You were saying . . ." "You say you have pain . . ." The incomplete sentence has a prompting quality, signaling the patient that he can go on—now or the next time—if he desires. Open-endedness seems to break down most often when the interviewer seeks to reassure the patient. A nurse might attempt to reassure a patient who seems to be anxious about his condition by saying, "You're going to be all right," or "You've got a good doctor," or "After a few more treatments things will be all right." This may be reassuring to the patient, but on the other hand it may make it difficult for him to go on and reveal what he is anxious about. In following the principle of open-endedness, the nurse might better say, "After a few more treatments it ought to go better, but let's talk about it if you feel this way again." Thus, the way is left open.

4. *The interviewer uses minimal verbal activity.* Most interviewers say more than is necessary, which tends to obstruct the patient's responses. If the patient asks a testing-out question, one need do no more than answer it. The principle of minimal activity tends to break down in health education. For example, nurses often use this kind of interviewing effectively up to the point at which health education is indicated. Then they tend to use maximal activity with explanation, description, and interpretation in order to get the information across. A great deal of this is lost to the patient unless he feels that the overactivity indicates that the nurse is extremely interested in him. With minimal activity, it is possible to get health education across more effectively by proper timing, giving only as much as is necessary at the moment.

5. *Spontaneity should be encouraged.* When the patient is talking spontaneously, he is more likely to bring out useful information. He may start off with a spontaneous account of an event and if he is prompted to keep talking, he will bring out all kinds of relevant material. We are often told that good interviewing is good listening. It is really not the listening quality that is so important. It is rather that by using minimal activity, the interviewer has

thrown the initiative to the person being interviewed, thus inducing spon-taneity.

6. *Interviewing should facilitate expression of feelings.* One can never really be sure where the nurse-patient relationship is unless the patient is able to express his feelings about some topic, person, or event. When feelings come through spontaneously, they bring clusters of facts with them.

7. *The interview must focus on areas which are emotionally charged.* Charged areas are problem areas involving interpersonal and social problems; they are areas of the person's life about which he is in some conflict. One can follow all the other principles of interviewing, but if the interviewer does not focus from time to time on what is important by indicating to the patient that he should go on in this or that area, the interview will yield diminishing returns and dwindle away. Focusing is one of the ways through which the patient knows that the interviewer and he are on the same wave length. For example, when a patient mentions his wife four or five times in a period of 15 minutes, we should realize that there is a problem which ought to be explored. The next time the patient mentions his wife, we should focus on the wife-husband relationship. At these points of focus, the interviewer takes the initiative.

8. *Movement in interviewing depends on picking up verbal leads, clues, or signals from the patient.* These may be words, facial expressions, acts, or gestures. There are certain key words which the patient may bring up and repeat several times, or statements which he may make very emphatically. If his face flushes as he speaks of another person, it may be a signal to an emotionally charged area that should be explored.

9. *The data must come from the content of the interview itself.* If the interviewer follows the interview as a bloodhound follows a scent, usually a great deal will come out of it. One does not pull questions out of the blue to ask the patient. Rather, one should attempt to introduce only material to which the patient has already referred and should focus on one or another lead which he has expressed previously.

The principle of minimal verbal activity is very important. It can be classified as low, moderate, and marked—which is to be avoided.

Low verbal activity can range from no verbal activity at all to part of a sentence, a short sentence, or maybe two sentences spoken by the interviewer. At the same time, the interviewer may nod, lean forward a little, or look a little more intent. When he does so, he is using a moderate type of nonverbal activity. Interestingly enough, a great deal of effective interviewing is done with a combination of low verbal and moderate nonverbal activity.

There are really two general purposes in low verbal activity: first, it prompts the patient and is a way of inducing spontaneity. Second, it is a mechanism for scanning for verbal leads. Anyone who is testing out the use of low verbal activity should feel free to use as much nonverbal activity as he wishes, since it is difficult not to be active in some way.

Low verbal activity is sometimes effected by repeating the patient's last word, with rising vocal inflection, or by repeating a significant word, groups of words, or complete or incomplete sentences. Another form of low verbal activity is the use of mild directives: "Tell me more about that," which indicates, "Go on in that area; that interests me."

The use of *moderate verbal activity* depends on the communication pattern of the patient. If he is not communicating well, or not at all, the interviewer cannot help but step up his own verbal activity. A poor communicator will eventually pull the interviewer into more and more verbal activity.

Moderate activity is often needed to focus on a certain topic and explore the patient's leads. As soon as the interviewer focuses on some event, some person, or some word that the patient has been mentioning, he takes the initiative. To do this, he uses more activity. Moderate verbal activity is used also whenever the interviewer focuses on feelings. He is being more active, going into something that is more personal for the patient when he says, "How do you feel about that?" "How did you feel when your child went to the hospital?"

Many times patients being interviewed will test out the interviewer with such statements as, "Are you married?" "How long have you been a public health nurse?" or "Did you ever have a patient with this kind of trouble before?" Minimal activity should be used here, the nurse answering in as few words as possible. Should the patient ask: "How long have you been a public health nurse?" the answer might be: "Why do you ask?" because the patient usually has some purpose in asking this. In this way the nurse focuses on the purpose. Responding to testing-out in this way becomes moderate verbal activity. Moderate activity is also practiced when several words are used in order to focus on something, such as, "Well, tell me—tell me more about that . . ." In this situation, the interviewer might lean forward as he says it, using nonverbal emphasis also.

Another technique is repeated focusing. In the case of the man who has problems with his wife, one may find that he mentions her and then goes on to something else. The interviewer should focus on the wife again when the opportunity arises and sometimes three or four times during a given interview.

Marked verbal activity—which is to be avoided—may take one or another of the following forms:

1. Activity for the sake of the professional person's own purpose—for example, wanting to get as complete a record as possible, wanting to get her job done.
2. Interjection of the professional person's private ideas, bringing one's personal self into the interview.
3. Very active reassurance which tends to cut off spontaneity.
4. Sharing experiences with the patient, which jeopardizes the nurse-patient relationship.
5. Socializing with the patient, again bringing oneself into the interview.
6. Giving unrestricted advice, saying more than one has to.
7. Over-ready verbal encouragement which may indicate anxiety on the part of the interviewer.
8. Active explanation and interpretation, such as giving health information prematurely.
9. Marked probing or forcing out of data, which tends to make the patient defensive and drive him away from a charged area.

10. Display of emotion by the professional person, in the words she uses, the way they are said, or even by her facial expression.
11. Premature discussion of the nurse-patient relationship—"Perhaps you could tell someone else a little more . . ."
12. Changing the topic to obtain facts for one's own interest, thereby interrupting the patient's spontaneity.
13. Defending other professional workers when the patient shows some hostility toward one of the "helping professions." This, too, cuts the patient off.

THE RATIONALE FOR INTERVIEWING

Deviousness of communication is one of the common characteristics of all illness. The acknowledgment, identification, or deciphering of what the patient is saying indirectly is carried out mainly through interviewing techniques.

There are many ways in which the patient may transmit messages connoting need. He may verbalize obliquely. He may act out in inappropriate or self-destructive ways. He may have a chronic medical disorder and attempt to communicate meanings through his somatic symptoms. For example, a patient may want to tell a nurse, "I have been forsaken and I am furious about it. Not only has my daughter forsaken me but you had to go and take the week end off," but be unable to. He may have an asthmatic attack instead.

What in the dynamics of human behavior lies behind this deviousness of communication? Any personal problem or charged life situation carries with it a drive for self-protection from the accompanying anxiety, guilt, and uncertainty, and a tendency to make it impossible for the unpleasant emotions to be repeated. A patient in such a situation will therefore guard against revealing this charged area, but will almost always reach out tentatively for help by broaching the subject in a devious and peripheral fashion. The helping person can best meet this situation by responding in kind, that is, by approaching the patient's communication peripherally as well. This in part explains the rationale for some of the principles of interviewing.

One must keep in mind that there are probably a limited number of emotional states which result from stress situations and lead to illness. Isolation is one in which the patient has experienced separation from an important person or rejection by him. Many of the problems of dependency and hostility which one meets in patients are probably based on the fact that they feel isolated. Interviewing techniques are one means of approaching the patient to bring him out of isolation.

Anxiety and guilt are other basic emotional feeling tones. These often result from the patient's fear of his own hostile feelings. Accordingly he will test the nurse to see if she will accept the kind of person who has such feelings. A nurse who allows even the briefest comments from a patient concerning anxiety and guilt is communicating with him.

Whatever mode of expression the patient uses, no matter how obscure, the nurse should keep in mind that he is motivated by unconscious forces over which he has little or no control. But he is expressing need. Interviewing, as a vehicle through which the nurse can determine this need, is an integral part of nursing function.

THE SETTING FOR THE INTERVIEW

Traditionally, interviewing takes place in a formal setting in which the interviewer and the person he is interviewing sit face to face and discuss for a determined period of time, usually one hour. In nursing, such opportunities are rare except in a public health service: even here the public health nurses' enormous case loads usually preclude the allocation of so much time to an interview.

Our results have shown, however, that the more the formal setting is approximated, the better are the returns. We have found notable value in having a nurse sit at the bedside, interviewing the patient behind drawn curtains, or sit face to face with him in a room to which she has taken him for the privacy of the interview. We have frequently recommended that the public health nurse, if necessary, control the setting by interviewing a family member in her car rather than in a crowded living room where children are running about.

Notwithstanding the advisability of optimal conditions, most nurses' interviews are carried out in quite different situations. Since any goal-directed contact between patient and nurse constitutes an interview, nurses can establish meaningful communication with patients while they are standing at a bedside for five minutes, or sitting at a desk in a busy clinic, or accompanying a patient from the hospital ward to the laboratory, or while giving physical care. In all of these situations, the principles and techniques of interviewing can be applied. Moreover, interviewing in nursing settings has certain advantages.

Physical contact seems to act as a powerful catalyst in communication. Nurses, in practicing their manual skills, have a legitimate reason to "lay on hands" and can put this feature to use in attaining their goals. We have encouraged nurses, therefore, not to dichotomize interviewing and manual skills but to use them simultaneously. Sometimes, in fact, the nurse's main purpose in rubbing a patient's back may be to strenghten the verbal interaction between her and her patient. Here again the value of nonverbal communication is emphasized.

In the helping situation, much more may be conveyed by tone or voice, movement, gesture, and bodily attitude than by words. A nurse may be completely unskilled in specific verbal techniques but at the same time be so masterful in nonverbal methods that her patient attains good results. Nonverbal effectiveness seems to consist of: (1) emphasizing physical proximity to the patient; (2) timing closer proximity to support him when he is exploring emotionally charged areas; (3) using minimal motor activity and gestures and facial expressions which emulate those of the patient; and (4) adhering to accepting and nonpunitive attitudes and feeling tones.

A particularly important nonverbal technique used by many experienced nurses is to respond with appropriate and corrective motor action to a patient's nonverbal cues. For example, the nurse may identify leads denoting somatic discomfort from the patient's position and attitude, and then may immediately carry out an appropriate corrective measure, without a word having passed between the two. This type of nonverbal interaction is a most effective avenue to a positive nurse-patient relationship.

THE GOALS

Regardless of where it takes place—whether in a counselor's office or at the hospital bedside—interviewing has certain specific purposes.

1. *Initiating and maintaining a positive nurse-patient relationship.* When the relationship between the nurse and the patient is positive and constructive, symptoms decrease, demands are lessened, and the patient moves toward health. There are many ways of initiating and maintaining a positive relationship, the most effective being the use of skilled interviewing techniques. A positive relationship results only when the patient recognizes that the nurse understands his needs at the moment. If the patient tries again and again to transmit a message of need by devious means—hinting at a subject or presenting symptoms—and the nurse does not have the techniques of approaching this need, a negative relationship will sooner or later ensue. If, on the other hand, the nurse approaches the patient's charged area by identifying leads and focusing on them, a positive relationship is the invariable result.

There is no assurance that once the nurse has recognized that the patient feels positively toward her, and accepts her, this state of affairs will be maintained. A positive relationship, like peace, must be worked at consistently, for the patient's specific need will be repeated several times during the course of nursing care. Interviewing acts as a barometer of the nurse-patient status and as an effective tool in influencing it. The patient's willingness to allow the nurse to approach a charged area and reveal meaningful material is in itself an excellent indication of a positive relationship.

2. *Determination of the nurse's role.* Another purpose of interviewing is to collect information which will help the nurse determine what role she is placed in by the patient. He may see her in the role of mother, daughter, sister, wife, or of a good or a bad nurse whom he has known in the past, or as an agent of the doctor, hospital, or public health department. Determining the role for which she has been selected so that she can either utilize the role or change it should be a consistent goal for the nurse.

3. *Collection of information on emotional crises.* Many illnesses are precipitated or influenced by an emotional crisis in the patient's life situation. Sometimes the patient will divulge this to the physician, but very often he won't. The nurse, because she is with the patient longer, often is in a position to receive information which identifies the emotional crisis. There are several reasons why she should proceed with gaining such information. Not only will it help the physician identify the diagnosis and plan treatment, but it will also increase the effectiveness of nursing function.

In the first place, their relationship is enhanced appreciably when the nurse and the patient share information about the crises. Secondly, the nurse gets clues from this information about the roles in wich she may possibly be placed. Thirdly, the nature of the crisis which precipitated the illness will reveal clues to the reasons why the patient experiences minor crises in the nursing setting—increased symptoms, constant demands, and variable emotional reactions.

4. *Identification and resolution of immediate crises.* Most changes in behavior and certain changes in symptomatology are influenced by something

that happens on the ward or in the family setting, which constitutes a brief emotional crisis for the patient. It usually indicates his sensitivity to particular types of interpersonal situations to which he reacts again and again whenever the stimulus occurs. Observation of nonroutine occurrences—the appearance of a new visitor, the removal of a neighboring patient to another room, the death of another patient, the doctor's failure to appear for rounds, or difficulty during a procedure—may identify the precipitating factor. If a stimulus is identified, its importance to the patient must be verified through brief interviewing. If the nurse cannot observe such clues, she should not overlook the opportunity to uncover the factor by communicating with the patient about the symptoms of the crisis. More often than not, the truth about it will out, and then the cause, rather than the symptom, can be considered.

The very act of eliciting the cause is in itself therapeutic, and is often more effective medicine for a headache than an analgesic, or better for asthma than aminophylline. Many of the difficulties nurses have with patients or failures in public health management can be reduced in the same way. This method of identifying brief symptomatic crises serves to keep the patient "on an even keel."

5. *Channeling feelings directly.* Devious displacement of feelings may account for patients' somatic and behavioral symptoms. Whenever new symptoms appear or old ones reappear, the nurse might explore the situation through a brief interview in the hope of directing the associated feeling toward the legitimate object. For example, a patient had a sudden nocturnal headache. When interviewed by the nurse, she immediately revealed strong antagonistic feelings toward her doctor who had made an evening visit to another patient and had merely nodded to her.

Another typical example is the tuberculosis patient who refuses care in a sanitorium and directs hostility and resistance toward the public health nurse. Interviews frequently reveal that such hostility may be intended for a wife whom the patient fears will become unfaithful if he leaves home, or toward an employer whom he suspects may not stand by him if he takes sick leave. A seemingly simple measure such as the interview may do more to enable the patient to follow recommendations than all the persuasion, coercion, and teaching the nurse can possibly do.

6. *Channeling communication.* Our studies have shown that meaningful communication between patients and professional personnel usually proceeds through predictable channels—from patient to ward aide to nurse to physician. Or, the patient will test out by revealing significant interpersonal and social data first to the aide, then to the nurse, and finally to the physician. The nurse's use of interviewing techniques can facilitate markedly the transfer of significant information to the physician. Also, the nurse can take advantage of this typical channeling by making the most of an interview when the patient reveals information with significance for nursing care.

7. *Preparation for health teaching.* Our data reveal that nurses practice health teaching with alacrity but also that the teaching they present is often premature and does not always yield the expected results. Obviously health teaching is not effective without adequate preparation for a positive nurse-

patient relationship. Purposive interviewing seems essential in establishing the kind of relationship in which health teaching can be effective.

WHAT LIMITS SHOULD BE SET?

What are the limits of interviewing for nurses? Is it not likely that the nurse will step over the boundaries into the areas of the physician, the psychiatrist, or the social worker?

Interviewing is no special prerogative of any one discipline; it is simply a method of interaction which occurs in every professional situation. Each discipline, however, has its own objectives when it practices these techniques. A major source of concern is to differentiate the nurse's purposes in interviewing from those of the psychiatrist. The general principles of the technique, as practiced by members of both disciplines, are the same, but the objectives in nursing are limited to nursing care alone, and do not extend to long-range alterations in maladaptive reactions. The nurse is concerned mainly with alterations in the patient's reactions in the *immediate* situation.

But might the nurse go too far? Naturally she is concerned with limiting her techniques so that the patient will not open up with material that neither he nor the nurse can handle. If the nurse keeps in focus the specific objectives of interviewing as they apply to nursing care, patients will rarely go too far. Secondly, her techniques should be confined to merely *approaching* charged areas from the periphery, not to exposing them. It is remarkable how frequently nurses can achieve their objectives by seeking merely to approach sensitive areas which are the patient's hidden agenda. Often they achieve desired results by recognizing and tentatively exploring leads without ever learning even a part of the full story. Rarely if ever do patients get out of emotional control as a result of interviewing by nurses, for the patient's protective devices serve as heavy armor.

Sometimes other problems arise which automatically place limits on interviewing when they should not. Nurses find themselves in a quandary when they are the only ones in the clinical setting who practice interviewing techniques and thus make discoveries about patients which supervising nurses, physicians, or public health officers do not understand. I know of only one way to meet this situation, and that is for the nurse to continue to give superior nursing care for the sake of the patient, come what may.

Another frustration which every interviewer—whether psychiatrist or nurse—meets is when he or she cannot capture the patient's meaning, or when the desired results are not obtained. Patients sometimes have defenses which defy all efforts, while with others it is necessary to continue one's efforts until the meaning emerges. Of course, certain interviewing methods may fail with one patient, and succeed with another. The nurse is fortunate if she has access to a more experienced interviewer with whom she can seek counsel, but even without such an opportunity, she can reap gratification through continuous practice with interviewing techniques.

There is one final problem. Nurses are with patients several hours a day. The purposive interviewing which I have described cannot be practiced continuously. If this is attempted, the interaction between patient and nurse becomes artificial and the relationship suffers. We advocate selective samples of interviewing to be done while physical procedures are being carried out, or at times of crisis. I sometimes call this "flurries of interviewing" to be performed at appropriate times. During the intervening time, the nurse can relax into superficial communication in which she makes no attempt toward meaningful expression, but holds her gains. For the public health nurse, the situation is somewhat different because her contacts with patients or family members are sporadic and so limited in time that she can use all opportunities for purposive interviewing.

10

Blocks
to Communicating
with Patients

Helon E. Hewitt and Betty L. Pesznecker*

Five categories of verbal errors are identified, which the authors believe nurses can use to examine their own responses to patients.

Nurses who genuinely want to comfort patients or help them solve their problems often fail in their attempts. Ineffective communication may be the reason and it is often the nurse's own words inadvertent though they may be which block communication between herself and the patient.

To help nurses study their own interactions with patients, we have identified five major verbal blocks to effective communication. They are: changing the subject, stating one's own opinions and ideas about the patient and his situation, false or inappropriate reassurance, jumping to conclusions or offering solutions to the problem, and inappropriate use of medical facts or nursing knowledge. The classification is based on an original system developed by Joan Bachand.[1]

Once a nurse identifies one of these blocks in her interaction with a patient, exploration of possible reasons, which may have precipitated the verbal error, can provide her with the insight she needs to achieve effective com-

*From *American Journal of Nursing*, Vol. 64, No. 7 (July, 1964).

Miss Hewitt (Emanuel, Portland, Ore.; B.S., M.N., University of Washington) was a research instructor in the University of Washington School of Nursing. She is education instructor at the University Hospital, Seattle.

Mrs. Pesznecker (St. Luke's, Spokane, Wash.; B.S., M.N., University of Washington) was research assistant professor at the University of Washington School of Nursing, Seattle, Wash.

[1]Bachand, Joan. *Problematic Verbal Patterns of Student Nurses in Initial Interviews with Psychiatric Patients; A Tool and Its Application.* Newark, N.J., Rutgers University, 1959. (Unpublished master's thesis)

munication. There are many reasons why she may have blocked her own good intentions. Her own anxiety, her attitudes about the patient, and her preconceived notions of how patients should behave are just a few. Before the nurse can deal with the underlying reason for poor communication she must be able to recognize when her own words cause the block.

CHANGING THE SUBJECT

In this category of verbal errors, the nurse shifts the focus of the conversation by directly changing the subject. Or she may shift the topic by responding to some insignificant aspect of the patient's conversation. The following example illustrates this.

Miss Brown: Good morning, Donald. How are you?

Donald: Hi (silence). Dr. Nash came in last night with Mrs. Robinson. He told me my mother died.

Miss Brown: I'm terribly sorry, Donald. Was she sick long?

Donald: Well, three months ago she told me her kidneys were all shot and the doctor said she had only three to six months to live. It was only three.

Miss Brown: It must have been quite a shock to you, Donald.

Donald: She was in the hospital when I had to come to the hospital, so I knew I might not see her again. (Donald began to cry.)

Miss Brown: I think maybe we'd better get started with your bath now, Donald. I'll get the linen to change your bed. (Donald continues to cry softly, and the nurse leaves the room.)

The nurse evidently could not respond to Donald's talk about his mother's death so she shifted to the safe topic of the bed bath. Perhaps her own anxiety concerning the subject of death was the cause.

Had Miss Brown been able to control her own anxiety, she might have been able to remain with Donald when he began to cry. Her physical presence could have conveyed to Donald that his feelings about his mother's death could be expressed freely. Verbal response from the nurse may not have been necessary at this point—just staying quietly with the boy.

In the next illustration, Miss Mills was not able to hear the patient's expression of concern because she was so preoccupied with a task she wanted to accomplish.

Miss Mills: Hello, Mrs. Long.

Mrs. Long: Yes?

Miss Mills: I'm Miss Mills. How are you feeling today?

Mrs. Long: Oh, pretty good. My back still gives me a lot of trouble.

Miss Mills: Oh. The doctor would like us to catheterize you for a urine specimen.

GIVING OWN OPINIONS

In this category, the nurse states her own opinions and ideas about the patient and his concerns in a way that hinders the exploration of the patient's problems. Such statements often have a moralizing tone.

COMMUNICATING WITH PATIENTS

In the following interaction, the nurse's ideas about how the patient should react to his hospital care blocked her from exploring how the patient thought and felt about his treatment.

Miss Lee: Good morning, Mr. Marsh. I will be taking care of you this morning. Would you like to wash before breakfast?

Mr. Marsh: Oh, I suppose (pause). I hope I don't get oatmeal again this morning. That is all they feed me for breakfast and I never get enough of anything.

Miss Lee: I know, Mr. Marsh, but you should be thankful that the doctors prescribed a special diet which will help you.

Mr. Marsh: I know! But it's no fun! I get hungry!

Miss Lee: Of course it's no fun but you'll be glad you kept on the diet when you begin getting well.
(After breakfast)

Miss Lee: Would you like your bath now?

Mr. Marsh: No, I want to rest. Besides, I don't want a bath. I don't need one every day. It takes too long to have a bath.

Miss Lee: It won't take long, Mr. Marsh. I'm sure you will feel much more comfortable and relaxed after you've had your bath.

Mr. Marsh: Oh yes, yes! Well, go ahead.

At first, Mr. Marsh was trying to express his feelings about his diet and some of the discomfort it caused. When the nurse implied that Mr. Marsh should appreciate the efforts of the doctors and nurses in his behalf, she stopped his expression of feeling. No doubt the nurse believed that all patients feel better after a bath. This attitude about patient care interfered with her ability to help Mr. Marsh talk about his need for rest and about the bath.

When Mr. Marsh said he never got enough of anything, Miss Lee might have explored this statement by saying, "Do you mean, Mr. Marsh, that you never get enough to eat?" This kind of question would have allowed the patient to further express his feelings about his diet or other concerns.

INAPPROPRIATE REASSURANCE

False or inappropriate comments made by the nurse can keep the patient from expressing his worry.

Mrs. Perry: Good morning, Mr. Cook, you look pretty fit. Feeling better today?

Mr. Cook: Yes, I just want to get out of this bed and go home. I can't take this lying around.

Mrs. Perry: Have you talked to your doctor about when you will be able to leave?

Mr. Cook: Oh, he doesn't say anything much. He keeps beating around the bush.

Mrs. Perry: Well, who knows, he may pleasantly surprise you soon. It probably won't be too much longer before you're on your way home. How about a bath, now?

Mr. Cook: O.K.

The conversation continued around the bath procedure and, interestingly, the patient did not again discuss his feelings about going home.

We can only speculate about the nurse's motivation. It is probable she sincerely wanted to relieve the patient of his anxiety. Perhaps this is often the reason for such inappropriate comments. Frequently, the nurse is unable to give an accurate answer to the patient's questions. Our data include many examples of nurses offering false reassurances and blocking communication with patients who question their prognosis, talk about death, or express fear of impending surgery. It is obvious the nurse cannot honestly answer a question about an uncertain outcome. These topics create a certain amount of anxiety within the nurse, and she sometimes feels more comfortable in cutting off the subject. .

The nurse might have responded to Mr. Cook's concern about going home as follows:

Mr. Cook: I just want to get out of this bed and go home. I can't take this lying around.

Mrs. Perry: You're pretty anxious to get home, Mr. Cook?

Mr. Cook: I've got to get home! I've been off the job two weeks now and I don't know how much longer I'm going to have to be off. If I just knew how much longer it will be before I can go back to work . . .

By focusing on Mr. Cook's concern about going home, Mrs. Perry encouraged the patient to express concerns which he might otherwise have kept to himself.

JUMPING TO CONCLUSIONS

Jumping to conclusions or offering solutions prematurely to the problem is another error in communication. The nurse responds to a part of a situation or problem expressed by the patient as if the entire situation or problem had been stated. When a nurse reaches conclusions without exploring what the patient is trying to communicate, she tends to propose a quick—and perhaps not the best—solution to the problem.

The nurse entered the room of a patient who had suffered a fracture of the right forearm and left side of the pelvis and was complaining thus:

Mr. Cox: My back hurts.

Mrs. Ray: Your back will feel much better if you can turn on your side.

Mr. Cox: Which side?

Mrs. Ray: Well, the doctor said either side, so why not the side that hurts the least. Here, let me help you.

Mr. Cox: Oh! I can't! The pain!

Mrs. Ray: You must get off your back so something can be done to help it besides medicine. A rub would help a lot.

Mr. Cox: No. No. I can't do it. Stop! Impossible!

The nurse seemed to be preoccupied with completing a nursing task or finding a quick solution to the patient's problems as she perceived them. This preoccupation interfered with her exploring and clarifying the problem from the patient's point of view.

We can only speculate what the real problem or source of discomfort was for this patient. The location of his fractures could interfere with a comfortable position in bed. The patient appeared to be unable to tolerate the pain of changing positions and was experiencing pain in the recumbent position. This is not an uncommon nursing problem. There are times when such nursing measures as positioning and turning the patient must be enforced. When giving the physical care, however, emotional support must be considered too.

The foregoing illustration has a tone of aggressiveness on the part of the nurse. The patient was not allowed to verbalize his feelings about turning. Nor was he given the opportunity to express his feelings about being in such a miserable condition. Frequently, if the patient is allowed to reveal his feelings without the nurse interjecting her own ideas, directing, or attempting to control the patient, he will be able to clarify his thinking and feeling, for himself and as a result, modify his attitudes and behavior.

Mrs. Ray might have been less directive, allowing the patient to express more clearly his difficulty. The scene might have been as follows:

Mr. Cox: My back hurts.

Mrs. Ray: Where does it hurt?

Mr. Cox: All over, but mostly in the middle. Can't you do something?

Mrs. Ray: You're probably pretty uncomfortable from being flat so long. Perhaps if you can turn on your side, I could rub your back.

INAPPROPRIATE USE OF FACTS

The inappropriate use of medical facts or nursing knowledge is a common error. In order to teach or tell the patient before exploring how he thinks or feels about the topic being discussed, the nurse may state facts. The premature use of nursing or medical facts was used most frequently by nurses in an effort to change the behavior or attitude of a patient. The tone may be argumentative, since the nurse may be directly opposing or ignoring the views or feelings of the patient.

In the following example, a nurse used facts in an effort to persuade a patient with tuberculosis to change his behavior to be more in accord with his prescribed treatment.

Miss Hill: Good morning.

Mr. Leaf: Good morning. How are you?

Miss Hill: Oh, fine. How would you like your bed straightened?

Mr. Leaf: Fine. (He hopped out of bed into a chair.)

Miss Hill: (She began to straighten the bed.) Sit down and rest.

Mr. Leaf: I'm getting too fat. I need more exercise.

Miss Hill: You shouldn't worry about getting fat now. Get all the rest you can, so you will get well faster. Then you can gradually increase your exercise to decrease your weight.

Mr. Leaf: I don't need that much rest.

Miss Hill: Oh, but rest is probably the most important treatment for tuberculosis patients. You see, by resting, the lungs can be at rest, too and, therefore, healing takes place more rapidly.

Mr. Leaf: I don't care. I simply can't endure lying in bed when I don't feel badly.

Miss Hill: Well, you think about it.

The facts the nurse told the patient were logical, but they did not seem to help the patient become more comfortable or accept the prescribed rest. The patient apparently was having difficulty in assuming the role of patient. Perhaps he viewed resting in bed as becoming dependent, which he could not accept at that time. Although he indicated a greater concern about getting fat than resting, the nurse explained the logic of his rest treatment.

This mode of interaction tends to weaken the relationship between the nurse and patient. By allowing the patient to express his feelings, rather than opposing his ideas, the nurse would have created a more positive climate and a more therapeutic relationship.

The nurse might have conveyed more interest in the patient's feelings by responding directly to his comment, "I'm getting too fat and I need more exercise," by saying, "You seem concerned about the lack of exercise you have been allowed since your hospitalization." This would have allowed the patient to express more of his feelings about hospitalization and the restrictions on his activities imposed by illness.

We believe that nurses can use these categories to examine their own errors in response to patients. Speculation about the reasons can help the individual nurse to improve her ability to provide therapeutic nursing care for her patients.

BIBLIOGRAPHY

Burton, Genevieve. *Personal, Impersonal and Interpersonal Relations; A Guide for Nurses.* New York, Springer Publishing Co., 1958, p. 230.

Roethlisberger, F. J. Barriers to communication between men. In *Language, Meaning and Maturity,* ed. by S. I. Hayakawa. New York, Harper and Brothers, 1954, pp. 61-66.

Rogers, C. R. Communication: Its blocking and its facilitation. In *Language, Meaning and Maturity,* ed. by S. I. Hayakawa. New York, Harper and Brothers, 1954, pp. 53-60.

11

Communication
A Factor in Meeting
Emotional Crises

Garland K. Lewis*

Because of what the nurse does and because the nurse has more time available to spend with patients, interpersonal communication must be a primary skill.

Communication has become an everyday household word, and has invaded every discipline—in the university, the business world, politics, labor and management—in fact, every facet of American life. It has become a major concern because of the nature of our society.

It is obvious that we are highly dependent upon our communication with each other in such an interdependent society. As our society has grown more complex, various symbols and codes have been devised to assist us in rapid communication. The Morse code, developed in 1844, was one of our early means of rapid signal communication.

Today, modern machines can send code messages from an office in Minneapolis to New York City via letters of the alphabet, dashes, and numbers, placing orders for various materials, such as steel, copper, aluminum, and oil. Highly skilled secretaries are needed to decode or interpret these symbols with the full knowledge that a transposition of "Ch" to "Wh" could cost an industry tens of thousands of dollars, or route a ton of copper to Australia instead of San Francisco, or even bring about some political holocaust.

*Reprinted from *Nursing Outlook,* August 1965, pp. 36-39, by permission of the author and The American Journal of Nursing Company. Copyright August 1965, The American Journal of Nursing Company.

Miss Lewis (Christ Hospital School of Nursing, Topeka, Kan.; M. S., University of Washington, Seattle) is associate professor and director, graduate program in psychiatric nursing, University of Minnesota School of Nursing, Minneapolis. She is well known as an author, lecturer, and teacher. This article is adapted from a paper presented at a workshop on "Nursing in Emotional Crisis" at the University of Kansas Medical Center, Kansas City, Mo., April, 1965.

THE CRUX OF THE MATTER

It may seem trite to insist that for the nurse communication is a significant factor in dealing with crisis intervention. We cannot expect the nurse to give the kind of support that some authorities believe a patient needs to alter his way of dealing positively with the crisis situation, if she does not know how to communicate effectively. Granted, she must have knowledge of and be able to recognize a crisis situation, but that knowledge alone is not sufficient, not unless she can intervene positively—can do something about the situation.

If we believe that only through communication we relate to another human being, it is imperative that the nurse understand this concept as well as be able to relate skillfully to patients in crisis situations. This sounds very simple on the surface, and I am certain that most nurses and, for that matter, most people believe they can communicate with others. Nonetheless, our feeling very certain that we are being understood and are understanding, that we mean what we say, and that those listening to us can actually sense what we mean is no guarantee against misunderstanding or misinterpretation.

How effectively do we communicate, and do we evaluate the results of our communication often and well enough to make us aware of our effect on the other person? In my experience, nurses and others in the health field tend to say, "The patient doesn't understand me," much more frequently than "I must not have made my explanation very clear, because the patient didn't understand my message."

Psychiatry, beginning with Freud, has been concerned with "talking" as a means of helping. Szasz says, "Psychiatrists communicate with patients by means of language, nonverbal signs, and rules."[1] Schramm describes communication as one of the busiest crossroads in the study of human behavior because communication is, perhaps, the fundamental societal process, and "without communication, human groups and societies would not exist."[2] Berlo tells us there is research evidence to show that the average American spends about 70 percent of his active hours communicating verbally—listening, speaking, reading, and writing, in that order. In other words, each of us spends about ten to 11 hours a day, every day, in verbal communication behaviors.[3] The scope of communication behavior is very broad and involves much more than most of us are consciously aware of.

Although only a small number of persons have devoted their concern to communication behavior exclusively, a great deal of information is available from the research that has been done in the communication field which includes *interpersonal* as well as mass communication. Berlo sees this age as one of symbol manipulation. "In our grandfather's day most people earned their living by manipulating things, not by manipulating symbols. Communication was important then, too, but it was less relevant to a man's career."[4]

According to Szasz, "[psychiatrists] analyze by means of verbal symbols the communication interactions which they observe and in which they themselves engage."[5] He believes that "from among the many different kinds of behavior, the verbal form—or communication by means of conventional language—constitutes one of the central areas of interest for psychiatry."[6] In *The Myth of Mental Illness,* he goes a great deal further in explaining his ideas relative to language and mental illness:

65

Although the concept of psychiatry as an analysis of communication is not novel, the full implication of the idea that so-called mental illnesses may be like language, and not at all like diseases of the body, has not been made sufficiently explicit.[7]

I will not attempt to describe here Szasz's theory other than to call attention to a new dimension of communication or language as he envisions the interplay between language and disease.

THE CONCEPT OF CRISIS

It has been my concern for some time that nurses should have more knowledge in the area of interpersonal communication in order to become helping persons. This applies to other health workers as well, but because I am mainly concerned with what the nurse does and because the nurse has more time available to spend with patients, I see this as her primary skill. In order for a nurse to communicate skillfully, other knowledge and attitudes are foundational. I will elaborate on these when I discuss specific situations.

Lindemann and Caplan have observed that an individual is usually in a state of relative equilibrium in relation to his milieu. This equilibrium is maintained by complicated interchanges between the individual and his environment, and is particularly dependent upon the interpersonal transactions through which he gratifies his emotional needs. Occasions arise, however, when the individual is incapable of solving the problems that have been brought about by his life situation, and the homeostatic mechanisms are unsuccessful in restoring his previous equilibrium. A more or less protracted period of emotional upset ensues which is called a crisis. The crisis is characterized by an increase in inner tension, unpleasant affect, and disorganization of behaviors.[8]

I think it is important here to focus on an aspect of this concept of crisis particularly significant to nurses—or any helping person—and that is the term "equilibrium." According to Lindemann:

In any ordinary life circumstances involving changes in the relation of internal and external psychic forces the person may temporarily fall into a state of unstable equilibrium but will spontaneously return to his previous state as a result of complex biopsychological control mechanisms. In a crisis situation, however, a special meaning of the environmental circumstances upsets the structuring of intrapsychic forces. During this period there may be a realignment of forces and this will lead to a new state of equilibrium which often differs from the former.[9]

Ackerman prefers "homeodynamics" to "homeostasis," explaining his discontent with the use of the term homeostasis as follows:

In the deepest biological sense, to stay the same is a certain warrant of death. I am suggesting that "homeostasis" or the principle of dynamic equilibrium, signifies the capacity for creative, fluid adaptability to change, which at the same time assures the measure of coordinated control that prevents the organism from being overwhelmed by a barrage of stimuli in excess of the organism's capacity to accommodate. The essence of life is change, growth, learning, adaptation to new conditions, and creative evolution of new levels of interchange between person and environment. In this context, life process cannot be secure and stable in any absolute sense; it is intrinsically fluid, changing, and unstable. . . . But this is a controlled "instability," controlled so as to offset a too rapid and destructive change.[10]

Becker also views the concept of homeostasis as inadequate when applied to human, symbolic behavior. He explains it thus:

On crude levels of organismic functioning the integration of organism and environment seems easily acquired. Each organism exists in a certain state of tension, a minus situation which it constantly attempts to overcome. No sooner is food ingested, waste excreted, satisfaction momentarily achieved, than the tension begins again to rise, and equilibrium to slip away. With the development of more complex receptors—sight, hearing—the scope of the animal's action is enlarged, and so also is the problem of satisfaction.[11]

I call attention to these considerations of homeostasis or equilibrium because if we are to become helping persons to individuals involved in crisis situations, we should not limit our goals to static equilibrium, but strive to assist the person to *dynamic* equilibrium.

The importance of communication in our society and concepts regarding crisis situations relate very specifically to what I believe is crucial in assisting patients and affect the nurse's communication with patients, that is, her ability to recognize and be aware of a person's positive strengths. We in nursing have been too long concerned with the abnormality, the disease, or the limitations —call it what you will—and have completely ignored the strengths the patient possesses. There are obviously many reasons for this, but we pay the person —labeled a patient—a disservice by concentrating on his "illness" and neglecting the "well" aspects of his functioning. For too long we have focused our observation of a person on finding out how sick he is—rather than looking at *both* his limitations and his strengths. We forget that some of his present limitations were not limitations in the recent past.

THE COMMUNICATION PROCESS

A young woman who requested admission to a psychiatric hospital did so on her own decision and against the advice of her parents, because she felt she needed help. The staff, however, viewed this patient as incapable of making a decision because she could not make the decision to ask her parents not to visit—even though she said in many indirect ways that she did not wish to see them. Without assessing the total situation, the staff had made a judgment which was based solely on the situation they had observed first hand. This illustrates what Caplan calls an "interfering theme" which influences our thinking about a person—a stereotyped expectation.[12]

Traditionally we have looked for or observed those symptoms with which the patient needs help—the sick symptoms. Nurses communicate to the physician such things as an elevated temperature, irregular pulse, and delusional, aggressive, or demanding behavior. Intervention is called for in all these instances, and for the majority of patients each of the above conditions is a temporary one. We tend to view the aggressive and delusional as being pervasive in nature. Perhaps we know less about the cause, and see this behavior as somehow clouding all of the person's other functions. We have not learned to assess these symptoms adequately in light of the person's total functioning. A person can be delusional and yet carry out many daily functions, just as the person with cardiac impairment can have adequate kidney function.

To give support to a person experiencing crisis, it seems imperative to me that we recognize the strengths of the person. Lindemann says that a most important factor in determining the outcome of crises is the behavior of the relevant human figures in the individual's life. He hypothesizes that even a very small influence exerted by a significant person during crises may be enough to decide the outcome, either toward mental health or mental ill health.[13]

Further, the nurse's attitude about the patient's means of coping with his problems will influence her communication with him. I once cared for a young man on a medical-surgical ward of a large general hospital where he was labeled "uncooperative" by the nursing and medical staff. He had had surgical removal of part of the bowel requiring a colostomy, impairment of kidney function, and cardiac involvement. He was and had been receiving intravenous saline solution for two weeks and had been on the critical list just prior to my arrival. It was reported by staff that he was holding the intravenous tubing against the cradle and slowing down the flow of the solution, and that if he did not stop this he would be given fluid intradermally.

I learned that no one had directly discussed this with the patient because, "He won't listen to anyone and its no use—he just complains." I observed the patient for a couple of hours while working with him and saw he was, indeed, slowing down the solution. When I asked him quite directly if he had a reason for doing this, he replied: "Yes, nurse. They told me when they started these that my heart would not take more than ten drops per minute, and now they have it up to 20 and I'm trying to slow it down." I explained that his heart had improved and that it was perfectly all right for the fluid to run at the present rate. He accepted the explanation, ceased manipulating the tubing, and seemed relieved to find his heart had improved.

Obviously there were many other variables operating in this incident, which I will not attempt to discuss. I have used this example to identify how the patient's means of coping with a situation was not understood by the staff and how this influenced their communication with him. They did not believe the patient could change, that their attitude influenced his behavior, and lastly, that they could communicate directly about his behavior, which is an indication of their belief that he lacked the ability to communicate. This had become a crisis situation for both patient and staff because the kind of intervention needed to resolve it had not been recognized.

CRISIS SITUATION IN THE HOME

Let us consider another example involving a student working in the home with a patient discharged from the state hospital. (Although the patient in this example was "mental," the implications regarding communication are not too different from those in any crisis situation.) The patient had been out of the hospital for almost a year, managing to carry out her responsibilities as wife and mother quite adequately until external factors in the family situation began impinging upon her ability to cope with the home situation. The main stressful event was the father's expulsion of the 17-year-old daughter from the home because she had refused to yield to her father's ultimatum to stop dating a boy who had been a patient in a mental hospital. One can readily see the implications for the mother.

During the nurse's first visit, the mother talked freely about the situation, but said nothing about her concerns for herself. The mother explained the daughter's presence in the home as an arrangement whereby the daughter came home while her husband was at work. This was being kept a secret from her husband. Several visits later, the mother began to talk about her relationship with her husband and his threats to send her back to the hospital for a variety of reasons, including her desire to have the daughter return home. She cautiously discussed how angry she was with him because of his treatment of the daughter, adding that she could not discuss it with him for fear of being sent back to the hospital and that she felt very guilty about being angry. The nurse did not attempt to deal with the angry feelings except to say that she could understand her anger, but pointed out to the patient various strengths she possessed: that she was capable of managing the household and family finances; that she had been able to plan and make a trip to another state; and that she was serving as chairman of a women's group. The patient seemed surprised, but acknowledged that these things were so.

During her fourth visit to the home, the nurse made a telephone call to a general hospital in reference to a matter which was not related in any way to the patient. On the fifth visit, the patient came to the door extremely angry, demanding to know almost immediately if the nurse had phoned the Minneapolis Federal Courts. Because the nurse had left the telephone directory open to the page on which the hospital number was listed, the patient had decided for herself that the nurse had called the courts, which were listed on the same page. The nurse assured the patient that she had not telephoned the courts, showing her the Minneapolis General Hospital telephone number on the same page with that of the Minneapolis Federal Courts. The patient then proceeded to question the purpose of the nurse's visits, whether the nurse really was coming to help her or just to observe her in preparation for sending her back to the hospital. The nurse explained again the purpose of her visits and asked if the patient was still angry with her. The patient was then able to discuss how angry she had been with the nurse and, further, her angry feelings toward the daughter's boy friend, something she had not discussed before. The nurse pointed out occurrences for which there were realistic reasons for being angry and those for which anger had been based on things the patient had assumed without really knowing.

The nurse worked with the patient for ten weeks, visiting once a week, and although the visits had many positive values, the most important was that of the supportive role to the patient in her development of a better relationship with her husband. The patient came to recognize how she had criticized him in front of his friends and how in many ways she had set the stage for him to threaten her. She very proudly told the nurse, in one of the later visits, how she had defended her husband in a situation and how surprised he had been. She was able to discuss the daughter with her husband much more realistically and, by the time the nurse terminated her visits, the husband was allowing the daughter to come home while he was there. Family relationships were much more congenial in all respects.

I think it is important to note that from the beginning the nurse looked for the patient's strengths and helped her see that she was not totally sick. Because the nurse knew how to communicate, she was able to work with the patient toward gradually looking at the performances which interfered with her relationships and set up situations that brought more threat to her. A higher level of equilibrium was achieved by the patient, I believe, in her ability to examine her functioning with her husband and deal with her angry feelings in a more healthy way.

OTHER CRISIS SITUATIONS

Several areas in the framework of public health services offer excellent opportunities for nurses to provide patients with assistance not commonly considered a part of the nurse's function. In the well baby clinic there is a perfect opportunity for the nurse to offer emotional support to mothers. An example comes to mind. A nurse saw a mother literally drop her baby on the table in the examining room and then go off to sit in a chair some distance away from the table. The nurse, highly incensed, scolded the mother for not watching her baby. What an opportunity the nurse missed by not attempting to find out from the mother the why of her actions.

An excellent film, *A Study in Maternal Attitudes,* which shows a portion of an attitude study project, strives to teach doctors and nurses how, in the limited time at their disposal, they can give each mother at least some of the help she needs.* The focus is on the mother and the purpose is to teach doctors and nurses how to listen, how to help a mother express her feelings, and how to provide an atmosphere in which her personality unfolds. By stressing individual differences, it teaches them to be more tolerant and less judgmental, and it emphasizes the principles that when mothers feel understood and appreciated, they are more receptive to their maternal role. Positive experiences can be provided in the same way in antepartal clinics.

I believe that one of our greatest drawbacks in nursing is due to what I call our "middle class values." Repeatedly I hear nurses criticize patients who do not share or hold our values of cleanliness, economic management, nutritional habits, child care, and a host of other daily living practices. We talk as though everyone had been educated in living in exactly the way we have been. I am reminded of one of my students who was highly critical of a mother in whose home the sink was always piled high with dirty dishes. The student, reporting her most recent visit, said that the mother was helping her boys prepare their camping gear for an overnight trip to the lake. She did not see that the camping trip meant much more to the boys than a clean kitchen until I questioned her assessment of values. Because of her concern about the dishes, she could not communicate any enthusiasm to the mother or praise her for helping her children with something they wanted to do.

Another nurse, visiting an antepartal patient (American Indian), had urged her on each of three visits, to go to the maternity clinic. Each time, the patient agreed to go, but never went. The nurse concluded that it was useless to continue encouraging the patient to go because "Indians never pay any attention to what white people say." During none of the visits had the nurse attempted to find out why the patient said she would go to clinic and then didn't, asked the patient if she had transportation, or explained that the patient's edematous condition was the reason for wanting her to go to the clinic. There could have been any number of reasons for the patient not following through on the nurse's advice, but it was as though the patient's concept of the clinic should have been the same as the nurse's.

*A Study in Maternal Attitudes. (Film) 1960. Available from the New York Fund for Children, 104 East 25th Street, New York, N.Y. 10010.

It is evident that effective communication is a primary and necessary skill in order for the nurse to become a helping person to patients in crisis situations. As previously stated, "crisis is characterized by an increase in inner tension, unpleasant affect, and disorganization of behavior." This statement demands that the nurse recognize the implications for intervention through her communication. She must understand that crisis situations can alter a person's behavior temporarily and, though the patient needs support and assistance, he is not necessarily "mentally ill." The nurse has a responsibility to identify the patient's strengths and to help him utilize these strengths.

We must evaluate our communication and whether it has been effective for the other person, and then be willing to assume the responsibility for correcting the error if we have not been effective. Caplan says, "It is remarkable to see the power that ordinary people have to adapt to reality, however unpleasant. They have a great deal more strength than we often give them credit for. Unassisted in a time of crisis, this strength may fail them. But, if we recognize it and build it up, we can help each other through times of trouble."[14] We must strive to assist the person to reach the highest level of equilibrium at any given point in time.

REFERENCES

1. Szasz, T. S. *The Myth of Mental Illness.* New York, Harper and Row, 1961.
2. Schramm, Wilbur, ed. *The Science of Human Communication.* New York, Basic Books, 1963, p. 1.
3. Berlo, D. K. *The Process of Communication.* New York, Holt, Rinehart and Winston, 1960, p. 1.
4. *Ibid.,* p. 4.
5. Szasz, *op. cit.,* p. 3.
6. *Ibid.,* p. 3.
7. *Ibid.,* p. 11.
8. Caplan, Gerald, ed. *Prevention of Mental Disorders in Children.* New York, Basic Books, 1961, pp. 309-310.
9. Lindemann, Erich. The meaning of crisis in individual and family living. *Teach. Col. Rec.* 57:315, Feb. 1956.
10. Ackerman, N. W. *Psychodynamics of Family Life.* New York, Basic Books, 1958.
11. Becker, Ernest. *The Revolution in Psychiatry.* New York, Free Press of Glencoe, 1964, pp. 33-35.
12. Caplan, Gerald. *Principles of Preventive Psychiatry.* New York, Basic Books, 1964, p. 224.
13. Lindemann, *op. cit.,* p. 310.
14. Caplan, Gerald. *Principles of Preventive Psychiatry.* New York, Basic Books, 1964, p. 193.

12

Orienting the Disoriented

Pauline P. McCown and Elizabeth Wurm*

Can a patient who has been disoriented for many years be helped to learn his name, respond to simple direct questions, and change some of his unpleasant personal habits? "Yes," say these authors and they describe the techniques they are using.

"Mr. Williams, it is time for your medication." This was the beginning. The beginning of a new approach to nursing care for the disoriented patient; the patient who is unable to tell you who he is, where he is, or to recognize the persons around him; the patient who is unable to find his room or his bed; the patient who soils his clothing, not because he is incontinent, but because he doesn't remember or cannot find the toilet.

Our unit is designated a special therapy unit—a unit where patients receive reality orientation. But, just what does such an approach mean for the staff and for the patients? We recognize reality orientation as a phase of rehabilitation for the mentally ill or the geriatric patient who is disoriented. It is an attempt to bring him from mental confusion to awareness and from vagueness to clarity.

Our techniques are tailored to the individual; some have proved effective, some have not. Our goal is to help patients regain their former abilities through reality-structured situations presented to them in a manner that will facilitate relearning or re-education. We have had to learn, through trial and error, the most effective ways of teaching each of our patients. Progress is

*From *American Journal of Nursing,* Vol. 65, No. 4 (April, 1965).

Mrs. McCown, supervisor of the Special Therapy Unit at the Veterans Administration Hospital, Tuscaloosa, Ala., is a graduate of the Birmingham Baptist Hospitals' School of Nursing, Ala.

Mrs. Wurm, head nurse on this unit, is a graduate of the Druid City Hospital School of Nursing in Tuscaloosa, Ala. Both authors have had many years of experience in psychiatric nursing.

slow and sometimes it is discouraging. But the moments of unexpected success always provide us with satisfaction and the impetus to continue.

Mr. Williams was 62 years old and had been hospitalized for 22 years when he came to our unit three years ago. He was preoccupied, showed little interest in his surroundings or in other people, smiled inappropriately, and was indifferent to his personal appearance. He presented a picture of marked regression with much childlike behavior. He required continuous supervision. He did not know the day, month, or year, and was unable to tell who he was, where he was, or who the people were around him. He wandered aimlessly about the unit, or paced back and forth singing loudly. He refused to participate in any planned activity. He was unkempt in appearance; his clothing was dirty and unfastened. He smoked continuously and when a cigarette became too short to smoke, he chewed it. Frequently, he would cough, expectorate in his hands, and then wipe his hands on his clothing. At other times he would expectorate on the floor. He ate fairly well but was underweight. He had to be reminded to swallow his food and his medicines.

The team members studied Mr. Williams' reactions and responses and decided that the first goal should be to reorient him to person. We recognized that progress would be slow and that we needed to focus on one point at a time. The group decided to begin by getting Mr. Williams to respond to his own name. All personnel were asked to use every available opportunity to call Mr. Williams by name and do so in a manner that called for a response. For example, when the nurse was ready to give him his medication, she said, "Mr. Williams, it is time for your medicine." In the beginning, he showed no outward signs that he recognized his name. After several weeks, he began to look at the nurse and reach for his medicine.

We then agreed to modify the approach and get Mr. Williams to state his own name. Mr. Williams was asked, "And what is your name, sir?" With patience, consistency, and much repetition, this approach was effective. In a few weeks Mr. Williams was able to state his name.

The team members believed that Mr. Williams now was ready to learn to call others by name. He did not know the name of the nursing assistant who was assigned to his care, so this learning was our next objective. For several months, Mr. Williams had incorrectly identified this nursing assistant as Mr. Burgess. Each time he was told, "No, I am Mr. Jacks" or "Mr. Williams, I am Mr. Jacks." This approach was not very effective. We tried a different approach. We agreed that all of us would continue to call the patient by name at every opportunity and wait for him to respond. His nursing assistant was to greet him each day with, "Good morning, Mr. Williams, I am Mr. Jacks." As he was told the nursing assistant's name he was shown the nursing assistant's name pin. Later, he was told the name, then shown the name pin, and asked to repeat the name. Similar approaches were used each day.

We did not expect an immediate response or an immediate change in his behavior, but it seemed to us that he would never respond. Finally, after several months, he called Mr. Jacks by name. Mr. Jacks was so surprised that he could barely maintain his composure. The other team members were just as elated. Our efforts were rewarded and we became enthusiastic and eager to continue the simple but continuous program.

Our present goal is to help Mr. Williams learn the head nurse's name and, gradually, the names of his fellow patients. He occasionally calls the head nurse by name, but usually he calls her "Mrs. Toppen." Is he saying Mrs. Top'en because she is a head nurse? We hope so, for this appellation will be easier to change than one adopted by misidentifying her. We are now using identification games to help Mr. Williams learn the names of his fellow patients. "Mr. Williams, throw the ball to Mr. Smith," and so forth.

We realize that the job of reorienting Mr. Williams is far from complete, but the team is pleased with the progress he has shown. His personal appearance, eating habits, and table manners have improved. No longer is he careless with his sputum; he responds to simple, direct questions, and he is able to identify at least two other patients by name. Our next objective will be to orient Mr. Williams to time and to place. We will focus on activities he attends and when he attends them.

During the time that we have worked with patients who have been disoriented for many years, we have learned approaches and techniques that have been effective. We have learned that reorienting patients who are forgetful or who are unable to remember recent events, names, or places, requires patience and consideration. Gains are not made with impatience or irritability. When a patient does not remember, remind him at regular intervals to go to the toilet. You may say, "It's time to go to the toilet, Mr. Jones" or, "Have you been to the toilet, Mr. Jones?" To help him remember when he eats, say, "It's twelve o'clock; where do you go now, Mr. Jones?" If he doesn't remember, say, "Mr. Jones, at twelve o'clock you go to lunch." If he is unable to find his bed, show him where he sleeps. "Your bed is the fourth one on this side: one, two, three, four; this is your bed."

Name pins, with both the patient's first name and his last name, may be made for each patient. The letters should be large so that patients who have visual impairment can read them easily. Encourage the patient who likes to reminisce to share his past. Learn all you can about his former interests, and help him relate the events of his past to those of the present. Perhaps he has farmed all of his life. Use this experience as a means of rebuilding his self-esteem and re-establishing contact with reality. Ask him to tell you how to plant cotton, corn, or potatoes, to tell you when these crops are planted, or to tell you when these crops are harvested.

To increase the patient's attention span, use small sea shells, blocks, or cards. Tell him and show him how to separate the shells. "Mr. Jones, put the white shells here, put the blue shells there." Later, ask him to separate the shells according to color and size. Show him how to separate playing cards according to suit (hearts, spades, clubs, or diamonds). Then, ask him to identify a card (queen of hearts, jack of diamonds, and so forth) or tell which of two cards is higher or lower in value. When he is able to do this well, add simple card games. As his attention span increases, gradually introduce more difficult games.

Many times a patient is unable to listen when others are talking. He loses interest quickly or talks in a rambling manner. To encourage listening, ask the patient to repeat what another person has said. Direct his thoughts to the subject being discussed. Ask him questions about another person's conversation, such as, "Mr. Jones, what do you think about Mr. Jacks' idea? Is that the way you would do it?" In the beginning, much repetition will be required, but as he learns to listen reminders may be decreased.

Frequently an older patient feels hopeless, helpless, alone, and unwanted. Patience, understanding, and acceptance will boost his selfesteem and establish good interpersonal relations. Respect his dignity and call him "Mr. Jones"; not "John."

Present plans or directions to the patient in a simple, direct manner and repeat them frequently. Tell him, "This is Monday—bath day; the bathroom is this way" (as you accompany him to the bathroom). Repeat this procedure until he knows where the bathroom is and when to take a bath. Use the same approach in other situations: going to bed, going to meals, going to the toilet, or going to activities. Place calendars with large numbers conveniently about the unit. Give him a billfoldsize calendar to carry in his pocket. Each day, ask him to find the calendar and mark off or write in the date. Help him until he can do it alone. Use a wall clock with large numbers to help the patient know the time of day and remember the hours his daily activities are scheduled.

An older patient gains security from knowing what to expect, or knowing what comes next. Post activity schedules on the bulletin board. Check the schedule with the patient to help him understand and remember what he is to do and when he is to do it.

A fabricated board with slots for the day, month, year, weather, next mealtime, bath time, canteen visits, and so forth is an effective tool. Assign the job of keeping the board current to a patient. Help him until he is able to do it without being reminded.

Maps or chalkboards help stimulate interest in places. Using a map of the state, ask a patient or an employee to point out the city where the hospital is located. Then ask the patient to point out his home town. Help him if he is unable to do it. He will begin to learn where he is now in relation to his home.

Reality orientation is more than telling. It is showing. The key is consistency in conversation and activities that are short, simple, and focused on one point at a time. Basic requisites for a good reality orientation program are personnel who believe in this treatment program, and who are patient, considerate, understanding, and accepting of the patient.

13

Talking with Patients

Hildegard E. Peplau*

Social chit-chat must be replaced by the responsible use of words if this process is to be productive.

Talking with patients is easy when the nurse treats the patient as a chum and engages in a give-and-take of social chit-chat. But when the nurse sees her part in verbal interchanges with patients as a major component in direct nursing service, then she must recognize the complexity of the process. Social chit-chat is replaced by the responsible use of words which help to further the personal development of the patient.

It is this complexity which distinguishes the verbal part of the professional nurse's work from the verbal approach a layman might use toward a sick person. The layman most often is actually a friend or a member of the patient's family; the nurse is a stranger to the patient.

There are marked distinctions between a layman talking to a friend and a nurse talking to a stranger who is a patient. The role of friend has its own requirements. Friends trust each other, exchange confidences, advise each other, lend one another money. Since it takes time for friendship to develop, two friends learn enough about each other so that behavior becomes predictable to a degree; one friend will begin to take certain actions of the other for granted. Acceptance of such assumptions is often the basis of meaning on which conversation between two friends is built.

The nurse and patient are not friends; they are strangers to each other. If the nurse does not see the patient as a stranger, about whom she knows nothing but can learn much, then she is distorting the facts of the situation.

*From *American Journal of Nursing*, Vol. 60, No. 7 (July, 1960).
Miss Peplau (Pottstown, Pa., Hospital School of Nursing; B.A., Bennington College; M.A., Ed.D., Teacher's College, Columbia) is associate professor of nursing and director of the graduate program in advanced psychiatric nursing at Rutgers University College of Nursing.

She can distort in different ways. She might look upon the patient as a friend, seeking in him familiar elements that she has previously experienced with friends in other nonclinical situations. Or she can look upon the patient in light of her own need or wish to have friends, thus relating to him primarily to fulfill her own wishes. Such wishes for friends ought to be realized in the social life of the nurse outside the hospital. Another distortion is for the nurse to see the patient as a disease category. In this situation she searches only for familiar clinical signs which help her to feel able, and she misses the unfamiliar, the unique newness of the *person* who is a stranger.

When the nurse treats the patient as a friend, she puts herself in the role of friend to him. The actions of the friendship role come to be expected of the nurse by the patient. Often the nurse burdens the patient with her biography, even sharing her secrets or seeking advice about her personal affairs. The focus on the needs of the patient is lost. Many nurses rationalize their actions along these lines, saying "it is good for the patient to take his mind off himself." If this be the case there are innumerable nonpersonal subjects of common interest which might be a more useful focus for social conversations with patients than the personal life of the nurse.

When the nurse sees the patient as a stranger, her first verbal task is to help him get oriented to her, to the hospital, and to the tasks at hand. Here, the layman in the nurse often gets in the way. To get oriented to a stranger outside the hospital, most people use social chit-chat at first. The questions go something like this: "Where do you live, Mrs. Jones?" "Have you lived there long?" "Do you know Mrs. Smith down the street?" "She went to Jersey High School, did you?" "I did too; did you take cooking with Miss Main?" and so on. The process is largely one of locating common if elementary interests and experiences as a base from which friendship might later develop.

This approach works well among laymen. The professional nurse, however, is offering a direct and specialized experience from which, hopefully, the patient will learn something of lasting personal value with regard to health. The professional nursing focus is the needs of the patient. The relationship, if it is to be governed by sustained objectivity in the interest of the patient's learning, will be time-limited by the duration of the illness—it is a temporary, often brief relationship. The approach to the stranger must therefore be different in the nursing situation.

THE PATIENT IN FOCUS

When the focus is on the needs of the patient, then the time of the nurse must be used purposefully in the patient's interest. This is not to say that the nurse does not have needs. Of course she does, for she is human too. But her needs are met outside the sickroom. Inside the sickroom, the focus is on the patient.

In getting oriented to the nurse, the patient needs to know her name, he needs to know that she is a registered nurse, what she may be called upon to do, the time limits which govern the duration and frequency of his contacts with her, and what she will do with information which she gets from him.[1]

---

[1]Peplau, Hildegard E. Principles of psychiatric nursing. In *American Handbook of Psychiatry*, ed. by Silvano Arieti. New York, Basic Books, 1959, pp. 1840-1856.

The patient may need validation of the self-evident. If he says "You have red hair" and the nurse has red hair, she can say "Yes, I do." But the patient does not need to know that all the women in the nurse's family for five generations back had red hair. If the patient notices a wedding ring on the nurse's finger and asks "Are you married," the nurse can reply "Yes, I am." But when she begins to describe the data and circumstances of the marriage this indicates pretty clearly that she is more interested in talking about herself that she is in the patient.

The nurse's biographical data is a burden to the patient who has no recourse but to translate the nursing situation into a social, chum-like one. Often the patient asks about the nurse's background primarily to test her capacity to focus on his needs and to find out whether she prefers instead to talk about herself. Since the patient must depend upon the nurse for many things, he will try to meet her needs so that he can feel safe with her. The nurse who can survive the patient's testing, and let him know clearly, simply, and directly that "this time is yours," will have offered the patient a unique experience with potential for learning.

Nurses should distinguish between a patient's demands and his needs. A demand is a request, a claim, or coercion to evoke some kind of response. In recognizing a need, on the other hand, the nurse draws her inference not only from such demands as the patient might make but also from her own observations and from other data.

A nurse does not meet the demands of a patient unless a valid need is represented in the demand. When a patient demands or asks persistently for biographical data from the nurse, she does not need to be pulled willy-nilly by these demands. She can say, quite simply, "Use this time to talk about you." Or she can ask gently, "What do you need this information for?" If the patient persists, the nurse might become more firm and ask, "Of what benefit to you would a review of my social life be?" or "I wonder what uses you would have for such personal information."

Of course, if the nurse is desperate for the patient's approval and uncertain about her professional role and its boundaries, then she will simply yield to the patient and answer any and all questions about her personal life. In a general hospital no great trauma will thereby accrue to the patient; only another opportunity for a patient to learn something of value about himself will have been missed. In psychiatric work, however, the nurse will have proved to the patient his belief that people are not interested in him—only in themselves.

If the nurse wishes to focus on the needs of the patient, then she must know how to listen and how to respond in ways that will further the patient's learning. There is a technique for creative listening. It is not just a matter of letting a patient ramble on as though the nurse had her hearing aid turned off. It is more like listening to music—for the themes and variations, for the nuances of meaning that are conveyed indirectly through sound or hint.

Teaching a nurse to listen can only be done in clinical seminars, where interfering factors in the individual can be revealed and looked at and, hopefully, deleted. But there are some general guidelines.

Patients frequently make such comments as "I'm not hungry," "I'm not sleeping," "I'm not feeling well," or "I'm not comfortable." In situations such as these the verbal response of the nurse should be used to help the patient describe what went on instead of opening further discussion of what did *not* occur. Comments such as "What did go on" (instead of sleep), "What do you feel," or "Are you saying you are uncomfortable" help the patient to think directly about what did happen or is occurring.

In these situations, the nurse often automatically asks "Why not?" More often than not a "why" question has an intimidating effect. It has a ring of familiarity and is frequently reminiscent of earlier experiences when mother or teacher reiterated "Why don't you do this" or "Why can't you tell me" or some similarly coercing "why" question. Moreover, if the patient knew why he wasn't hungry or sleeping or comfortable, he would most probably deal with the situation. A "why" question asks for reasons which the patient is not likely to know immediately. He can discover them with help. But, in order to discover them, the patient requires some raw data—he must recall, for example what actually went on, instead of sleep. The reasons can be generalized from these data; then the "why" question can be answered.

PERCEPTIVE DESCRIPTION

In order to understand the reasons for the patient's behavior, both the nurse and the patient must have descriptions of the patient's experience. Such descriptions are not as easy to secure as many nurses assume. A great many people are singularly lacking in skill, especially in describing personal perceptions of experience.

Many nurses themselves do not describe what they observe but record instead stereotyped clichés which condense and classify rather than describe their observations. Valuable data from which fresh insight about illness could be drawn are lost this way. Verbatim descriptions given by psychosomatic and psychiatric patients would provide nursing with a far more useful base for determining nursing practice than the current tendency to translate doctors' findings into nursing knowledge.

Such words as "what," "where," "when," and "who" will assist the nurse to elicit useful description. A few highly serviceable clichés like "Tell me about that," "Then what," "Go on," and "You will remember" will be convenient when a direct question seems inappropriate. Except in rare instances, the nurse will find patients eager to talk about themselves; when a patient is reluctant or definitely not eager, the nurse can show respect for privacy of thought and silently await initial comments from him.

Words such as "how" or "why" are quite challenging ones. Nurses who really consider their meaning use them sparingly. The nurse who asks a patient "How do you feel" really asks, in effect, "In what manner or by what process do you have a feeling?" It would be simpler and more direct to ask "What are your feelings this morning?" The phrase "how come" is a cliché that communicates even less about what the nurse is seeking. In general, "how" and "why" questions require the patient to analyze the data of his experience and to respond with a generalization about it.

QUESTIONS AND ANSWERS. A "how" question asks for the process, the operations, the steps by which something has occurred. A "why" question asks for reasons, causes, explanations, or conclusions. If a person has adequate information, and analytical abilities as well, then he can answer a "how" or a "why" question directly. If, on the other hand, a patient does not fulfill these two basic requirements, then a "how" or "why" question is a nonsense one which leaves him feeling inadequate, helpless, or powerless. The patient who is well educated and is quite aware of the cliché usage of "how" and "why" questions is more likely to consider as unknowing the nurse who uses these clichés.

One problem common to many patients in both general and psychiatric hospitals is the problem of self-identity; their answers to the question "who am I" have not yet been formulated. This problem is reflected in what the patient says. Through her responses, the nurse can further stalmate the patient in his struggle with this problem or she can assist in its solution. Self-identity is in part reflected in the use of personal pronouns. To speak for oneself requires use of such pronouns as "I," "me," "mine." When a patient speaks of himself as "you," or "one," the nurse ought to inquire about the referents. "You said 'one,' to whom does this refer?" In this way the nurse can help the patient to refer more directly to himself—to use the pronoun, "I."

TROUBLE WITH PRONOUNS. "We," "they," and "us," are similarly troublesome pronouns. Of course, there are group situations in which the group members know one another and, as "togetherness" evolves, they use "we," "us," or "they" to indicate they are speaking for others present or absent. When asked, "Whom do you mean by we" they can probably name the referent. That is, the speaker can tell you that he and Tom Jones were included in his use of "we."

But there are many patients who use these pronouns in a global way— they either have some difficulty or are completely unable to say whom they mean when they use "we" or "us." When a nurse is working with a patient who has this particular difficulty in self-identity, she has two tasks. First, she needs to raise the question, "Whom do you mean by we" (or us, or they). Secondly, she must be sure to speak only for herself and keep her identity clearly separate from that of the patient. In this instance, she would not use "we," "let's," or "our," as in the proverbial "We will now have our enema." Instead, she would say, "I have brought the enema you are to have."

Here is an example of a nurse reinforcing a patient's difficulty through the use of language:

A nurse said to a patient, "Let's go over what's been said and see if we have anything particular for us to discuss." The patient replied, "Oh, well, let's see what we'll see. Shall we watch for whether we are anxious between now and next week?" The merging of identity of nurse and patient—so that neither has the status of an independent person—is clear in this verbal interchange.

Magical or automatic knowing causes another communication problem. Magical knowing refers to knowing automatically—without asking, investigating, or finding out. Such phrases as "I know," "I see," "I understand" are included in this category when they precede rather than follow inquiry into a situation. Value terms such as "nice," "good," "bad" can also be used in such a way that consensus as to their meaning is assured rather than determined. For example, a patient said, "Well, last time my visitors were nice."

The nurse responded, "Maybe today will go as well." This kind of verbal exchange shows the same limited communication inherent in such meaningless transactions as "Hello, how are you" to which the equally noncommunicative reply is "I'm fine, and you," and the final response is "I'm okay." Nothing has actually been said; these are merely words in juxtaposition.

The use of "they" as a pervasive global reference in which the identity of the referents is lost is typical of the patient diagnosed paranoiac. If you ask, "Who are they" the patient not only cannot tell you but may become quite anxious. If the nurse persists in asking, the "they" will become "other people," then a class of people as "my family" or "nurse" or "doctors," and finally names of particular people. Nurses should help more people become aware of the tendency toward loss of the referents by questioning "Who are they" whenever this pronoun is used.

SUMMARY

Talking with patients becomes productive when the nurse develops awareness of her own verbal patterns and then decides to take responsibility for her part in verbal interchanges with patients. When nursing is seen as an opportunity to further the patient's learning about himself, the focus in the nurse-patient relationship will be upon the patient—his needs, his difficulties, his lacks in interpersonal competence, his interest in living. What the nurse chooses to talk about during the relationship will be guided by her understanding of the scope and boundaries of nursing practice as a professional service.

14

Communicating with Schizophrenic Patients

Alice M. Robinson*

Communication is the most prodigious problem in schizophrenia. Yet it is this barrier we must penetrate if our efforts to nurse these patients are to be successful.

There is no other illness, physical, emotional, or spiritual, which is as profound, malignant, perplexing, and frustrating as schizophrenia. Despite complicated and lengthy research, we are still without answers to the many challenging questions which arise in our own minds as we struggle to help this group of lost human beings.

For almost a hundred years, since Kraepelin first differentiated what he termed "dementia praecox" from other types of emotional aberration, learned men and women have wrestled with the problem. We now know a great deal about the dynamics of schizophrenic behavior, about the symbolism, the hereditary and the organic factors, but we are still faced with the enormity of "why" and "what to do."

While psychiatrists and allied scientists have come to grips primarily with the technical aspects of schizophrenia, nursing has gone through a number of phases in dealing with the *practical* aspects.

For many years, nurses were so baffled by the number and complexity of the problems of caring for the mentally ill that the schizophrenic was just part of the vast melee of filth, denudativeness, assault, din, and fear. Following this period, years of hydrotherapy, electric shock, restraints, seclusion, and adherence to a rigid routine of bare essentials comprised the nurse's "duty."

---

*From *American Journal of Nursing*, Vol. 60, No. 8 (August, 1960).

Miss Robinson (Duke University School of Nursing; B.S., Catholic University of America; M.S., Boston University) is director of nursing education at Vermont State Hospital. She is also chairman of the ANA Conference Group on Psychiatric Nursing Practice.

Today we are faced with a far greater challenge and its promises to increase. Drugs and a profusion of qualified personnel have brought us face to face and eye to eye with patients—and most particularly, with schizophrenic patients. They still outnumber other types of patients, and they are still a vast enigma of perverted communication, stunning withdrawal, and personal deprivation of an amazing breadth and depth!

Nurses have, in essence, learned to cope with certain of the basic problems involved in caring for the schizophrenic patient such as bathing, feeding, elimination—the physical aspects. But we have only begun to scratch the surface in our approach to the most prodigious problem—communication. In order to be reasonably successful in our efforts to give individual nursing care to schizophrenic patients, this is the barrier we must penetrate. To say that it takes limitless patience, abysmal insight, and a great deal of warmth and love is, at best, an understatement.

COMMUNICATION PROBLEMS IN GENERAL

The crux of successful interpersonal relationships lies in successful communication. Successful communication is seldom immediately accomplished, even in the so-called "normal" world of human relations. It is usually the result of long acquaintance, individual comfort, and acceptance. If one maintains an attitude of realism in relation to schizophrenia, this tenet would obviously hold true in interpersonal contacts with these patients as well. A basic fear—born of many (often untold) experiences with others—the fear that what is communicated may be "dangerous," "threatening," or might produce rejection, provides the foremost barrier to human understanding. The schizophrenic experiences double the impact of this very personal fear. We must approach the schizophrenic with a minimum of judgment and a maximum of tolerance, for he is looking for the impossible. Yet he recognizes that he can control the situation by exercising the power of his everpresent weapon—withdrawal.

THE POWER OF SCHIZOPHRENIA

For many years, I held the considered viewpoint that the schizophrenic is a lonely, pathetic, troubled, and lost soul—to be pitied, loved, and nurtured, regardless of behavior. Although I still hold this opinion, in essence, the feeling permeates, more and more, that the schizophrenic is really a masochistically powerful person who "keeps everyone at bay," neatly, and by a number of defensive mechanisms. In other words, the schizophrenic, with full knowledge, holds us in his power, behaves any way he likes, seduces us through his asocial acting-out, and keeps us well in hand—the way he wants us to be! Even though this creates for him tremendous personal deprivation, the schizophrenic seems to enjoy it.

Recently, while acting as a consultant at one of the VA hospitals, I was shown a patient in the medical-surgical building who was recovering from his fourth fractured jaw. The medical staff had ordered a faceguard for him much the same as that worn by a football player or the goalie in hockey. I inquired further about him, finding out that he had created an attitude of fear among all the personnel associated with him, that when his name was mentioned, a general cry of dismay arose, and that he excused himself by saying, "I can't help it. The impulse just comes to strike out at someone, and I can't control myself." The broken jaw, the awe and fear in which he was held all contributed to the sealing of his private world.

I began to look at the schizophrenics in my home hospital more acutely. The one who can talk but successfully frustrates by clamping her teeth and lips and making half-intelligible sounds, the one who sits day after day and smiles and mumbles incoherently when she is approached, the one you try and try to convince of your faith in him and love, who simply ignores your words, clinging tenaciously to ludicrous delusions. The latter, when he sees you slipping away, says something lucid and meaningful and once again you are hopefully trapped.

What kind of an approach can we employ to reach through this power, to be able to love the patient well enough to convince him that the love is "unequivocal"? How can we *show* him that we are prepared to give enough to crumble the walls, to stop the fists, to help him to produce words?

Obviously, telling him is not enough. Indeed, for a nurse to consider only verbal communication in her individual nursing care of patients, and psychotic patients in particular, would be very remiss. The simplest gesture, the subtlest facial expression, even the most insignificant odor, are meaningful to the patient. Many times what we *say* and what we *do* with patients are in complete discord. This is confusing to the average person. To the schizophrenic it can be chaotic.

I believe that the nurse who intends to work with schizophrenics should go through a minute personal appraisal of her own symbolic and kinetic characteristics. What is the sound of my voice, my laugh, my emphasis? How do I look? How do I walk? How much personal physical contact do I have with patients—the hand on the shoulder, the "elbowguiding," and the like? Do my movements belie my words? What do I do with the emotional response I experience in relation to people—and to patients in particular? Following such an appraisal, it behooves the nurse to examine how she interprets the painful world of symbolism contained in the nonverbal communication of the schizophrenic.

Sylvano Arieti in his *Intrepretation of Schizophrenia* says that "Schizophrenia is a specific reaction to a severe state of anxiety, originating in childhood, re-experienced and increased in some later period of life." I believe that this original experience would have been profound in nonverbal communication.

Let us look briefly at the classic example of the mother who calls her son across the room saying, "Come here, Johnnie, and kiss Mommie." Johnnie, in the perilous innocence of youth, rushes toward this love, but just at the point of contact, Mommie unconsciously and almost imperceptibly stiffens in her innate ambivalence toward Johnnie.

Johnnie is caught in the crossfire of love and hate, and must make a choice. He is capable of choosing love, and usually does. The preschizophrenic may not be capable of this positive choice. While enmeshed in a full-blown psychosis in his later years, he may be forced by a nurse into the same "double-bind." She may greet him, verbally, with a warm and meaningful, "Hullo, Johnnie. How does it go?" But then in the next second, she glances at his soiled shirt or his open fly and she too, almost imperceptibly stiffens in her innate ambivalence!

LOVE AS A TOOL

Perhaps it would be prudent, at this point, to define love as a specific and potent nursing tool and a skill which can be developed with warmth and understanding.

Smiley Blanton, in his book, *Love or Perish*, has done a superb job of analyzing the emotion as subtracted from passion and envy and sexuality, as such. The positive, constructive influence of love (as against the frightening, negative, and destructive influence of its counterpart, hate) has inestimable value as a therapeutic agent in the individual nursing care of the schizophrenic. The schizophrenic can accept unequivocal love—nothing less—and responds, tediously to be sure, to the extent that he can get a fingerhold, and begin to pull himself away from the mire of his pathology.

How does the nurse give this kind of love? What are the guideposts? How does she get it across to the patient?

The giving and receiving of love, at any level, requires first of all *self-acceptance*. Until this is achieved, the average person is too fearful of this warm gift and of the response it evokes. Nurses are average people, generally conditioned as individuals to fear rejection, the bugbear of human relatedness. It is necessary, in the nurse-patient relationship, to see this in its true perspective, from both sides of the fence.

The uncomplicated love which the nurse can give to the schizophrenic contains the all-important elements of *warmth, acceptance, consistency, tolerance,* and *firm limit-setting.* This simple version of Rosen-theory can hold the key to recovery from the acting-out stage, or, in other words, it can get beneath the overt symptomatology.[1]

When such a relationship has passed through the stage of nurse-giving and schizophrenic-taking, and becomes more *equalized* in terms of give and take, the opportunity for working through the fundamental dynamics of the illness has arrived. Here is where the qualified psychiatric nurse—always with supportive supervision from the psychiatrist—can begin working with the talking out, the interpretation, the understanding—work which the patient is now more ready to share.[2]

To illustrate the effectiveness of this theory of individual nursing care, the following examples are cited from personal experience:

Pat was a 16-year-old patient who was admitted with a tentative diagnosis of mental retardation. Whether or not this was a functional retardation remained to be seen.

My first contact with the patient was during rounds on the admitting wards (I was then director of nursing in a large, metropolitan state hospital). She was standing awkwardly with both toes turned sharply inward, very un-

---

[1]Rosen, J. N. The treatment of schizophrenic psychosis by direct analytic therapy. *Psychiat. Quart.* 21:3-27, Jan. 1947.

[2]Here, the inexperienced nurse gives over the "interpretation" to the psychiatrist (or other trained therapist), nonetheless continuing her supportive relationship with the patient.

tidy, and with the defeated blank expression so characteristic of the catatonic. She appealed to me immediately in the sense that, for no particular reason which I could discern at that time, I felt acutely optimistic about her ultimate recovery. I knelt to tie her undone shoelaces, and she followed me throughout the rest of my trip through the ward.

I decided to return later that week, and I found her with two attendants who were attempting to give her a shower. She was wailing loudly, drooling copiously, and resisting, with amazing physical strength, every attempt to get her to shower.

It was difficult to make any contact with her through the din of crying, but at one point I managed to ask her if she would like a bath in the tub. The response was amazing. She quieted down and allowed us to give her a bath without further ado. The attendants and I were curious, and I went immediately to read her record. The answer was there. During a previous brief hospitalization, she had been routinely given a shower, preceding electroshock therapy. Her rank terror of EST was intimately associated with showering.

For many, many weeks I visited Pat whenever I could (usually two or three times a week) and had lengthy conferences with the ward doctor about her. We went through the initial period of positive transference during which she was clinging and infantile and communicated virtually nothing except her hunger for attention.

The period of negative transference lasted much longer, and was, at times, almost finally discouraging. She began by being verbally abusive, drifted toward physical abuse, delighted in picking dried, old food from her dress and eating it, or soiling or wetting herself almost as soon as I reached the ward. Her psychotic awareness of my personal problem with compulsivity became quite clear, and I was cognizant, not infrequently, that I was communicating my disgust and intolerance in many nonverbal ways.

In response to this "acting out" on my part, she withdrew further and further into bizarre, negativistic, noncommunicative behavior. Despite all she would do, however, I continued to return, even though there were many times when there was a complete lack of verbal response from her. After eight months, she was transferred to a "back ward" of about 70 deteriorated, very ill schizophrenic women.

One evening I went to the ward just as the patients were returning from supper. During this pre-drug era, as I look back on it, this was an appalling sight. The one attendant assigned to the evening shift was presumably still in the cafeteria lining up stragglers. I sat down next to Pat and she maintained her stony, untidy silence. The patients, as they arrived, one by one, lined up against the wall and took off, over their heads, their ungainly "state dresses" and stood naked, their long unattended shapes grotesque in the evening light. In their strange, caste system, each had a spot and if anyone else ventured near it, a battle ensued.

Several patients, noting me in the white uniform, came over and threatened me, some shaking their fists, others shouting angrily. One even spat at me. After one or two such semi-assaults toward me, Pat got up and walked a few feet away, then turned and stared at me. I felt some resentment at this desertion, and after 20 minutes or so, I got up and went over to her and said, gently, but not without evidencing limits, as a mother might say to a child: "Pat, I've never let you down, no matter what. Tonight you let me down." And then I left.

For some reason or other, Pat said later, she knew then, with certainty, that I would ride out her illness with her, and she felt, somehow, clear and inordinately well mentally. (This, we know, is not uncommon in the course of a schizophrenic illness.) She felt that she could trust me, that she could tell me some of the fears, the pathos, the unhappy experiences which had inevitably forced her into the retreat of mental illness. This event occurred in late winter, and by the next Thanksgiving, Pat managed a two-week home visit successfully.

The second illustration concerns a 32-year-old woman patient named Lillian, a full-blown paranoid schizophrenic who, when I met her, had been actively ill for 11 years. She had just been readmitted to our hospital, hostile, homicidal in her brutal assaults, alternately sweetly sarcastic and miserably lonely and tearful.

Only one or two people could approach her without personal danger—an attendant who cared for all her physical needs, and the ward doctor, a very tall, heavy man, gentle and tender in his relationships with patients. Again, I was making rounds and ventured to the door of her seclusion room, having been duly warned by the attendants.

She greeted me in a friendly way and I asked her why she was in seclusion. Her reply was: "I belong here right now." I asked her if I might come in and sit with her a while and she replied: "I don't know you." I did not pursue my request but told her I would return.

I came back three days later and found her sitting, leaning against the ventilator, humming softly to herself. She beckoned for me to come in and I asked the attendant to lock the door after me, but to please stay near by. This seemed to surprise Lillian and she asked if I wasn't frightened. I assured her I was, giving her back her words to me: "I don't know you." We talked briefly and then she seemed to become not angry but tense, so I left. For several weeks thereafter, I repeated these seclusion room visits, and she talked at length, almost completely in delusional patterns. She misidentified me many times, frequently mistaking me for her sister (who had also been hospitalized for mental illness).

She became worse toward the end of her third month on the admitting ward, and one day when I went into seclusion with her and sat on the floor, she paced angrily and finally turned to me and said, in a flat level tone: "Get out of here, Alice. Get out." Foolishly, I offered the banality: "Why? What's wrong, Lillian? I don't feel like leaving." Of course, she attacked me, savagely, and did considerable superficial damage before someone came to my rescue.

Considerably shaken, I pulled myself together, combed my hair, replaced my cap and went back to her seclusion room. The door was locked, but her angry face peered from the open window. I simply looked at her, and I said, as gently as possible: "The next time you attack me like that, Lillian, I shall have to defend myself." I knew intuitively that she would interpret this, in her schizophrenic way, just as I meant it—"the next time you attack me Lillian, I'm going to fight you back." She never touched me again, and—as with Pat—this episode seemed to be a turning point. She was soon transferred to a "chronic, disturbed" ward, and although she remained deeply delusional, she was no longer hostile and assaultive toward others.

I continued to see her, and began to take her out occasionally, as the warmth and rebirth of Spring came. One day I ventured to take her for a drive. She seemed uncomfortable as we entered the car, and soon asked to be taken back. She was very upset that evening, and, since I happened to be working late, I returned to the ward before she went to bed. She was able to tell me that she had been extremely upset as a youngster of 11 at being present during the home-delivery of her sister. "There was so much blood, Alice! It was terrifying! I hated it and I had so many questions about my mother and father and the conception of babies. *The red upholstery in your car* brought all that back so vividly!"

The tranquillizing drugs came into favor about this point, and Lillian was put on 100 mgm. of Thorazine four times a day. She was able to leave the hospital six months later, and to my knowledge, has not returned.

These two meaningful experiences in the individual nursing care of schizophrenic patients are selected from about seven in my limited experience. Administrative and educational pressures sometimes frustratingly limit one's availability to give individual nursing care!

CONCLUSION

Despite the "power of the schizophrenic," despite the personal inadequacies of the nurse, there is much to be said for this tool of "love" in overcoming the problem of communication in the relationship of the nurse and the schizophrenic patient.

For many years, on a definitely unformulated basis, love has been the answer in the individual nursing care of the schizophrenic patient. There is no reason to believe that it cannot continue to be therapeutic; there is no reason to believe that it cannot be taught. To quote Professor Pitrim Sorokin, in a "Lenten Message" which appeared in the *Boston Globe:* "Someday—perhaps soon—mankind will learn what individuals have always known: that love is the only true creative force in the world."

Developing Therapeutic Nurse-Patient Relationships

15

When Nurses Interview Patients

Sidney Berengarten*

The success of any interview, whatever its objective may be, depends primarily upon the nurse's ability to establish and maintain a sound interpersonal relationship with the patient.

Do nurses interview? The answer depends on your definition of the term. In its simplest form we have the basis for an interview whenever two people talk things over. In order to differentiate between interviewing and ordinary conversation, however, we should add the requirement that the interview must be a purposeful discussion directed toward some goal of action for the person who wants something for himself or is in need of help.

Interviewing is thus used extensively by all the "helping" professions, including nursing. Regardless of their specialized fields, all nurses do interviewing. It is through the interview that the clinic nurse obtains necessary factual information from the patient before his first medical examination; the bedside nurse determines the patient's reaction to his hospitalization and treatment; the public health nurse gives emotional support and sound health instruction to the young mother.

INTERPERSONAL RELATIONSHIPS

In professional nursing education increasing recognition is being given to the importance of interpersonal relationships which are based on regard for the patient as a *feeling* person as well as a thinking and physical being. Frequent reference is made to a new approach in medicine and nursing which

---

*From *American Journal of Nursing*, Vol. 50, No. 1, (January, 1960).

Mr. Berengarten, who is an assistant professor at the New York School of Social Work, Columbia University, also teaches an orientation course in social work for graduate nursing students at Teachers College, Columbia.

is patient- rather than disease-centered. The medical and nursing professions are becoming more aware of the role of the emotions in illness and are more readily acknowledging the effect of the patient's attitudes and feelings toward the illness as factors in retarding or promoting recovery. In many situations they recognize that medical treatment and nursing care alone are not enough to restore the patient to good health.

This shift in emphasis, with the emotional components in illness granted equal recognition with the organic, is also bound to be reflected in communication between nurses and patients. In addition to making her basic contribution to the patient's well-being through properly ministering to his physical needs, the nurse can be a vital therapeutic agent in the patient's mental health. Her method of communicating is recognized as being no longer essentially physical but is rather a combined physical-verbal-visual means of working with him. This is accomplished through the medium of interpersonal relationship. We shall briefly discuss several significant factors in the nurse-patient relationship as they relate to interviewing.

The nurse, as she is frequently reminded nowadays, is called upon to temporarily assume a psychological mother-substitute role—a function which results from the patient's normally regressive behavior during illness. The man who is literally flat on his back and is dependent on others for his physical care is often emotionally supine. He comes to the hospital with the combined fear about himself and his illness and also of what may be in store for him in the course of treatment. His anxiety, which is realistically warranted in part but which is also reinforced by fantasies about his condition and his future welfare, frequently interferes with normal recuperative processes. By her demeanor, attitude, and approach the nurse may either intensify his fear and anxiety and thus possibly prolong his illness or help drain off tension and thereby accelerate his return to physical health.

Present-day educational programs for nurses do not allow time or provide the content needed if nurses are expected to acquire a profound knowledge of the psychodynamics of behavior. However, the nurse should at least be oriented in this area and should be able to contribute to the patient's ease and emotional well-being.

How can the interested nurse make constructive use of the psychological knowledge she does possess, of her good personality equipment, and her impulse to help people who are in difficulty?

Her first and most fundamental obligation is to establish a positive relationship with the patient. The attainment of such a relationship is largely based on the nurse's warmth, sensitivity, sympathetic understanding, and her objectivity. It requires particularly the ability to feel deeply with the patient but still retain her own identity and not become personally overwhelmed and enmeshed in the patient's problems. Because the nurse is herself an individual having unique personal feelings, attitudes, beliefs, and biases like all people, the Socratic admonition of self-knowledge is most important for her if she wishes to help others.

Our attitudes, feelings, and behavior toward those whom we wish to help have been largely conditioned by our own life's experiences and relationships. Among other things, the age and sex of the patient as well as his physical and personal characteristics often activate certain feelings and responses which may have no basis of reality in our experience with the particular patient. We may find ourselves liking or disliking him and, if called upon to explain, would have difficulty in giving a logical reason. Most likely, we are attributing and displacing on him our own feelings which stem from identifying him, usually unconsciously, with someone extremely close to us, very often a parent, brother, or sister. In the process of growing up emotionally no one has entirely resolved his conflicting feelings toward key members in his family group and this is often reflected in the way in which we relate to others in our personal and professional relationships.

This explains to some extent why some nurses derive little satisfaction in working with elderly patients, while others react less positively to children. Others find themselves tense and ill at ease with patients who are their contemporaries. Some nurses are less responsive to women patients, others to male patients particularly. Generally there are limits to the range of our capacity to relate positively to others.

NEED FOR SELF-AWARENESS. In order to prevent her intuitive reaction to the patient from getting in the way of establishing a sound relationship, it is most important that the nurse be able to recognize and not deny her feelings toward him, even though she may be unaware at the time of the origin of such feelings. This self-awareness is the first step in arriving at a more complete self-understanding. It will help her to achieve the ultimate self-discipline and control of her feelings which permit the patient to accept the fact that here is a warm, permissive, understanding person in whom he can invest his confidence and feel free to express his preoccupying feelings about himself and his condition.

To illustrate this principle, a supervisor in public health nursing cited a situation involving a new staff nurse. The latter repeatedly discharged her diabetic patients after they had mastered the technic for administering insulin, but without teaching other factors involved and failing to determine whether their adjustment to the illness was adequate.

The nurse was extremely defensive when the supervisor first tried to discuss the basis for her premature withdrawal in those cases. The nurse was equally concerned, however, about her apparent resistance to diabetic patients and with the supportive, understanding help of the supervisor was later able to share the fact that her mother's diabetes had been discovered several years previously. Ever since, her mother had allegedly "played invalid" and demanded constant attention. The nurse's father, to whom she had been strongly attached, capitulated to her mother's demands. When he died suddenly several months after the onset of the mother's illness, the nurse felt bitter toward her mother and held her responsible for her father's death. She resented having to provide for her mother's maintenance and medical expenses. Her supervisor commented, "As she grew more secure in the field she was able to accept these feelings as the basis for her dislike of diabetic patients. It was a realization to which she finally came unaided and, although she has not yet entirely gotten over her feelings, her visits to diabetic patients are among the most thorough and independence-stimulating that I have seen."

ACCEPTING THE PATIENT. In illness the patient's threshold of tolerance for frustration frequently is low. This fact gives the nurse another opportunity to offer the patient tangible evidence that she likes him as a person and accepts his feeling toward himself and his condition. Denial or slowness in meeting his demands is often interpreted by the patient as lack of interest on the nurse's part, and his resentment is touched off quickly. He may express this verbally or convey it in his attitude and behavior.

The nurse who is personally secure tries not to respond subjectively to the patient's negative feelings. She consciously guards against reacting with similar hostile feelings or in using punitively the authority her position affords. Perhaps more than anything else, her ability to accept the patient despite his expression of resentment helps convince him that she truly understands and accepts him.

Like everyone else the nurse wants to be liked. When this is an excessive need, however it imposes an undue strain on the patient to suppress his feelings in order not to offend her, resulting in increased tension and personal distress for him. The nurse who has this exaggerated need for personal acceptance is usually insensitive to the emotional pain accompanying the patient's physical pain. Surprisingly, some nurses have said in all sincerity that they could recall few instances in which a patient was hostile toward them. Because these nurses are unable to tolerate hostility, they have had to obliterate any such experience from memory. Their approach to patients is often characterized by an attitude which seems to convey that they "love everybody," and in turn they expect unconditional reciprocal affection.

Instead of responding to the patient's own feelings about this condition, they often tend to be overreassuring, and there is nothing more irritating and annoying to the patient than to be advised that he has nothing to worry about when in reality the situation may well warrant his anxiety and fear. He becomes confused, bewildered, and resentful when there is any attempt to minimize or deny his feelings. Reassurance and encouragement must be given only when there is a valid basis for it. Otherwise it is regarded as false and is interpreted by the patient as further indication of the nurse's insensitivity and failure to appreciate how he feels.

TEACHING THE PATIENT. In addition to their traditional functions, which chiefly concerned the physical care of sick people, nurses are accepting increasingly greater responsibility for disease prevention and health maintenance. This is particularly true of the public health nurse who now has the dual role of nurse and educator. However, she can fulfill her educational role properly only if her relationship with the patient is meaningful to him.

The most expert teaching methods and technics are of no avail unless the patient's emotional resistance to the nurse and her instruction is minimal. The patient may frequently understand and intellectually assimilate the content being taught. He is unable, though, to convert the knowledge into a skill or practice if he has not integrated it emotionally. He may be highly defensive and may not have permitted the nurse to reach him except superficially. This defensiveness may stem from a number of causes. We can comment on only a few characteristic patterns.

Like the nurse in her initial reaction to the patient, he is also conditioned by his past experiences and relationships with others who are symbolically like her. If his past experience with parent figures and authority has been emotionally charged with overt conflict, one would anticipate a poor response to the nurse and her teaching. However, if she accepts him as an individual and is not the controlling, authoritative person he may have anticipated, he has less need to resist her in her educational and helping role.

There are also patients at the other extreme who may have been deeply dependent on parents or persons in authority. Their repetitive pattern is to attempt to recapitulate the same relationship with all persons in authority. As in the case of the patient whose illness is emotionally satisfying because it permits continued dependency, the resistance they manifest to learning the principles and practices of proper health care and management often arises from their underlying reluctance to assume responsibility for themselves or others. Unless the nurse is quick to appreciate the significance of such behavior when it expresses itself in surface compliance, she will mistake it for mature receptivity.

A frequent problem for many nurses, particularly in public health work, is how to meet the patient's request for clarifying information about his illness. This is an area in which the nurse rightfully feels secure in her professional knowledge, and she often tends to respond literally to the patient's expressed desire for such an explanation. There may be times when a direct and precise answer to such a question is desirable. One must determine, however, whether the patient is really seeking and can use a literal explanation or whether the request may not stem from exaggerated fear of his illness and upset feelings about himself. Thus the patient with a disease like tuberculosis often feels personally and socially ostracized. He may react to his condition with a feeling of unworthiness and his primary worry may be whether his family and friends reject him.

Like the doctor the nurse also symbolizes society to him, and, through her regard and acceptance of him, his own self-esteem becomes enhanced. Until he is comfortable in his relationship with the nurse and is able to express the feelings which preoccupy him, his anxiety may prevent him from intelligently understanding or using the factual knowledge requested.

It is not easy for the nurse to restrain her impulsive wish to give explanations and interpretations to her patients. However, when she learns the importance of effective listening in order to understand more adequately what is involved in the patient's situation, she will find that the patient is often willing and appreciates the chance to share with her his concerns if he is permitted to do so at his own pace and in his own way. He will then be truly receptive to her explanations and interpretations.

THE PATIENT'S RELATIVES. The role of the patient's relatives in contributing either positively or negatively to his recuperation must not be minimized. He is affected profoundly by their attitudes and feelings. The nurse often represents the same parent figure to them as she does to the patient, and she should anticipate similar displacement of their feelings. It may be more difficult, however, for the nurse to tolerate from them the same manifestations of hostility, guilt, dependency, and indifference which she is able to accept in the patient. Apart from the realization that the patient's negative behavior is induced in part by the stresses of his illness, the nurse is naturally more sympathetically responsive to him than to his relatives. Without knowing the conditioning influences it would obviously be hard for her to understand why the relatives often seem so ready to divest themselves of responsibility for the patient's care, are insensitive to his pain, or respond with excessive anxiety to his condition. In any event, unless the nurse is capable of conveying her warm acceptance of them and of showing that she appreciates their feelings—even though they are negative toward the patient and his illness—she may be thwarted in her efforts to help him. The nurse can provide for the relatives a rare opportunity to express their feelings to someone who is understanding and is not critical or moralistic. This benefits the patient as well. When the nurse recognizes that the relatives are having a difficult time and lets them know that she understands, she is giving them emotional support which, added to her function in sharing or relieving them of the burden of physical care, increases their ability to meet the patient's demands for personal support and reassurance.

A FEW POINTERS ON INTERVIEWING

1. To elicit pertinent data
2. To impart information
3. To provide an opportunity for the patient to ventilate his feelings and thus release tension
4. To motivate the patient in the direction of understanding and resolving his own problems and feelings.

Any interview may include one or more of these objectives.

Regardless of the specific objective, the verbal-visual medium of communication between nurse and patient is the cornerstone of the interview. In this connection it should be noted that the nurse's physical expression is vitally important in furthering a good relationship. Speech alone does not transmit depth of interest and feeling. If the nurse is truly sensitive to the patient and his feelings, she will appropriately express her concern and regard for him. She will not assume a so-called neutral appearance, which could be described more accurately as impassive and Sphinx-like.

An appropriate control over feelings is required, however. Overresponding, whether verbally or facially, is as detrimental to the relationship as being unresponsive, since it only serves to intensify and color the patient's feelings and attitudes, thus adding to his emotional burden.

It is advisable to examine ourselves carefully to detect and control any characteristic mannerisms or expressions which tend to convey subjective feelings or critical attitudes. For example, the arching of an eyebrow, the furrowing of the forehead, the narrowing of the eyes, the rigid set of the jaws all reveal the interviewer's feelings. An expression reflecting warmth, friendliness, sincere interest, and sympathetic understanding helps to induce a favorable response.

A general atmosphere of personal relaxation and freedom from pressures has the anomalous effect on the patient of being both a sedative and stimulant and speeds the establishment of a satisfactory relationship. The public health nurse who is considerate of the patient's time and schedules home visits or office appointments at his convenience helps to reduce pressures for him so that he too is at optimal ease in the interview. The office interview, if it can be arranged, often has many advantages since it insures proper privacy and freedom from distractions found in the home.

Regardless of the setting, as little attention as possible should be directed to the mechanics of the interview. Patients are usually more relaxed and freer in their responses when notes are not recorded during the discussion. Note-taking may be necessary to insure accuracy of factual data, as in a registration interview. The nurse's mastery, through practice, of the ability to record unobtrusively and simultaneously stimulate the flow of discussion through her warm interest, sustained attention, and supportiveness helps to offset the anxiety aroused by the recording.

There is a difference, of course, in the extent to which the various groups of nurses engage in interviewing as a formal process. Fundamentally, however, the same factors which are basic to good interpersonal relationships are also basic to successful interviewing. Any form of interviewing between a nurse and her patient, whether its objective is essentially education, therapy, or information gathering, must depend primarily on the nurse's ability to initiate and sustain a relationship that fosters the patient's personal growth and movement toward self-direction.

16

What's Wrong
with
Getting Involved?

Marguerite J. Holmes*

We need to reconsider whether any work with patients can possibly be so separated that we do not get involved, or, even more, whether we really wish to disengage ourselves from patients.

Why is it that "involvement," when it refers to student-patient or instructor-student relationships, is considered wrong, almost immoral, especially in psychiatric nursing? Students are cautioned by instructors not to get "involved" with their patients, and new instructors are cautioned by older instructors not to get involved with their students, but few persons bother to explain what this dreadful thing actually is or why it is to be feared. Beyond saying that the student-patient or the instructor-student relationship must be "professional"—another overworked and little understood term—very little explanation is given about a relationship which basically must be involved by its very nature.

In the discussion of involvement and professional relationships considered here, student-patient situations are being used as illustration, but the same material applies equally well to instructor-student situations.

How many student nurses are greeted each year, particularly as they begin their clinical psychiatric nursing, with some sort of a warning about not getting involved with their patients? The clichés flow hot and heavy as ambiguous and contradictory advice falls on the ears of the students: ". . . learn to relate to patients . . . interact with them in a therapeutic manner

*From *Nursing Outlook*, Vol. 8, No. 5 (May, 1960).

Miss Holmes (B.S., M.N., University of Washington School of Nursing, Seattle) is assistant director of the NLN Seminar Project for Teachers of Psychiatric Aides, and had majored in psychiatric nursing before working in the project.

. . . don't become involved . . . communicate with them . . . strive to understand their needs . . . give the patient a feeling of 'togetherness' . . . don't become involved. . . ." Interesting, that relating is suggested in the same breath with not getting close to persons, isn't it? Difficult, too.

The subject of overworked and ill-defined psychiatric jargon and stereotyped clichés whose meanings have long since been forgotten is too large to consider here except to point out that much of this terminology must leave new students hopelessly confused—especially if the instructor is not exactly sure what she is trying to say. My major concern here is an attempt to define "therapeutic student-patient relationships" and to relegate to their proper places the terms "professional relationship" and "involvement."

Rollo May discusses participant observation as a tool or technique used by the psychotherapist or psychoanalyst. It is used, also, by nurses. If we substitute "nurse" where May used the word "therapist," what he says applies equally well to both groups. The whole concept of participant observation places emphasis upon the

. . . significance of the therapist in the relationship with the patient. The fact that the therapist participates in a real way in the relationship and is an inseparable part of the "field" does not, thus impair the soundness of his scientific observations. Indeed, can we not assert that unless the therapist is a real participant in the relationship and consciously recognizes this fact, he will *not* be able to discern with clarity what is in fact going on? (1)

If this is true, and if these ideas about participant observation can be applied to nurses, and I believe they can, it becomes apparent that if a nurse is to be of any help to the patient she must become involved with him. Surely if she "participates in a real way in the relationship and is an inseparable part of the 'field,' " she is involved.

We can look at it in another way. What are the things nurses are supposed to do for patients? Tend to their physical needs for one. A nurse can do this without necessarily experiencing any kind of emotional "involvement" with the patient. But what if she does some of the other things nurses are also supposed to do while she tends his physical needs? What if she accepts him exactly as he is, respects him as an individual, allows him to express his feelings to her, concerns herself with him as a person rather than as a set of symptoms, observes him in an honest attempt to understand why he does the things he does, responds as best she can do to his attempts to communicate with her, helps him learn to deal with problems as they come up rather than avoiding them, and helps him curb his behavior when necessary? Can she do any of these and feel nothing for the patient, not "get involved" with him? Could he be helped in the same way by some sort of wonder machine to carry out these activities rather than being given the care by a slightly blundering nurse who cares what happens to him? I think not. And this, I believe, is the substance of nurse-patient involvement. It is not a bad thing. It is the interest, the feeling of compassion, the concern, the desire to help, or whatever else you may call it, which one human being feels for another.

To return to May, he also says that the therapist must consciously recognize the fact that he is a participant in the relationship. " . . . anyone in a therapeutic relationship, or any person observing others, for that matter, must clarify very well what his particular emotions and involvement are in the situation" (2). This, perhaps is where some nurses have difficulty. It is not easy to scrutinize one's own emotions and involvement in a situation. It is easier and less painful to avoid becoming involved with a patient, simply not to allow oneself to care about the patient as a sick and needy human being.

We get around that by maintaining a "professional relationship," whatever that is, with the patient. Too often, "professional relationship" is used to avoid any kind of relationship. The nurse who hides behind the term usually has built up a wall of defenses which allows her to perform her nursing functions perfunctorily, routinely, mechanically, without even seeing the great need around her, without feeling the pain and anguish her patients are experiencing—without humanity.

A professional relationship need not be cold and detached. It can be warm and gentle and tender, while the nurse maintains an awareness of her own emotions and involvement in the situation. The true professional relationship must be geared toward meeting the needs of the patient, not the needs of the nurse.

An individual must be mature to relate to a patient in such a way; she must be able to give something of herself, her time, her concern, her interest —without demanding anything in return. She must be able to keep a check on her emotional lability, and be constantly aware of her feelings about the patient and his relatives. She must be able to allow the patient to need her less as he moves toward health, rather than to bind him closer to herself. The nurse must not wear apron strings. She must be able, also, to seek out supervisory help when she finds her emotions interfering with her work: causing her to reject the patient or to smother him and stifle his efforts to grow away from her.

Nursing students are rarely sufficiently mature to be able to assume full responsibility for their relationships with patients, and particularly with psychiatric patients. No doubt, this is why instructors warn them not to become involved. Perhaps we instructors would do well to examine our vocabularies to see if we are using terms which have no meaning or have altered their meaning through misuse. We need to get acquainted with students well enough to estimate their individual abilities to relate well to patients, and we need to help them individually rather than warn them collectively. Those students who are rather immature need more than usual guidance and direction in their clinical experience. We can help them see the pitfalls before they fall into them; if we fail that—and we do fail at times—we can learn to profit from their mistakes, rather than punish them or permit them to continue mistakenly. In short, we can help students if we show them the positive side of the picture. We can show them, by teaching and by example, what a helpful relationship is, rather than frightening them away from any kind of relationship.

REFERENCES

1. May, Rollo, and others, eds. *Existence; A New Dimension in Psychiatry and Psychology.* New York, Basic Books, 1958, p. 27.
2. *Ibid.*

17

Dependency in
Nurse-Patient Relationships

Hellene N. Jensen and Gene Tillotson*

Nurses can create a therapeutic environment for patients who express their conflicts through excessive demands, withdrawal, or disrespect.

In the process of growing up in the American culture, a constant struggle exists within the individual between the desire to be dependent and the necessity to be independent. The struggle is between what is considered an acceptable dependence for a given stage of life and the striving to be an individual entity. The characteristics of dependent or independent personalities evolve with the process of growing up.

One can note many areas of behavior in our culture in which a child is expected to become proficient at an early age and those in which independence is postponed. A high degree of independence is expected of a child in early control of elimination, learning to walk, in feeding and dressing himself, and acquiring speech.

At the same time there is an element of dependence introduced in the limitations imposed. Where he walks, how and what he eats, which clothing he puts on, and what he says are rather rigidly controlled. This element of dependence in itself is not necessarily bad. Unfortunately, close adherence to these limitations is often a basis for parental acceptance or rejection of the

*From *American Journal of Nursing*, Vol. 61, No. 2 (February, 1961).

Miss Jensen (General Hospital School of Nursing, Everett, Wash.; A.A., Everett Junior College, Everett, Wash.; B.S., University of Washington, Seattle, Wash.; M.A., Columbia University) is director of nursing education at the Mental Health Institute, Cherokee, Iowa.

Miss Tillotson (B.S., University of Minnesota, Minneapolis, Minn.; M.N., University of Washington, Seattle, Wash.) is an instructor at the Veterans Administration Hospital, American Lake, Wash.

child himself. In such cases the child becomes highly dependent upon parental approval. He learns to conform and exhibits little individuality.

In schools of nursing, there is still considerable autocracy prevalent in nursing instruction, despite the fact that democratic principles are widely voiced. General learning conditions to which nurses are exposed foster conformity rather than creative activity.

The nurse who is a product of the autocratic atmosphere is not free in her mental activity. She has been "taught" that there is a premium on conventional behavior rather than on individuality. The potential capacity for self-expression in each individual needs release through collaboration and experimentation with new ideas. Individuality is compatible with high standards in professional skills. The freer one is to be one's self, the more professional growth is fostered.

The cultivation of sensitivity to the feelings of others is important to the personal growth of the nurse. The good nurse is the one who can sense what the patient thinks, what he needs, what he feels, through a consistently warm and eager study of her patient. Through observation and practice, she recognizes day by day how to serve the patient's needs without having to prod him constantly to spell them out for her. Learning to be consistent and to listen with warm, emphatic feeling facilitates this understanding.

Actually, it is more a matter of self-study and self-development than of teaching. The nurse must understand her own weakness, her own assets and abilities, before she can accept herself as an individual. Acceptance of herself is essential before she can know and accept her patient. If patient situations are viewed critically, one can often see evidence of hostility and the conflict with dependency impulses which can be perpetuated or alleviated according to the staff's concept of the problem.

A DEMANDING MAN

Mr. Case was a 28-year-old single man, hospitalized for the treatment of a bleeding peptic ulcer. In addition, arthritis in his left knee prevented ambulation. His orders included a Sippy diet and amphojel, with food and medicine alternated every hour, and continuous hot packs to his knee. During the first week after admission, he was cared for by the regular hospital staff.

The daily reports portrayed him as a demanding and complaining patient. Each time any member of the nursing staff passed his bed, he complained either of discomfort or of the care he received, or he requested some special service. When personnel were not available, he spent most of his waking hours complaining to other patients in the ward.

He continually voiced complaints of neglect and inadequate attention. His reiterations proved disrupting to the morale of the ward.

Supplies for the Sippy diet and the amphojel were left on the bedside stand, so that he could help himself at the prescribed times. He refused to minister to himself and demanded the assistance of a nurse. He was heard to remark, "Where is that nurse? It's time for my amphojel."

Frequently, he was sarcastic, "I don't know what good they think this cold pack is doing for my knee." He demanded a bed bath every day, although a bath every other day was routine. If he was not the first patient attended he would blurt out, "Do I have to wait all day for my bath?"

Occasionally, his unpleasantness was overlooked by the busy personnel, but more often they retaliated with, "You're not the only patient on the ward, you know," or, "You know you were instructed to take your amphojel yourself. You can tell time, can't you?" Another scolded, "I suppose you know you are upsetting the entire ward," and again, "I have only two hands and two feet!"

These rebukes were of sparse comfort to the conflict-ridden patient. Although the nurses believed they were giving adequate nursing care, the attention given was based on their concept of what he needed. No attempt was made to interpret what he really was trying to communicate through his accusations and resistance to routines.

TRYING TO UNDERSTAND. At the beginning of the second week a nursing student was assigned to the patient. Customarily, the nursing students spent four hours a day, five days a week, for two weeks with three patients. On the first day, Miss Maxwell gave him his prescribed daily care and studied his history, the report of his progress, and her patient. She observed that his behavior over the past week had alienated him from everyone in the environment. Other patients did not include him in their conversation, and personnel avoided him. The nurses remarked that they were glad to have someone else take care of him.

Miss Maxwell's previous orientation had been directed toward giving comprehensive nursing care to individual patients. This technique included an awareness of patients' emotional and social as well as physical needs. Mr. Case, however, was her first patient with a peptic ulcer.

At the end of the first day, the student felt that while she had the skills to provide for the physical needs of the patient, she could not help resisting his insistent emotional demands. Her uncertainty about how to handle the problem prompted her to seek suggestions from the clinical instructor. Together, they decided on an approach which they thought could alter the situation.

Miss Maxwell organized her morning activities so that Mr. Case received a bath each day and was cared for first. She listened to his complaints without retaliation, responding from time to time with such comments as, "It's pretty hard to stay in bed and have others wait on you," "I can imagine how you must feel," or, "I'll do all I can while I'm here to make you comfortable."

She anticipated his requests and made provisions to meet them before he could ask. Each time a medication was due, she was present to pour it and offer it to him. The hot water bottles in the hot packs were changed before they cooled. Each time she passed the bed, she indicated that she would be nearby and would return soon to continue with his care. At no time during the two-week period did she criticize either the patient or the nursing staff.

During the 10 days of actually caring for the patient, Miss Maxwell had frequent discussions with the instructor to clarify the interactions taking place between herself and the patient. She wanted to evaluate the changes in behavior of the patient and the staff. The student's natural acceptance and understanding attitude obviated the friction that previously existed between the patient and staff members.

The patient's complaints and demands gradually decreased until, toward the end of the period, they were no longer evident. On the seventh day he actually offered to take the medicines from the bedside stand for himself. Other patients by now occasionally included him in their conversation. He was even observed to show real humor and laughed at their jokes.

MIND AND BODY. Resistance to being dependent is seen in Mr. Case's overbearing, demanding attitude. The unconscious motivation to have his dependency needs satisfied was communicated to the nursing staff and other patients by disrespect. His needs were so all-consuming that he was quite unable to show consideration for those around him. His disturbing behavior was met by resentment on the part of some patients and withdrawal on the part of others to show a like attitude.

The patient's initial belittling and critical attitude was a threat to each nurse's self-esteem, both as an individual and as a professional person. The anxiety engendered in the nurses resulted in their becoming defensive in order to ward off threats and protect their own adequacy. It is common for nurses to expect patients to conform to hospital routines rather than to feel that they should make the adjustment to patients. If the patient does not cooperate, the nurse loses status by being unable to control the situation.

When Miss Maxwell arrived to care for Mr. Case, it would have been easy for her to follow the same pattern of behavior. In her contact with the patient, she was aware that she was inclined toward reactions similar to those of the hospital staff. She realized that her nursing care objectives and her resistance to the patient were incompatible. With help, she outlined a plan that might lessen the tension of the patient.

WHY SHE WITHDREW

Mrs. Shelby was a 26-year-old woman who had been hospitalized for two months in a tuberculosis sanatorium. She was in a private room and still on bed rest. The nursing service personnel considered her a definite problem because of her extreme, uncooperative behavior.

She kept herself isolated from all other patients by having her door closed and the shades drawn. She objected strenuously to following any hospital routines. Each day, it was impossible to give her more than minimal care until almost noon. She specifically refused streptomycin injections when other patients received theirs at nine-thirty in the morning. She demanded it in the evening.

Her behavior provoked considerable hostility in the day staff. One day while making her report to the evening nurse, the head nurse remarked, "You don't have to give Mrs. Shelby her shots at night. She can just have them when we give the others. There's no need for her to have a special routine."

The evening nurse, Miss Blake, was a young graduate who had had about three years experience. She consistently displayed considerable understanding and acceptance of the behavior of all patients. Her reply was quiet, "But you won't change her. I don't mind giving the shots at night."

Miss Blake utilized the period of giving the medication to demonstrate her acceptance of the patient by a warm, friendly attitude. She had only a limited amount of time to spend with Mrs. Shelby but consistently encouraged her to express her feelings. Bit by bit, the patient began to verbalize her concerns about the illness and about her husband and child at home. Miss Blake passed this information on.

Gradually, the staff showed acceptance of the patient. After several weeks, the change in the patient's attitude was noticeable. She talked more with the personnel, but the most apparent change came when she put her window shade up and shortly after that had the door left open. Eventually, she even enjoyed greetings from ambulatory patients.

The willingness of Miss Blake to go along with Mrs. Shelby's demands indicated her awareness of the patient's emotional requirements. Moreover, it indicated her belief that the patient's individuality is more important than hospital routines. The exact time of administering the medication was not vital to the patient's welfare. It was important only that she receive it once a day. When the staff relented and adopted a more friendly interest, Mrs. Shelby relaxed and was cooperative.

When conformity to routines was no longer forced, she had no need to fight for her independence. The conflict between her drives for dependence and independence was reduced. As long as Mrs. Shelby experienced disrespect from the staff, she could be expected to respond disrespectfully by withdrawal and nonconformity. Miss Blake, trained not to be the authoritarian, was the first to alter the pattern of disrespect. She not only could accept the patient's behavior but also could refrain from attacking the hostility of the staff.

Among the patients in a tuberculosis hospital, a wide variety of reactions to their illness is observed. Some studies which have been made indicate that these reactions in part may be related to a conflict between dependence and independence.

ON THE BACK WARD

Mrs. Ishimoto was a 41-year-old American-born, Japanese woman, diagnosed as a schizophrenic, hebephrenic type. She had been in a state mental hospital for 12 years and had spent nearly all the time on a ward for disturbed patients.

During the years, she exhibited extremely disintegrated behavior. Any attempts to approach her or to converse with her were met by giggling and laughter. Ward personnel described her as mute, for she never responded verbally to them nor talked to other patients. She was able to follow the routines of the day and created no major problems in ward adjustment.

She could care for her personal hygiene with a minimum of encouragement. The attention given to her amounted to mere "custodial care," since all personnel considered her extremely "deteriorated" and completely out of touch with reality.

Every three months, Mrs. Ishimoto was presented in a classroom to the group of student nurses who affiliated at the hospital for experience in phychiatric nursing. For many years she was used routinely as a demonstration case of "typical" hebephrenia. From her ward across the hospital grounds, she was taken to the building where classes were held. There she waited with other patients and a nursing instructor in a small anteroom next to the class-room.

During these waiting periods, the nurses were polite to Mrs. Ishimoto, but they paid little attention to her. They never attempted to talk to her, knowing that they would get no appropriate response. When she was brought before the doctor and his class, the patient's symptoms and behavior were discussed in her presence. This was not a malicious procedure; for the doctor was firmly convinced that Mrs. Ishimoto comprehended nothing that was said to her.

Almost invariably during the waiting period, Mrs. Ishimoto would leave her chair and edge restlessly toward the door as though anxious to leave. She offered no resistance, however, when she was told it was not time to go yet and was guided back to her chair. Then sitting on the chair she voided through her clothing so that the back of her dress was always wet as she was taken into the classroom. Little ever was said concerning this behavior, although the nurses' disapproval was evident.

Even though over the years several different nurses were responsible for supervising these patients, the same attitude prevailed toward Mrs. Ishimoto. Eventually, Miss George, a nurse having considerable psychiatric nursing experience and training, assumed this responsibility. The first time Miss George assembled the patients for the class, Mrs. Ishimoto behaved as usual.

After the patient had voided, wetting her dress, the nurse felt concern about the patient's appearing in class in this condition. She found a surgical gown in a nearby room and put it on Mrs. Ishimoto, saying, "It is too bad this happened, but we can cover it up so no one will notice." She did not register disapproval.

The nurse by now sensed that the patient might be reacting to the necessity of appearing at class. She made it a point to remain nearby until time for the patient to go in. After Miss George accompanied the patient back to her ward, she inquired as to whether Mrs. Ishimoto usually was incontinent. The head nurse stated that she always went to the toilet by herself.

AN UNDERSTANDING NURSE. Three months later when it was again time for the class, Miss George called at the ward for Mrs. Ishimoto. She greeted the patient by name and explained where they were going. During the walk to the waiting room, the nurse gave the patient direct attention and made a few comments, even though she expected no answer.

Because she was now cognizant of the general opinion about the patient, the nurse made a special effort to observe her behavior for indications that she was aware of her surroundings. In the waiting room the patient again was restless. Remembering the former incontinence and hoping to avoid a repetition of it, Miss George spoke quietly, asking, "Do you need to go to the toilet?"

Mrs. Ishimoto looked at the nurse, shook her head positively and said, "No! No!" so emphatically that it appeared as if she had understood the question. In a few minutes she left her chair, moved near to the wall and, with her feet apart, voided.

Again the nurse's attitude was accepting. Uncomplaining, she wiped up the puddle and checked the patient's clothing. Only her panties were wet. The nurse took the patient to the next room and had her remove them. During the rest of the waiting period, Miss George sat beside Mrs. Ishimoto. They looked at a magazine together, the nurse making an occasional comment. Mrs. Ishimoto looked at the pictures most of the time and frequently nodded when the nurse spoke, although it did not often appear that the nods were actual affirmative responses to the comments made. On the way back to her ward, the nurse spoke to the patient assuming that she understood what was being said.

The third time Miss George went to bring Mrs. Ishimoto to the class, she approached her with the same friendly attitude and again explained why she was there. The nurse noticed that Mrs. Ishimoto was wearing new shoes and commented on them. It seemed as if the patient evidenced some pride in the shoes and that her smile was appropriate to the occasion. In the waiting room, she was helped out of her coat, which then was placed in an adjoining room. No reference to voiding was made this time.

In her behavior, the patient seemed a little more alert. She held her head erect and looked at the other people in the room. The nurse frequently directed her attention toward Mrs. Ishimoto with comments specific to happenings in the environment. This time, the patient was not incontinent prior to her appearance before the class. Following the class period her behavior seemed to be more appropriate than before.

As Miss George was about to remark that it was time to return to the ward, the patient spoke, "Time to go now?" Slight movements and glances toward the other room indicated that she remembered where her coat had been placed. The nurse held the coat and helped her into it, and the patient responded with a distinct, "Thank you." On the way back to the ward she voluntarily took hold of the nurse's hand and held it tightly all the way.

THE MEANING OF INCONTINENCE. Researchers have explored the meanings of incontinence in various kinds of situations. Several investigations have taken place in psychiatric settings. From these, it is apparent that one of the main causes of incontinence is underlying hostility. Mrs. Ishimoto's incontinent behavior seemed directly related to a specific situation. On the ward, she needed no reminder or encouragement to use the toilet; even during the night she did not wet the bed. She knew, when she was brought to the class, that toilet facilities were available in the area.

This situation demonstrated changes which can take place in a patient's behavior when the attitude maintained by the nurse is consistently one of acceptance, even though the meetings between patient and nurse may be infrequent and of short duration. Actually, Miss George saw Mrs. Ishimoto for approximately two hours every three months. Behavioral changes were noticed in the class situation by the end of three visits, although no changes were seen on the ward. It seems quite probable that the patient was aware of the different attitude of this nurse toward her.

FEELING RESPECTED

The emotional problems demonstrated in the foregoing illustrations are largely based on difficulties with interpersonal relationships. Although the problems had their inceptions much earlier, they were exacerbated through the added trauma of illness. Illness reestablishes a position of dependency. If one has not resolved his dependency needs prior to the illness, strivings for independence may become extreme. The conflict created results in anxiety and a threat to a person's adequacy and self-esteem. As one's self-respect has not been established, lack of respect from others is unconsciously anticipated.

In the three examples discussed, it was seen that when the nurse had no understanding of the needs being communicated by the patient, a non-therapeutic atmosphere prevailed. The common ground of communication was disrespect, which was manifested by withdrawal, avoidance, rejection, and hostility. One or more of these methods were demonstrated by both patient and nurse.

Conversely, when the nurse showed respect through acceptance, freedom from control, regard for individual rights and feelings, and empathy, the patient responded with similar attitudes.

18

The Nurse-Patient Relationship

M. Audrey Kachelski*

The patient brings his need for care and comfort, the nurse her need for job satisfaction. In the relationship described here, the needs of both were met.

The nurse-patient relationship is a bond between two people, one a nurse, the other a patient. Both bring something to that relationship; both need something from it. The patient brings his discomfort and needs some kind of caring from the nurse; the nurse brings her professional skills and her need for a measure of success and satisfaction in carrying out her role. When the needs of both patient and nurse are met, it becomes a mutually satisfying relationship and one in which each becomes a stronger person because of the experience that brought them together.

Patients do not choose the nurse-patient relationship. They enter into it because of an accident, a heart attack, childbirth, the necessity of losing a part of their body, or because living has become too frightening or too overwhelming. Each patient brings to the relationship a deep concern about what has happened as well as what is to happen to him—and he brings with him the loneliness of pain and illness. The nurse may give a hypodermic; she may teach a patient how to care for a colostomy with which he must learn to live; she may sit in a rocking chair with a one-year-old child who has awakened at night crying; she may guide young parents in their first awkward

*From *American Journal of Nursing*, Vol. 61, No. 5 (May, 1961).

Miss Kachelski (B.S., University of Wisconsin School of Nursing; M.S.N., Catholic University of America) is assistant professor in psychiatric nursing at Indiana University School of Nursing. She was assistant director of the Seminar Project for Teachers of Psychiatric Aides, a project co-sponsored by the National League for Nursing and the American Psychiatric Association, and financed by the National Institute of Mental Health.

attempts at handling their infant; or she may sit in silence with a patient who is too frightened to talk with her. These are ways in which the nurse communicates to patients the fact that she is caring.

With the psychiatric patient, it is often difficult for the nurse to communicate that she is caring. All nurses deal with emotions and feelings to some extent, but for the psychiatric nurse this area is primary because it is the area of the patient's greatest difficulty and discomfort—and his primary reason for being in the hospital.

A review of some aspects of a nurse-patient relationship that extended over a two-week period for five days each week might be helpful in seeing how one nurse established a meaningful relationship with one patient. The nurse was with the patient each morning from 7:00 A.M. to 11:00 A.M. and then wrote daily interaction notes which included what she would recall and what she considered important in her relationship with the patient.

The patient, Kathryn Jones, was a young lady of 23 who had come to the state hospital for the first time 10 months before this nurse met her. The nurse knew the patient was receiving Thorazine; that she complained of feeling pressure in her chest; that she stayed by herself much of the time but would talk with others if approached; that she could go off the unit with the nurse; and that one of the main problems she presented on the ward was that she did not keep her underclothes clean.

Note how the nurse and patient are getting acquainted in their first meeting and how the nurse responds to what the patient is trying to communicate to her in such a way that her response facilitates the patient's communication.

FIRST DAY

This patient is a rather tall, attractive white female with long blonde hair and fair complexion. She wore a yellow dress, a blouse tied around the dress, and white high-heeled pumps. The dress and blouse were soiled and the shoes dirty. There was also a body odor about her. Her legs were not shaven and her teeth needed cleaning. Her nails were short, from biting them, and were partly covered with red nail polish.

After we were introduced I asked her if she would like to sit down with me. After finding chairs and getting seated, she said, "My name is Kay."

Nurse: Is that what you would like me to call you?

Kay: Yes.

Nurse: I'm going to be with you until 10:30 this morning and every morning for two weeks.

Kay: What am I supposed to tell you, everything?

Nurse: We can talk about anything you feel comfortable in talking about.

Kay: Well, it's just this feeling in my chest, which is really silly, and isn't anything at all.

Nurse: Would you like to tell me more about it?

During this time, she displayed much anxiety, crossing and uncrossing her legs, shuffling her feet, and working with her hair and the collar of her blouse. Her eyes would dart from side to side, as if she expected someone to be there.

Kay: Oh, it really isn't anything, it's so foolish.

Nurse: It has made you uncomfortable, though.

Kay: Oh yes. (*slight pause*) It started about a year and a half ago, and it was only in the mornings. I can't describe it, except it's a heavy feeling in my chest, and it makes my eyes look funny. Guess it was just a nervous breakdown, but I'm O.K. now, it's really nothing.

Nurse: What did you do when it first started?

Kay: Nothing. I finally went to a doctor and he told me that there was nothing wrong with me, that it was my nerves.

Nurse: How did you feel about this?

Kay: Terrible. (*slight pause*) It's all so silly.

Nurse: No, this isn't silly, because it makes you uncomfortable and it's something you need help with.

Kay: Are you here to help me?

Nurse: Yes.

Kay: Really, I don't think I need any help. I'm O.K. now.

Nurse: What kind of work do you do?

Kay: I was a receptionist and typist, but after I got this feeling in my chest, I felt I couldn't do a good job and everything I picked up felt masculine instead of feminine. I was embarrassed to be around people and wanted to get away from them.

Nurse: Do you live alone or with someone?

Kay: My father. He lives here in North Carolina and my mother is in Ohio.

Nurse: Does your father come to visit with you?

Kay: Yes, every Sunday. (*Occupational therapy personnel came on the ward*) Oh, there are the O.T. people.

Nurse: Do you usually go to O.T.?

Kay: Yes.

Nurse: Would you like to go this morning?

Kay: Well . . . (*hesitating*) maybe I'd better not.

Nurse: If you would like to go, I'll go with you.

Kay: No, I'd rather stay here this morning.

During this time she had left me five times saying, "Excuse me, I'll be right back." She would go to the bathroom, get a drink of water, and stand in front of the mirror, straightening her blouse and running her hands through her hair.

Nurse: Would you like to show me the ward?

Kay: Yes.

We walked up and down the hall and she showed me the different rooms. When we came to hers, the door was closed and all she said was, "That's my room."

She carried an oversized pocketbook and a notebook with her at all times.

Nurse: What do you have in your notebook?

Kay: Oh, just a lot of junk.

I asked her what time they ate breakfast and made plans to meet her the next morning and go to breakfast with her.

At times I sat quietly by her not saying anything and she would usually start the conversation again. About all she would talk about was the terrible feeling in her chest and how it made her look different from other people. When I asked about hobbies or friends, she said she had none now.

Her anxiety did not decrease while I was with her, and she left me about eight times, but always came back. I think that she feels very insecure and that anything she might do is insignificant to others and of no concern.

I felt nearly as uncomfortable around her at first as she did around me, and rather helpless as to what to do to begin to help her with this problem. She gives you the feeling she wants help, but feels so insignificant she cannot accept it.

Let us take a look at this first day in more detail. What was going on in this relationship? After being introduced the nurse took the initiative in asking Kay to sit down. On this first meeting the nurse and patient were getting acquainted. Together they established what the nurse would call the patient and clarified their role together. Both were actively involved in this clarification. The nurse informed Kay of the time limits of their relationship, and Kay was able to ask for clarification about what was expected of her in the relationship. ("What am I supposed to tell you, everything?") When she received an answer that did not put pressure on her ("We can talk about anything you feel comfortable in talking about.") she was able to proceed.

The nurse noticed the patient's anxiety, lived through some of it with her, and then, when it seemed to be intolerable for Kay, gave her an "out" by asking her if she would like to show her the ward—thus moving from a more to a less personal, less anxiety-producing involvement.

When Kay said about her chest symptom, "It's really nothing, it's so foolish," the nurse sensed her embarrassment and emphatically shifted the focus to Kay's discomfort saying, "It has made you uncomfortable, though," to which Kay immediately responded, "Oh, yes." One can almost sense her relief. Could Kay, who may have wondered if anyone could understand her, have felt that *maybe* here was someone to understand? Would she feel less hopeless about herself, less alone with her feelings—and would this be enough incentive to help her try again for more satisfying human relationships? Would she again have faith in the legitimacy of her own observations and her recognition of her own needs and feelings?

When the nurse began questioning Kay directly rather than responding to her feelings she received answers without much elaboration—like the answers to a questionnaire. Kay also shifted the discussion from her father to the occupational therapy people. The nurse sensed Kay's indecision, but although the nurse helped her to make the choice, it was Kay who made the decision to stay on the unit.

Toward the end of their time together, when the nurse was feeling uncomfortable and helpless, she seemed to "clutch" at anything to ask the patient—for example, about her notebook, friends, hobbies, none of which Kay was ready to talk about. When Kay indicated that she was not ready, the nurse did not press her, retaining her sensitivity in spite of her own anxiety and discomfort. The nurse was able to recognize and write about her own feelings in the time she spent with Kay.

111

SECOND DAY

When I first entered the ward this morning, my patient was standing in front of the mirror straightening her clothes. The first thing I noticed was how nice she looked. She had on a clean dress and a black sweater and sandals. After greeting her, I asked her what time the patients would be going to eat breakfast.

Kay: Soon, and I hope I can hold together. This is the time I always feel the worst. Is it because I'm so nervous that you're going with me?

Nurse: No, I'm just going to be *with* you.

Kay: Oh, O.K.

She ate a good breakfast and drank three cups of coffee. Upon returning to the ward she excused herself and went immediately to brush her teeth and to spend a few more minutes in front of the mirror. Then she came back and said, "Do you suppose we could go out for a walk now?" I said, "Yes, we can and it's such a nice morning out."

Not knowing my way around too well, I asked her to show me the way out, which she did, showing for the first time a little enthusiasm and less anxiety. We went first to the canteen where I bought her a pack of cigarettes and we sat down for a cup of coffee.

Kay: Really, I feel so silly about feeling this way. You must think I'm stupid.

Nurse: No, I don't because when things bother us or frighten us it's of much concern to us.

Kay: Yes, it really is, and I'm so frightened of everything, and that's my whole trouble, I've been running away and retreating for so long that I don't know how to do anything else. Really, it's nothing.

By this time our first cup of coffee was gone.

Kay: Would you like another cup of coffee?

Nurse: Would you like another cup?

Kay: Yes, if it's all right with you.

We drank another cup of coffee and more people started coming into the canteen. Her eyes darted from one to the other, and she appeared to be more anxious, so I suggested we go for a walk. Before leaving, she said, "Would you please get me another cup of coffee to take with me?" After walking a short distance we came to some benches.

Kay: Shall we sit here?

Nurse: This is fine.

Kay: This happened to me once before when I was in the seventh and eighth grade, and my teacher told Mother to take me to the doctor. I didn't want to be around people, and withdrew from my friends, but I kept up my school work, now I can't even do that.

Nurse: Does it worry you that perhaps this will happen to you again after you leave the hospital this time?

Kay: Yes (*very anxious expression*), do you suppose it will?

Nurse: That's something I can't answer because so much depends on the person herself.

Kay: You're so right, but I'm just not going to let it happen to me again.

Nurse: What did you do about it the last time that made you start feeling better?

Kay: I just talked with my friends and with Dad.

Nurse: Do you and your dad have a close relationship?

Kay: Yes, I could always talk to Dad, but not my Mother. Oh, I shouldn't say that, but she has an awful temper and really I do love her, it's just that . . . .

Nurse: Perhaps you could try the same thing this time, by finding someone that you can really talk to and tell your feelings.

Kay: Well, yes, I used to believe in love and God, but now I'm not sure, I'm just all mixed up. I know what my problem is, but I just can't do any-thing about it. I used to be pretty, but you'd never know it to look at me now.

Nurse: You still are pretty.

Kay: Do you really think so?

Nurse: Yes.

Kay: I was planning on going to California to work and if I'd gone, every-thing would have been O.K.

Nurse: Do you feel that by going that far away from your problems it would have helped, or would you not still have your problems in California?

Kay: I'm sure I'd still have them, but maybe I could have coped better with them in California.

Nurse: Do you hear often from your mother?

Kay: Yes, but I didn't write her for a long time after I came here because I was afraid of what she'd think of me for being in a place like this, and I really love her and don't want to hurt her.

She kept talking as she had the day before, about "how silly" all this was. She also said that she felt people were watching her and would know how inadequate she was. I tried to point out to her that this was a feeling that came from within herself, and that people really didn't feel this way about her.

When it was close to 10:30 she said, "I guess we'd better be going now, because you have to leave at 11:00." On our way back she said:

Kay: Would you do me a favor?

Nurse: Certainly, if I can.

Kay: Would you buy me another cup of coffee?

We went into the canteen and sat down. Another nurse came and spoke briefly to us and when she left Kay said, "I wish I could be like her. I used to be, but now I feel so low and so dirty all the time."

Nurse: I know you feel that way now, but these feelings will change as you get well.

Kay: I sure hope so.

We walked back to the ward and she thanked me, said it was just won-derful to get outside, and could we do it again? I assured her that we could.

Kay: You've helped me with one thing today.

Nurse: What is that?

Kay: You've helped me to understand that a lot of my feelings are coming from within myself.

113

Nurse: I'm glad that I have, because I want to try and help you while I'm here.

Kay: You already have.

We said good-bye and she went into the bathroom. When I got to the nurses' office I found that I had to turn her cigarettes in, so I went back into the bathroom to ask her for them. She was sitting with two other girls, looking at a magazine, which pleased me very much because this was the first I had seen any interaction with others.

I felt much more comfortable this morning, and I feel the patient did, too. She was more relaxed, didn't act as caged and could talk about more things to me.

The first thing the nurse noticed was a change in Kay's appearance—this had happened without any comment about it from the nurse.

Today Kay had someone with her at a time she "feels the worst." She was still wondering why the nurse was with her and asked for clarification. ("Is it because I'm so nervous that you're going with me?")

The nurse was able to follow through on Kay's request to go to the canteen, and it was while they were having coffee and a cigarette together that Kay was able to share with the nurse some of her embarrassment about her illness, and a concern about what the nurse thought of her—perhaps wondering how someone could like her. The nurse was able to shift the focus from "being stupid" to what troubles or frightens people as a cause for what they might do—a meaningful shift which Kay responded to immediately. Because the nurse seemed to understand her, Kay felt safe enough to reveal more about what was hurting her.

Then Kay shared with the nurse her deep concern about what her life might be—would she always be like this? What could she look forward to—a life spent in a mental hospital or might there by something else? Dare she even allow herself to think in terms of what others her age often think about—dates, engagement, marriage, home, family? Would she be O.K. for a while and then would it all start over again as it did once before? Would she have the courage to continue if this was what was in store for her?

The nurse did not give her a definite answer, but helped her look at her own experiences in her past and try to make use of the more helpful ones, like talking with people. Kay then talked of her relationship with her mother—a relationship in which she seemed torn between her duty to love her mother and her mother's "awful temper." Kay continued to tell the nurse how mixed up she was, that she was different than she had been (not sure if she could believe in love and God, "used to be pretty"); how discouraged, hopeless, and helpless she felt ("I know what my problem is, but can't do anything about it"). The nurse, without overemphasis, reminded her she still was pretty. Kay asked for verification, and apparently could accept the nurse's "Yes" as sincere. This was acceptable because the nurse had established her interest and so her answer did not seem to be an isolated remark meant merely to bolster morale.

Kay continued to share her thinking with the nurse—that if she had gone to California things would be different—wishful thinking, perhaps, but when questioned she felt the need to defend herself somewhat ("I'm sure I'd still have the problems, but maybe I could have coped with them better in California"). She was conveying to the nurse her search for an answer to the question, "Why am I like this?" There is hopefulness in Kay's "maybe." She was not *convinced* that she could have coped with her problems better in California, only *maybe* she could have. Her defense system was not yet a rigid one, and in experience of a safe human relationship, her own questioning was weakening it. She was seeking change in the direction of more satisfactory human living and she was open to influence.

The challenge to the nurse in this situation is to help Kay move in the direction Kay would like to move in, not only in the direction the nurse would like to see her move. Helping Kay to deal realistically with her daily living is one way the nurse can help her. And the nurse's own deep respect for the right of people to be different can help them both.

When Kay was talking about coping with her problems better in California, the nurse brought the conversation back to her mother. Was this the nurse's need to find out more about her relationship with her mother? If so, why? Was it curiosity? Or, was it that the nurse did not know what to say to respond to Kay's talking about California and felt she had to say something, anything? Was this due to the nurse's anxiety at this point? Is this what she felt she should ask about in order to be a good psychiatric nurse?

However, to Kay this question did not seem "out of order." Apparently it helped her share more of her feelings about being ashamed of being in a mental hospital—afraid to write her mother because of what her mother would think of her for being "in a place like this."

Later, she shared more of her feelings—that people were watching her and would know how inadequate and stupid she was. The nurse gave her something to think about—not only telling her that all people did not feel this way, but, after accepting Kay's feelings as real, explaining where such feelings came from.

Kay asked for another cup of coffee (and how many of us reach for the coffee cup and cigarette when we are anxious!) and when the nurse met her need without a lecture on the number of cups of coffee she had already had, she was able to tell the nurse how she felt about herself—personal and hurtful things. When Kay talked about "feeling so low and dirty all the time," the nurse accepted her feelings, but also gave her tremendous reassurance that as she got well her feelings would change. What meaningful words! No denial of how she felt, but the calm reassurance that things can change and the hopeful expectation that they would.

As they returned, the patient again let the nurse know how desperately she was searching for understanding, and pointed out spontaneously and with gratitude to the nurse how she had already helped her.

When the nurse learned that she was to turn the cigarettes into the office, she went back to ask Kay for them. It would have been possible for the nurse to report that Kay had the cigarettes and let someone else ask her for them, but she chose to handle this herself.

THIRD DAY

When I entered the ward this morning, my patient was down at the end of the hall on a sofa doing shorthand. She looked very nice in a stylish striped cotton dress and her white high-heeled pumps which were still quite soiled, but she looked cleaner than yesterday and appeared glad to see me. She began to talk about when she used to have dates.

Kay: I used to dress up and wear hats but I don't even keep clean now, and I've got to start thinking something of myself and keeping myself clean.

I don't even care about keeping my underwear clean, and that's awful.

Nurse: Perhaps this is something I could help you with.

Kay: Well . . . maybe, but it's really not important.

Walking back to the building she said again that she would like to see her mother.

Nurse: Have you written your mother about how you feel?

Kay: Yes, but I'm afraid she'll be ashamed to come and see me.

Nurse: These feelings you have about being in the hospital bother you a lot, don't they?

Kay: Yes, they do, but I know I need to be here and I need help.

I feel more comfortable each day, and the time really passes fast, but I worried some today for fear she might feel she had revealed too much about herself to me and how will this affect our relationship? I feel much empathy for this patient, and can understand better how miserable and utterly helpless she feels in this situation.

These excerpts indicate that Kay's appearance was continuing to improve; that she felt safe enough with the nurse to talk about the problem of her personal cleanliness. She was not yet ready to accept help from the nurse in this area. The nurse indicated her willingness to give help but did not press Kay into accepting it. This indicated her respect for Kay and perhaps conveyed that when Kay was better this would no longer be a problem for her. The nurse responded to Kay's feelings about being in the hospital and facilitated her communication—and what Kay communicated was a shift from "It's silly," to "I know I need to be here and I need help." Was this easier for her to say because the nurse let her know that she did not think it "silly"?

The relationship established in the first three days continued. The remaining excerpts were selected either because they are related to the nursing problem Kay presented, or because they illustrate how the nurse helped Kay become more comfortable in their relationship.

FOURTH DAY

Kay again told the nurse how "low and dirty" she felt, and also said, "I'm really very lonely."

FIFTH DAY

The patient had been putting on nail polish.

Kay: I like that. It's so pretty. I think I'll go and put on a sweater. It will look better than this blouse. Could you let me in the clothes room?

We went into the clothing room; she got out a brand new coral colored slip-on sweater that had never been worn before. She showed me her clothing bin.

Kay: I've got a lot of dirty clothes that need washing, but I'll do that this afternoon after you leave.

She then got all the dirty clothes and put them in a paper sack.

SEVENTH DAY

Kay: You know, I felt very uncomfortable and anxious around you.
Nurse: I know. How do you feel about it now?
Kay: I still feel somewhat uncomfortable at times.
Nurse: Are you able to tell me what it is that makes you uncomfortable?
Kay: Well, sometimes I get the feeling that you don't think I have a mind.
Nurse: That must make you feel very uncomfortable.
Kay: Just sometimes with you.

EIGHTH DAY

When I entered the ward this morning, my patient was sitting in the day room with some other patients. I greeted her and she seemed pleased to see me, and said she felt much better this morning, except she had not slept too well last night because she had "all these things" on her mind. She looked fairly neat but not quite as much so as previous days. She had on a skirt and blouse and although she still hadn't washed her hair, she had done it up.

After breakfast, we sat down to talk. She had brought her notebook along and opened it up for me to see for the first time, and she didn't make any comments about it being "silly." She went over all the things in it, and told me where she had gotten everything, and some of it she had made up herself. Most of the contents were typewritten and pertained to mental health and psychology. We read them over one by one, and she read to me, which she seemed to enjoy. She made several comments.

Kay: Oh, just look at this dirty notebook. I hate dirty things, and this is terrible. I've always been used to keeping things clean and neat.

At the canteen she said:

Kay: Oh, I just feel like a tramp, and I look like one, too. I've just got to start and keep my personal appearance up. I never used to be like this. You probably think I was but I wasn't.
Nurse: No, I don't because if you were like you were before all this happened to you, you wouldn't be here.
Kay: You're so right! Oh, you just don't *know* how low and miserable I feel. I'm lost, like a man without a country, and I have no one to hold onto, and I'm so confused.
Nurse: I don't know *exactly* how you feel, because I'm not you, but I can try and understand how you feel and try to help you.
Kay: I appreciate that, really I do, and are you sure that everything I tell you will be confidential, what I mean is, you won't go back to the ward and tell the aides?
Nurse: No. If you tell me anything that I feel the doctor should know, I would have to tell him for your good, but otherwise, our conversation is confidential.
Kay: Good, because I don't want just everybody knowing about what I've told you.

Before we left the canteen Kay bought some cold cream, perfume, potato chips, coffee, and candy, then said, "Now I'm going back and start making myself look better, I feel better already." Upon returning to the ward she went immediately to the bathroom, combed her hair, put cold cream on her face and put on some perfume. She brought the perfume out to me to smell, and said, "Oh this is so good, doesn't it smell good?" We sat and talked some more.

Kay: I used to feel half dead in the mornings and couldn't get out of bed.

Nurse: What sort of a feeling was this, of being half dead?

Kay: Oh, I really don't know. I know but I can't explain it, it's so miserable.

Today for the first time she took more of an interest in me personally, asking about my husband and children, wanting to see their pictures.

TENTH DAY

When it was time for the nurse to leave, Kay said:

Kay: I certainly do hate for you to leave and just wish that I could express my sincere appreciation for what you have done for me.

Nurse: I have enjoyed knowing you and being with you these two weeks, and will continue to be interested in how you are getting along after I leave.

Kay: You won't be back tomorrow?

Nurse: No.

It was not easy for Kay to see the end of her relationship with this nurse. The nurse wrote: "I said good-bye; she looked at me rather wistfully; tears came into her eyes, and she walked into the bathroom."

It is obvious that this nurse was a very sensitive person. What is it that she did that helped Kay?

One of the first things was to accept Kay exactly as she was—unkempt and not especially clean. She did not ask Kay to dress up for her, but instead, focused her concern on Kay as a person, not on her symptoms of uncleanliness. Soon Kay was able to tell the nurse how she felt about herself—"low and dirty" and "like a tramp." Her appearance was an expression of how she felt about herself. The nurse did not press her to talk about her feelings, but Kay did when she was ready and felt safe enough with the nurse to do so. Once she had shared these feelings she seemed able to move toward the next step—that of doing something about them. Her behavior changed with her feelings about herself. Also the nurse believed in Kay's potential for change.

The nurse had to recognize her own feelings about being with Kay—her anxiety, her feelings of uselessness and helplessness at times, her eagerness to see Kay more comfortable with herself and with others, her feelings about Kay's greasy hair. It wasn't until the ninth day that Kay's hair was washed. The nurse had had the support of her supervisor in waiting it out until Kay was ready for a shampoo. She was not made to feel that she was "less good" a nurse because she did not "get" Kay to wash her hair. On the contrary, it often takes more skill to help a patient reach the point where he can change his own behavior than it does to get something done.

By attempting to understand and respond to what Kay was trying to convey through her behavior and her conversation, the nurse facilitated Kay's communciation with her. The nurse did not interpret Kay's behavior to her because she was not prepared to do so. Instead, she focused on their present relationship and helped Kay get some of her current situations clarified. Most nurses are not prepared to interpret behavior, but they can try to respond to the patient's feelings and his perception of his situation, even if they do not know the cause of those feelings or if they see the situation differently than the patient does.

Just how can nurses help patients get some of their current situations clarified? What kinds of questions should we ask patients? First of all, we might ask ourselves, "What do I want to find out—and why? What will I do with the answer? Nurses ask questions all the time—often personal and hurtful questions—and sometimes wonder why patients do not answer them. The uniform does not give any prerogatives—they must be earned. If the nurse conveys to the patient her interest, concern, understanding, and willingness to do what she can, he will tell her what he is able to tell her when he is ready. This does not mean the nurse asks no questions—she asks many.

The following example indicates how the nurse's questions helped Kay examine her own feelings.

Kay: I just get the feeling that people don't want me around here.

Nurse: Do you feel it is the personnel or the patients?

Kay: Both, I guess.

Nurse: Do you just feel that they feel this way, or have you heard them say it?

Kay: I think I've heard them say it. I don't bother anyone, but I know they don't want me.

Nurse: I know you feel this way, but the personnel are here to help you, and all the patients are here because they need help in one way or another, just as you do. But I know you still feel this way.

Kay: I get the feeling they think that it's all physical, and sometimes I think it is, too.

Nurse: This is what you'd rather it would be, instead of emotional?

Kay: Yes, because it was hard for me to accept that it was emotional.

When Kay had an opportunity to talk about her feelings, she discovered how unsure of some of them she was—she "guessed" it was both patients and personnel who didn't want her around and she "thought" she heard them say they didn't want her around.

The nurse observed Kay's behavior and reactions and was especially sensitive to Kay's anxiety level. The nurse used her observations in her suggestions to Kay—to show her the ward, for example, and to leave the canteen. Perhaps eventually the nurse would have been able to discuss some of her observations with Kay, for it is by sharing her observations and feelings that the nurse can help the patient become aware of what is going on in his relationships with people.

The nurse faced with Kay the incidents that came up in their relationship —such as asking for her cigarettes and helping her examine her thinking and feelings. Their relationship did not suffer; on the contrary, the nurse-patient relationship can be strengthened by facing what goes on and helping the patient to deal with what comes up rather than avoid it.

When Kay said, "I've been running away and retreating for so long I don't know how to do anything else," she was pointing up one of the most important aspects of our work with patients. Behavior is meaningful and what a patient does at a particular time is the best he is able to do—if he could do it better he would (1,2). In that same statement Kay might also be saying to the nurse, "Help me learn another way to do things. My way is not satisfactory—see where it has gotten me. I am willing to try but I don't know how to start." She is also pointing out some implications for the nursing role. In what ways can the nurse help her and be understanding of her hesitation, her awkwardness, her failures as she tries again? What experiences can the nurse plan with the patient so she can learn what she will have to learn in order to believe that she can live again with people?

When Kay tells the nurse that she cannot describe how she has felt because there are no words to tell of the misery she has experienced, she conveys her utter aloneness. The suffering of the mentally ill person cannot be communicated, and therein lies some of his loneliness, isolation, and separation from people—which is only part of his misery.

In this nurse-patient relationship, several principles of psychiatric nursing were evident:

The nurse respected Kay and accepted her exactly as she was; she allowed and facilitated Kay's expression of her feelings; she let Kay set her own place in working with her problems: she centered her nursing care on Kay as a person, not on control of her symptoms; her observation was directed toward trying to understand Kay's behavior; her communication with Kay involved attempting to understand what Kay was trying to express and responding to Kay's communication; she recognized her own feelings about being with Kay; she recognized that Kay responded in a situation in relation to whatever or whoever was in it with her—imaginary or real; and she dealt with the issues that came up in their relationship rather than avoiding them.

When these principles are applied and the patient's needs are met, the patient experiences a satisfying human relationship and the nurse experiences satisfaction in carrying out her helping role.

The illustration given referred to a psychiatric patient but these principles can be applied to all nurse-patient relationships, for all nurses work with people in discomfort and stress of some kind. It is only the particular expression of that stress that takes the patient to a medical, surgical, obstetric, pediatric, or psychiatric unit.

REFERENCES

1. Peplau, Hildegard E. *Interpersonal Relations in Nursing*. New York, G. P. Putnam's Sons, 1952.
2. Brown, Martha M., and Fowler, Grace R. *Psychodynamic Nursing*. Philadelphia, W. B. Saunders Co., 1954.

19

Separation Anxiety

Jeanette Nehren and Naomi R. Gilliam*

Feelings of loss may be expressed in many ways when a patient-nurse relationship ends. Reasons for these reactions must be understood if a nurse is to manage her own feelings and help patients resolve theirs.

The termination of an interpersonal relationship can be a problem to any or all of us. The feelings we encounter when someone we treasure leaves us can cause a type of pain that cannot be relieved by a hypodermic injection, tranquilizer, or even a pleasant "good-bye." The impact of the termination process on patients and nurses is not limited to psychiatric situations. We have observed this phenomenon in other clinical services.

We have noticed that if the nurse-patient relationship has been intensive or the patient's hospitalization has been extensive, both the nurse and the patient may experience feelings of loss when the patient is discharged or when the nurse leaves the nursing care unit. The feelings centering around this object loss may be expressed in many ways. Because of our cultural orientation, they arc not likely to be verbalized and may not always be recognized.

Patient: Well, I'm all packed. I guess I'm ready to go now.
Nurse: Did you get your medicines from the pharmacy?
Patient: Yes.
Nurse: Check with the business office?

---

*From *American Journal of Nursing*, Vol. 65, No. 1 (January, 1965).

Mrs. Nehren who is assistant professor, School of Nursing, University of Washington, Seattle, is a graduate of St. Vincent's Hospital School of Nursing, Indianapolis, Ind. She earned a bachelor's degree at Indiana University and a master's degree at the University of Colorado.

Miss Gilliam holds a B.S.N. degree from the University of Mississippi School of Nursing in Jackson and currently is a candidate for a master's degree in psychiatric nursing at the University of Washington School of Nursing.

98069

Patient: Yes.

Nurse: Yes, you are ready to go. I'll get an aide to help you with your luggage.

Patient: You have been very kind during my illness. I want to thank all of the nurses. I know I've been a difficult patient for you to handle.

Nurse: You've been here a long time. Let's see, it's been three months. Gee, I'll bet you will be glad to get home.

Patient: Yes . . . that's great I guess. (He smiles wanly and turns away. The nurse watches from the nursing station as he slowly walks down the hall.)

Every nursing practitioner has witnessed or participated in interactions similar to this one. How often do we stop to ask what is happening? Why is the patient so hesitant about leaving? Why does the nurse seem so interested in his medicines and business matters, but show so little interest in him? Why does she keep him from venting his feelings?

The phenomenon of separation anxiety was first identified by Freud in 1905. He related it to the reaction of the loss of a loved object and the pain of mourning. Otto Rank believed that separation anxiety first occurs at birth when an infant is separated from his mother but, according to Klein, a child first experiences separation anxiety at the time of weaning, thus creating in the child feelings of depression and persecution. As a result of these theories we now place greater emphasis on experiences in the early developmental years (1).

The degree of anxiety and depression created at early separation experiences will determine how the individual will manage future separations or termination of friendships during his entire lifetime. The love, security, and trust the mothering figure gives to the infant and young child at these crucial periods of emotional development help prevent feelings of rejection, depression, or guilt, and the need for punishment in future separations.

Probably another major separation experience by a child is separation from the family to the school and its significant people. Again in middle-class America the end of the teens usually is a time when separation from the family to college, a job, the military services, or to marriage occurs. In the healthy person, this is a time when dependency on parents ceases—a time when anxiety and depression may occur. An individual does not always move from one emotional developmental level to the next with adequate feelings of love, security, and trust from those persons who are significant to him at these particular times in his life. For instance, the loss, through death or divorce, of one or both parents during a crucial developmental stage of life may occur without love and support from another person. The loss of other significant persons in his life—teachers, classmates, and friends—may also affect a person's later capacity to manage separation anxiety. The sense of loss may be the same regardless of who does the leaving, and the loss may be perceived as a feeling of rejection, loss of a loved object, or the need for punishment.

The nurse seldom knows—nor is it important for her to know—all a patient's experiences of early separations from significant people. But, in order to understand a patient's feelings and behavior, she does need to know that his feelings are primarily a revival of feelings of earlier separations and terminations. These feelings transferred to her may be either conscious or unconscious. The nurse also needs to recognize her own feelings about a pending separation. Frequently, she may need help in identifying her own feelings and the manner in which she expresses them. A teacher, co-worker, doctor, or supervisor may help her do this. Such persons can provide an opportunity for her to express her feelings of anger or loss and help her relate her feelings to separation anxiety. Increased self-understanding may evolve which may help her to help the patient.

In order to cope with separation anxiety, both patient and nurse will utilize defense mechanisms which they have found useful in maintaining their self-esteem in past experiences. However, these unconscious responses to perceived or actual object loss may not always be effective under stress situations and the nurse can help the patient find other mechanisms for expressing his anxiety.

Theoretically, termination for the patient begins for him at the time of his first contact with the nurse, doctor, hospital, or community agency. At this time the staff should focus their health teaching upon the day when the patient no longer will be dependent upon them. For instance, when a nurse teaches a patient with diabetes to give himself injections, she is preparing him for the time when he must take care of himself.

Preparation for termination may not be the same for all patients. For example, a patient who has had an appendectomy and is hospitalized for five days will have different feelings about leaving the hospital than the patient with a chronic illness who has had a long hospitalization. As with other interpersonal relationships such specific variables as the physical or mental health of the patient, former separations, the person who is leaving, the intensity and length of the nurse-patient relationship, and the patient's current relationships in the family and the community determine the degree of anxiety present.

When a nurse structures a continuous relationship with a patient he is entitled to know what expectations the nurse has for him and what expectations he may hold for her. In the initial contact, she should tell him how often she will see him, the length of time she will stay with him, and how long she will be working with him. Many times the nurse does not know all these details in the beginning but she should keep the patient informed when she is able to do so.

A patient's initial response to being told that the nurse will be leaving him or that he is being discharged may be denial. This reaction may be a denial of the pending separation or a denial of any significance in the separation. It may be expressed in behavior or in words. If the patient can be helped to recognize the meaning of his behavior he may be able to manage a healthy resolution of the separation anxiety. The following example from a process recording shows a nurse confronting a patient who had denied that his nurse was leaving although he had been told several times that she would leave him.

Patient: I look at people as an accounting problem. Some of them are listed under credits or debits. If I like them and they seem to like me, they're an asset. If they don't like me, they're a liability. But the columns keep changing.

Nurse: If people you care for do something that you don't like, what happens then?

Patient: They go under the liability column.

Nurse: I will be leaving March 13. I wonder what kind of feelings you'll have about me.

Patient: Well, I won't commit suicide, if that's what you mean.

In the interaction the nurse again confronted the patient with the fact that she would be leaving. At this time, he could no longer deny the fact, but could deny its significance.

A nurse may also deny her feelings about the separation or deny her own importance to the patient. In doing so, she may prevent his expressing positive or negative feelings toward her. She may encourage him unconsciously to keep conversation on a superficial level. Failing to mention that she is leaving or failing to mention the patient's pending discharge exemplify her denial or repression.

A patient may be overwhelmed by a sense of hopelessness or helplessness when denial is no longer effective. Anger and hostility may be a means of coping with these feelings. The patient may be angry with the nurse for leaving him or may feel that she is making him leave. These feelings may be expressed in various ways. Anger may be directed toward the nurse but may be focused on some incident other than the termination. More often, the anger may be directed toward another member of the staff, his own family, or another patient. If an open display of anger is alien to the patient, he may resort to being late for appointments, attempting to terminate the nursing interview early, or telling the nurse how "good" other personnel treat him. Finally, the patient may make use of projection as a defense against his anger. He may perceive that the nurse or another person is angry with him.

The nurse who is aware of the dynamics underlying such anger will respond to the patient's feelings of hopelessness and helplessness by being supportive. Becoming angry with the patient only would reinforce his feelings of rejection. Accepting his behavior as something to be explored with him enables him to start resolving his anxiety. If the nurse is not able to cope with her own feelings related to the termination, she may respond with such forms of anger as forgetting promises to the patient, cutting down the amount of time she spends with him, or by including other patients in their conversation.

Withdrawal is another device which the patient may employ during the termination of a meaningful relationship. He may not keep appointments. He may not talk to the nurse or, if he does, he may keep the conversation on a very superficial level. Nurses also use this mechanism.

Frequently, the patient who is awaiting discharge has little contact with the nursing staff. Although the physical care needed at this time may be minimal, the patient's psychological discomforts may increase.

Separation anxiety may be so intense that regression occurs. The psychiatric patient may return to his delusional system. The surgical patient may experience pain and request his postoperative medication. The medical patient may have a recurrence of symptoms. The public health patient may telephone for another visit. The nurse may begin to feel guilty for leaving the patient or the doctor may reconsider the discharge order. Because of her guilt, the nurse may allow the patient to manipulate her. She may have set aside an hour to be with the patient, but may stay longer. She may ignore phases of the patient's behavior with which he would ordinarily be confronted; for example, breaking his diet. Failing to set limits may, as a matter of fact, increase the patient's anxiety and reinforce his dependency needs.

Recognizing that the resolution of separation anxiety is not a constant, ongoing process, the nurse should reinforce the healthy components of the patient's personality at this time. She should be consistent. She should continue to evoke the exploration of feelings, to point out the significance of relationships, and to teach mental health principles. She also should constantly remember that backsliding may occur in any termination process. The process which enables the patient to use the healthier features of his personality varies with each interpersonal relationship. It is dependent upon the treatment goals for the patient, his self-awareness, and his ego strength.

Although a patient may have shown infantile idiosyncrasies in the early stages of termination, often the healthier features of his personality are mobilized for the final leaving. The hospital environment does provide a measure of security and permits the expression of feelings on a regressed level. The outside world is less tolerant. Rationalization, a socially accepted defense mechanism, is an aid in preserving ego integration at this time. A surgical patient who had not been prepared for termination and had been informed of his pending discharge on the day prior to this interaction aptly demonstrated his ability to rationalize in the following:

"Well, then it's O.K. So, today's the day, huh? I been thinking about it and I figure I'll be better off at home, anyhow. Around my own things, eat some good Italian food, and get my strength back. So, it's all for the best. I'm ready to go at any time."

A patient who has been able to manage his separation anxiety may identify with the nurse. He will be able to relate the feelings and experiences he has shared with the nurse to those in other significant relationships. If the nurse-patient interaction has been important, he may have learned new and more effective techniques to employ in other interpersonal relationships. In the following interaction, the nurse used the book, *The Little Prince*, as a teaching aid when she discussed termination with the patient (2). His response shows how he identified with the nurse.

Nurse: It's almost time for me to leave. I am thinking now of the fox in *The Little Prince* who said, 'I'll cry,' when the prince left. The little prince told him that it was his own fault if he cared. The fox was the wiser of the two, for he knew that even though the little prince was leaving, their relationship had been meaningful. He could look at the wheat fields and see the gold of the little prince's hair. I hope, Mr. Crowly, that our relationship will help you to relate more easily to other people—to apply the things with them that you have learned with me.

Mr. Crowly: Yes, it has been meaningful. I have been able to talk. I even find it easier to talk to my sister now. It has helped relieve my anxieties and tensions. Maybe you've learned something from me, too. You are studying about this, aren't you?

If she understands the psychodynamics of feelings in the termination of a meaningful relationship, the nurse, hopefully, can manage her own feelings, accept the patient, and guide him toward resolving some of his feelings during this critical time. The patient may feel rejected, hopeless, helpless, or worthless as he is faced with leaving or being left by someone who has listened, understood, accepted, and assisted him in solving his own problems in daily living conflicts. This separation, though, may well be a less painful experience than experiences he may have encountered earlier.

Nursing interventions are influenced by the nurse's knowledge of the behavioral sciences, her application of interpersonal skills, her self-understanding, her ego strength, and her frame of reference. In planning for the termination processs, the nurse's primary objective is to help the patient to sustain his integrity as a human being when he is experiencing the loss of the nurse as a significant person in his life. This will result in a prepared rather than a perplexed termination.

REFERENCES

1. Bowlby, John. Separation anxiety; a critical review of the literature. *J. Child Psychol. Psychiat.* 1:251-269, Feb. 1961.
2. Saint Exupery, Antoine De. *The Little Prince*. New York, Harcourt, Brace and Co., 1943.

20

Interpersonal Techniques
The Crux of
Psychiatric Nursing

Hildegard E. Peplau*

The counseling role, not a half dozen other subroles, is the heart of psychiatric nursing, says this expert. She then goes on to explain how the kinds of techniques it demands can be developed, taught, and used.

The time is past when a nurse could become, in one lifetime, an expert in all clinical areas. Advances in all fields of knowledge and within nursing science itself point to the inevitability of clinical specialization.

When you begin to think about specialization, however, you think not only of a focus in a particular area but of considerable depth. As the scope of the specialists' work narrows, the depth intensifies at, I submit, the point of the uniqueness of the clinical area. The unique aspect of a clinical area is twofold: it is that which occurs in other clinical fields but is not emphasized to the same extent and it is that which is almost entirely new—the uncommon, promising developments which result from thinking deeply about a particular facet of work in just one area.

Each of the areas of nursing practice has a particular clinical emphasis. This emphasis does not preclude attention to all the other aspects of the workrole of the nurse practitioner, but more time, effort, and thought are given to this particular facet. For example, nurses in public health programs emphasize health teaching, not to the exclusion of the technical aspects of

*From *American Journal of Nursing*, Vol. 62, No. 6 (June, 1962).

Hildegard Peplau (Pottstown, Pa., Hospital School of Nursing; B.A., Bennington; M.A., Ed.D., Teachers College, Columbia University) is professor of nursing at Rutgers University and chairman of the advanced program in psychiatric nursing in which graduate nurse students are trained for clinical specialization in psychiatric nursing.

nursing practice nor of the supportive, reassuring, mother-surrogate type of nurse activities. But, by and large, nurses who visit patients in their homes spend a proportionately larger part of their time teaching. Medical-surgical nursing emphasizes technical care; pediatric nursing emphasizes the mother-surrogate role; in this paper I want to consider the particular emphasis of psychiatric nursing.

I have indicated various subroles of the workrole of nurses. Briefly, these include mother-surrogate, technician, manager, socializing agent, health teacher, and counselor or psychotherapist.[1]

Psychiatric nursing emphasizes the role of counselor or psychotherapist. It is true that this idea is not a universally accepted one in all psychiatric facilities. But note that I say "psychiatric nursing," not "nursing in psychiatric units."

There are two levels of professional nurse personnel practicing in psychiatric units—general practitioners (general duty nurses) and specialists (psychiatric nurses). Let me clarify the difference. A general practitioner is a nurse who has completed only her basic professional preparation. From my viewpoint, a "psychiatric nurse" is a specialist and at this time specialist status can be achieved by two routes—experience and education.

Before the passage of the Mental Health Act in 1946, experience was the route by which a nurse earned the title "psychiatric nurse"; since 1946, however, some 25 graduate level, university-based programs in advanced psychiatric nursing have been established. There are stipends available for study in these programs. Any nurse who can qualify—because she has completed her full basic professional preparation and has the intellectual and personal qualifications for graduate study—can secure a stipend for graduate study toward becoming a clinical specialist in psychiatric nursing, that is, a "psychiatric nurse." From my point of view, then, the route of clinical specialization for any nurse who was graduated since 1946 is through a university-based graduate level program.

I realize this is a status problem but the profession of nursing will strengthen its position in relation to all other professional disciplines when it recognizes the culturally accepted fact that university education is the route for clinical specialization. There is good reason for this. Theoretically the university is free of the service commitment of the hospital—it can take objective distance, look dispassionately at the work of nurses, and dare to consider gross changes in the workrole.

When you are employed in a service agency, on the other hand, you become a participating member in its social system, ties of friendship and loyalty becoming binding as well as blinding, and dispassionate inquiry is greatly lessened. There is another reason why universities have culturally been charged with graduate education: the scope of established and newly formulated knowledge represented in a university faculty is ever so much wider than that represented in a professional staff group. It is access to this

---

[1]For a more complete discussion of subroles see Peplau's "Therapeutic Concepts" in *The League Exchange*, No. 26, pp. 1-30, published in the National League for Nursing, New York. 1957.

knowledge and its application to clinical observations that transform the student into an expert clinician.

There is clear distinction then between nursing in a psychiatric unit (what a general duty nurse does), and psychiatric nursing (what an expert clinical practitioner does). This distinction should be kept in the foreground for in this paper I will refer to nurses and nursing, when speaking of the common and basic elements, and to psychiatric nurses and psychiatric nursing when speaking of the more specialized clinical functions.

A psychiatric nurse is first of all an expert clinician. She may also be a teacher, supervisor, administrator, consultant, or researcher, but underlying all these functional positions there should be advanced clinical training. Such clinical expertness revolves around the field's unique aspect or emphasis, in this case, the role of counselor or psychotherapist. I want to develop the importance of this idea for the general practice of nursing in a psychiatric setting, but, first, I wish to pinpoint why other aspects of the work in a psychiatric unit are not the central focus of psychiatric nursing.

The emphasis in psychiatric nursing is *not* on the mother-surrogate role. Some nurses believe that the unmet needs of a patient's infancy and early childhood can be met by the nurse taking on various mothering activities. This belief assumes that the corrective experience is largely an emotional one resulting from a relationship in which the nurse complements a need for mothering of the patient, by supplying its counterpart—need-reducing mother-surrogate activities. This is analogous to the notion that when calcium deficiency produces tooth decay, supplying the calcium will fill up the cavities! A patient needs love, warmth, acceptance, support, and reassurance —not to supply the unmet needs of the past but for current reasons; having these emotional experiences makes it possible for the patient to come to grips with the earlier unmet needs on intellectual rather than on experiential grounds.

The notion that a made-up "good mother" experience will correct the patient's pathology is based on the assumption that the patient has not moved ahead in other areas compatible with chronological development— for example, language, vocabulary, and thought develop despite emotional deprivations.

To give mother-surrogate activities the central emphasis would be to de-emphasize these tools which have developed and can be utilized.

There is another inescapable fact; the small number of professional nurses in psychiatric facilities has for a long time required that the necessary mother-surrogate activities—the bathing, feeding, dressing, toileting, warning, disciplining, and approving the patient—be taken over largely by nonprofessional nursing personnel. I do not foresee that any great benefit would accrue even if the supply was such that professional nurses could take on fully these mothering activities. Note that I have not said that a nurse never bathes or feeds or dresses or warns a patient in a psychiatric unit; what I have said is that these mothering activities are not the central focus.

The emphasis in psychiatric nursing is *not* on the technical subrole. Some nurses believe that the cause of mental illness will ultimately prove to be some biochemical or otherwise organic problem, identifiable by the results of various laboratory test procedures and correctable by some technical manipulations analogous to the injection of insulin in the therapeutic management of a person diagnosed as diabetic. Other nurses in the past and present have believed that technical expertness in giving tubs, packs, coma insulin and care in the pre- and post-phases of electroconvulsive therapy or lobotomy would lead to solutions to mental illness. Technical expertness in giving medication or carrying out procedures associated with nursing is, in my opinion, not the desirable emphasis in psychiatric nursing.

CUSTODIAL ACTIVITIES

The emphasis in psychiatric nursing is *not* on managerial activities. Historically, these have been aspects of custodial care with restraint, protection, cleanliness, and order the dominant themes. Many of the housekeeping activities associated with these themes have been shifted not only to nonprofessional personnel but to work details made up of working patients as well. The housekeeping activities have given way to a host of clerical and receptionist activities, which nurses have taken on, and which presumably have to do with the management of the patient's environment in the interest of his care. I submit that the time is near at hand when administrators will recognize that these clerical and receptionist activities can be performed far better and more cheaply by a high school graduate; that these are not "professional" activities but instead are largely busywork which keeps the nurse away from direct contact with patients.

The emphasis in psychiatric nursing is *not* on socializing-agent activities, such as playing cards and games with patients, taking walks and watching TV with them and the like. In some basic schools of nursing, students are taught that these activities are central in the work of the nurse; I submit that the preparation of a nurse is not required for such activities; that the use of a nurse's social experience as an interesting diversionary activity in the patient's daily life is not the best use of the time of a professional nurse. Nonprofessional nursing personnel, volunteers, and visitors can do this game-playing just as well as a nurse can. The professional education of the nurse is wasted; it is not needed to perform these activities which most laymen learn some time during their "teens."

Group activities along these lines might better be planned and carried out by the recreational department or some department other than nursing service (or nursing education since students are largely "used" for this purpose). I have not said that a professional nurse *never* plays cards with patients; however, these activities are not the central emphasis in psychiatric nursing and at most should take a bare minimum of the day's time of a professional nurse.

The emphasis in psychiatric nursing is *not* on health teaching although this subrole, in the workrole of the nurse, is an important one which needs to be developed further. I have pointed out that this is an important part of the work of nurses in public health. But the patients in the case load of these nurses are more often immediately able to use information than are patients in the psychiatric setting. Even so, teaching psychiatric patients about diet, nutrition, grooming, sex, and the like, may be very helpful. There has also been one promising study reported in which psychiatric patients were taught a concept of anxiety to apply to their own experiences; several similar studies are now under way.[2]

The emphasis in psychiatric nursing is on the counseling or psycho-therapeutic subrole. This generalization is based upon the assumption that the difficulties in living which lead up to mental illness in a particular patient are subject to investigation and control by the patient—with professional counseling assistance. It is also based on a second assumption: that formal knowledge of counseling procedure is absolutely essential for the more general type of approach which may be useful in very brief relationships with patients. Further, these general approaches are in the nature of "interpersonal techniques" useful in relation to specific problems—such as withdrawal, aggression, hallucinations, delusions, and the like—and these are the crux of psychiatric nursing.

There is being developed in psychiatric nursing a theory and procedure of nurse counseling. This development is proceeding along two lines:

1. A "surface type" of formal counseling procedure, such as a general nurse practitioner might use with patients in all clinical areas, is being described. Many schools of nursing already are beginning to teach interviewing —of a therapeutic in contrast to a biographical type—as a basis for counseling. A companion result of this development will surely be the identification and description of a variety of general approaches to specific problems—interpersonal techniques—which nurses can use in everyday brief contacts with all types of patients.

2. Depth counseling, such as might be employed by a psychiatric nurse specialist who had completed two years of master's level clinical training, is also being described. Several nurses are now employed in situations in which they are doing long-term counseling of patients, utilizing the competencies secured through such clinical training. It is conceivable that in another decade or two nurses will share offices with psychiatrists and psychologists and social workers for the private practice of psychiatric nurse counseling, although now there are no publishable instances of such practices.

TEACHING STUDENTS

In many basic schools of nursing, students are being taught counseling technique in connection with nurse-patient care studies, particularly in the psychiatric setting. I have talked with a number of teachers in these schools and their general conclusion seems to be that when the student has an opportunity to work directly with one patient—say in one-hour sessions twice a week over a period of ten weeks—a great deal of learning takes place.

The student gets more than a textbook picture of pathology; she gets a full view of the complexity of the difficulties of a psychiatric patient, of the variations which occur in particular patterns of behavior. Many students find out, for example, that there are infinite variations of the pattern of withdrawal and that observed changes in the behavior of a patient are more

---

[2]See "Teaching a Concept of Anxiety," by Dorothea Hays in *Nursing Research*, Vol. 10, pp. 108-113, Spring 1961 issue.

likely to be changes from one variant to another of a central pattern that persists. Thus, a patient who uses gross withdrawal—by muteness, for example —can, as a result of a nurse-patient relationship, eventually, begin to speak; the verbalizations, however, are also classifiable as a variant of withdrawal, particularly when the patient talks but doesn't communicate anything descriptive of his difficulties.

In a carefully guided nurse-patient relationship, the nurse learns the art and science of counseling technique. She discovers that the art part of it is intuitively based—it is a clinical judgment which she herself makes, minute by minute, that this maneuver or that maneuver might conceivably be useful to the investigative effort. The student also learns the value of knowledge and procedures for their application to explain observations; this is the scientific part. The student gradually ceases to use such terms as anxiety, conflict, dissociation, and the like, as mere labels for behavior; she begins to use these concepts as scientific tools to guide her in assessing the investigative effort under way and in getting more information. Both the nurse and patient need as much descriptive information about the patient's life experiences as can be obtained without making the patient too uncomfortable. It is this information which will be worked over by the nurse and patient together so that the patient can understand and benefit from his previous experiences in living.

ANOTHER BENEFIT. Another important learning accrues from teaching counseling in the nurse-patient relationship. The student learns detachment; she learns—with the help of her teachers—how not to usurp the counseling time to meet her own needs; how to use the time instead, to help the patient formulate and meet his needs. She learns to make clearer distinction between techniques that are useful to her socially, outside the professional work situation, and those specifically useful in a clinical situation.

Moreover, the student learns a lot about herself as she begins to understand her reactions to the patients' behavior and verbal content, her own need for approval, the points at which she is particularly vulnerable. Patients have a way of unwittingly locating the vulnerabilities of students—be it their need for approval, their sensitivity to their appearance, their embarrassment in discussion about sex, or any one of a host of similar problem areas.

Once a student nurse has had successive counseling interviews with a particular patient, and has responsibly reviewed her nurse-patient data with an expert psychiatric nurse teacher, she is able to transfer—or generalize—the learning products to much briefer relationships with patients. Students invariably report that learning about counseling of one patient helps them to use to better advantage the two-to-three-minute contacts they have with patients in the ward setting. Nor do I know of any other way for a student to achieve these understandings except as a result of talking with one patient about the patient's difficulties, in designated, time-limited sessions occurring over a period of time, and following each session by a substantial review of what went on with an expert psychiatric nurse. You can't tell students what to do along these lines and then expect them, magically, to be able to do it. The student must not only experience this day-to-day process but she must have interested and active help in examining, bit by bit, the interview data which she thus collects.

One result, then, of the nurse-patient inquiry is the ability to transfer a substantial amount of learning toward more generalized interpersonal techniques. I believe that such techniques are the crux of psychiatric nursing and it seems to me that it ought to be possible for psychiatric nurses to develop specific interpersonal techniques useful in intervening in specific patterns of pathological behavior of patients. And it is possible; several nurses I know are currently involved in developing and testing such techniques.

STEPS TO ABATE ANXIETY

One of the major difficulties of most, if not all, psychiatric patients is anxiety. We need a simple interpersonal technique which would be of value in the productive abatement of severe anxiety in patients. What might the steps of such a technique be? Could these steps be carried out by nonprofessional nursing personnel under the supervision of professional nurses who would have a deeper insight into the merits of the technique based upon the emotional experience of the nurse-patient investigation?

The steps are simple:

1. Encourage the patient to identify the anxiety as such. This is done by having all personnel help him recognize what he is experiencing at the point when he is actually anxious. Such anxiety is observable. In other words, the patient may well be unaware of his anxiety but another person—particularly a trained professional person—can observe the effects of anxiety and therefore infer its presence. So, a professional nurse would determine that a particular patient was anxious and unaware of it. Her behavior toward the patient and her supervision of the relationships which nonprofessional personnel have with him would be guided by the aim: to help the patient identify the anxiety as such. This would be done by saying to the patient, for as long as it takes to achieve the recognition, "Are you uncomfortable," "Are you nervous," "Are you upset," "Are you anxious?" With most psychiatric patients, it may take an amazingly long time to get a "Yes" answer, that is, to get him to recognize his anxiety. In many instances, the patient's responses will follow a sequence, beginning with "No" to "Sometimes I am," "Maybe," "A little," and finally, "Yes, I am uncomfortable (or anxious)." When such "Yes" responses are obtained, the nurse can assume a modicum of awareness of anxiety; then, and not before then, the patient is ready for the second step in the interpersonal technique for utilizing anxiety constructively.

2. Encourage the patient to connect the relief-giving patterns that he uses to the anxiety which requires such relief. The nursing personnel focus their efforts on maintaining the patient's awareness of the anxiety and connecting it to his anxiety-relieving behavior. Thus, the nurse might observe that a patient was anxious. The nurse would ask, "Are you uncomfortable now?" If the patient replied, "Yes," the nurse would ask, "What do you do to get comfortable again when you are anxious?" This step would be repeated until it was clear to the professional observer that the patient did, indeed, formulate the connection between his anxiety and the anxiety-relieving behavior he uses. Describing this behavior, he might say, "I cry," "I swing my foot," "I pace," "I talk to voices," "I worry about my family," and the like.

Working in this manner with a particular patient, one graduate nurse student had the experience of hearing a patient say, "Yes, I am anxious right now, I am very anxious, I feel terrible, and I'm going over there and rock myself on that rocking chair good and hard and then I'll come back." A bit later, the patient did return to the nurse and commented, "Now I'm not so anxious; that rocking chair sure helps but I need to find out why I am anxious."

3. Encourage the patient to provide himself and the nurse with data descriptive of situations and interactions which go on immediately before an increase in anxiety is noticed. Once he has connected his anxiety-relieving behavior with his anxiety, the patient is ready for this third step: beginning the search for precipitating causes of the anxiety. Here the nursing personnel might ask, "What went on just before you got so uncomfortable?" The aim is to get the patient to describe the situations or interactions in which he was involved immediately preceding the developing increase in anxiety. Such description provides the nurse with a range of data about the patient so that she can begin to speculate (for herself) on probable causes of the anxiety.

Here, the application of the concept of anxiety—which defines areas of causation—would be useful for the professional nurse. It cannot be over-emphasized that in this step the patient is not searching for immediate, situational causes of the increase in his anxiety; he is merely providing a description of experience from which such causes can later be inferred.

4. Encourage the patient to formulate from the descriptive data the probable immediate, situational causes for the increase in his anxiety.

In Step 3 the professional nurse can begin to speculate as to causes; helping the patient to formulate his own view of the reasons for his anxiety is Step 4. Step 4 makes use of the descriptions which have accumulated out of several days of talks between the patient and the nursing personnel. The professional nurse might ask such questions as, "What have you noticed going on before you get anxious that might increase your discomfort?" Questions of this type encourage the patient to notice and to formulate cause-effect relations on his own.

Any patient who is able to utilize these four steps will show improvement in his ability to cope not only with living in the ward setting but with his pathology as well. Such a patient is most likely ready for a fifth step—referral for intensive counseling so that the causes of anxiety involving the connections between remote past experience and immediate situational experiences can be identified.

It is my premise that interpersonal techniques—such as the one I have indicated here—can be devised and utilized by nursing personnel in relation to problematic behavior patterns of psychiatric patients. I believe that these interpersonal techniques, rather than modifications of medical-surgical nursing techniques, are the crux of the practice of nursing in a psychiatric setting.

21

Themes in
Nursing Situations—Power

Hildegard E. Peplau*

This is the first in a series of articles describing themes that recur in nurses' relationships with their patients. One of these themes is power.

THE THEMATIC PHASE OF PSYCHIATRY

Three important phases in the continuing development of psychiatry have recently been identified (1). The first phase is *descriptive psychiatry* in which peculiarities of behavior are listed and grouped into categories which are used in making diagnoses. The second phase is epithetic or *typological* psychiatry in which the primary focus is the identification of types of individuals, and placing them in such categories as schizoid, extroverted, ectomorphic, overactive, and so on. This labeling of "kinds" of people has also influenced lay and professional people's attitudes and has in some instances led to the use of these labels as epithets with which to derogate people. The third, the *thematic* phase in psychiatry, is a trend that has recently gained prominence. The psychiatrist, or any other worker, who is interacting with, and studying his relations with a patient, becomes concerned with the focal problems, recurring patterns, or central themes in the patient's past or present experience.

Each of these phases—descriptive, typological, thematic—is part of the gradual evolution of a mature theory in psychiatry that explains observations and guides practices in this area of health service. When another phase

*From *American Journal of Nursing*, Vol. 53, No. 10 (October, 1953).

Miss Peplau (Pottstown, Pa., Hospital School of Nursing; B.A., Bennington College; M.A., Ed.D., Teacher's College, Columbia) is associate professor of nursing and director of the graduate program in advanced psychiatric nursing at Rutgers University College of Nursing.

emerges that explains or guides psychiatric practices more productively, it too will be identified. This is the nature of theory—ever changing, being revised, reconstructed, and made more useful. Focusing on the thematic phase of psychiatry does not obviate the importance or simultaneous use of what is offered from the descriptive or typological phases, or of what is being produced in continuing explorations, such as in biochemical research.

WHAT IS A THEME? A theme is a generalization, a summarizing characteristic, an abstraction of an event that actually consists of many details that are best summarized as this theme. The word is used in the thematic apperception test in which individuals are shown various pictures and asked to tell a story about each one. One of the values of this test is that it gives a general view of the abstract themes that recur and indicate the individual's mood, or thoughts, or actions.

In music we speak of a theme as a "melody constituting the basis of variation, development, composition, or movement." In the continuing nurse-patient relationship, do we find outstanding themes that occur again and again in many different variations? Do these themes recur so as to characterize either the process, or the event, or a substantial part of it? In dream analysis, the therapist may take the dream as it is told and the secondary elaborations of it and try to abstract recurring threads or themes, from the way the dreamer tells it, from the explanations he gives, and from the dream itself. These recurring threads indicate dominant concerns which the dreamer cannot reveal to himself directly; only under the conditions of sleep can disguised messages about these concerns be made available to him.

Anthropologists, in casting about for ways to study industrialized societies, are using the thematic approach. All institutions can be studied from the standpoint of universal themes such as *power*. Or particular institutions can be studied from the standpoint of particular themes such as the influence of *profit* upon production. Industrial engineers are interested in how the theme *compensation* affects labor unions, workers, and industrial management. These are recurring themes that characterize institutions and affect the interpersonal relations within them.

Perhaps the importance of a thematic approach can be made clearer if we touch on one theme that seems to affect psychiatric institutions, doctors, nurses, their patients, and the public. This theme is *hopelessness*. It seems quite apparent that many individuals view psychiatric patients as "hopeless." The public's apathy in providing funds for their care is probably one aspect of the effect of this theme. Of course, we do not have any all-out studies of its effect on institutional and public behavior, and so there are no specific data that we can use to combat it with a more productive theme such as *hope*. But certainly the recurring pattern of this theme in the behavior of nurses, doctors, patients, families, and others causes many of the stalemates in clinical practice. Does hopelessness overshadow our work in such an insidious way that it handicaps our therapeutic efforts quite seriously? How do we offer incentives that hold out hope of satisfaction and recovery for patients?

THE IMPORTANCE OF RECOGNIZING THEMES. It is impossible for anyone to continuously recall or to keep in mind all of the intricate details of an interpersonal event. The mind of man does not work this way except for the few who have so-called "photographic memories." We get instead a general impression—or theme—concerning what went on. If we merely characterize an interaction as "disappointing" or "good" we have no cue to remind us of some of the details out of which a theme arises.

One purpose for getting at the themes of interaction is to find out, qualitatively, what goes on between us. When we are aware of what goes on—and by awareness we mean, when we have taken in the details in such a way as to make more and more correct and useful inferences about them—then the situation becomes amenable to control. This opens up the possibility of creating favorable changes here and in other situations as awareness leads us toward shifts in the way we take part in these situations.

A second reason for wanting to know the themes of interpersonal events is the economical communication they afford. Much transpires in an interpersonal relationship, through both verbal and non-verbal communication. If we have some generalized inferences—or themes—about the situation, then we have a basis for recalling, expanding, and clarifying what needs to be remembered. We also have a basis for determining practices and for structuring modes by which the nurse intervenes in particular kinds of situations. For example, if the theme *dependence* characterizes a patient's participation in a situation with us, and if this theme occurs over and over again, its variations give us clues to what this patient needs. If, on the other hand, *mutual dependence* characterizes the nurse-patient relationship, then it becomes clear that the nurse must take a different part (2).

This need to have inferences is likewise true in developing background information about patients. A case history reveals details of events as they have been recalled by various reporters and as they have been heard by various recorders. It also contains inferences, correct and otherwise, that have been made about those events.

There are, in state hospitals, reams and reams of case histories, and yet little is known about schizophrenia. Suppose we were to have a way of getting at the recurring themes that characterized the relationships of 100 schizophrenic patients with the significant persons in their lives—and also data about the interactions of nurses and these patients—from which themes could be abstracted. What themes would we find? At the very least, we would have something to work with that is not now available. We would also have an economical way to communicate and come to grips with the dominant features of these patients' past and present relations with people.

Using the interpersonal themes from a patient's past experiences as a hypothesis for studying his present relations, makes it easier for professional workers to study how their present responses might be reinforcing trends laid down long ago. It also permits them to steer away from traumatic events. It provides a frame of reference—which is open both to revision and validation—in talking things over with the patient and in making new observations. Helping the patient to discover the recurring threads in his attempts to relate to people is an important aspect of psychotherapeutic nursing, but to do this the nurse needs to have hypotheses with which to work.

A third reason for abstracting themes from interpersonal events is the basis they provide for comparing one situation with others. A blow-by-blow comparison of details is obviously unwieldly, and past experience shows that it does not help us much in finding out what we need to know. Our total impressions are more useful to us as a basis for referring back and forth from actual relations with patients to data in case histories, and for comparing what goes on in one situation with what went on in another.

A fourth, and perhaps the most important, reason for wanting to generalize from interpersonal data is that it provides us the opportunity to use our most human capacity—reasoning. Professional nurses operate in situations in which inferences and judgments must be made so that sound practices can be planned and carried out. Learning to make inferences is quite different from developing technical and manual skills, which much of our earlier nursing education focused on. The ability to reason and to arrive at useful inferences, judgments, or themes requires intellectual capacity that is developed slowly in a professional education program.

Judgments are the products of reasoning, they are abstractions from the details of a particular event or, from the details of a relationship between events. A professional person is able to formulate concepts from past and present observations and to infer the consequences of present actions in the foreseeable future. To become more creative in what we contribute, it is necessary to make some judgments about what can be observed. This is true for each nurse-patient relationship. It is just as true for the relationships in a nursing team or for any other intraprofessional as well as interprofessional relations. In fact, we might say that it is the moral task of the maturing adult and the obligation of the professional person to make ever more useful inferences about what goes on in relations with people, and to use these inferences or themes to foster favorable changes in situations.

THE USE OF POWER

One theme that cuts across all areas of living is *power*. Power is a theme in industry, in politics, in public and social life. It is also a theme in all nursing situations. Nurse-patient relations can be studied from the standpoint of the way power operates—how each individual uses it in the interactions of an interpersonal situation.

The purpose, meaning, and goal of power operations in interpersonal relations concern psychiatric nurses who wish to function therapeutically with patients. Personal power, and its counterpart—powerlessness—are important aspects of the recovery process which patients undergo. The ways in which doctors and nurses, as well as patients, seek and use power affect psychiatric ward situations. How do nurses' ways of using power, for instance, interact with power-seeking and power-using patterns of doctors and patients? If we identify these and gain some understanding of what actually goes on, we can consider how more democratic balancing of power can be effected in psychiatric ward situations.

Power can be defined in various ways. We might look at it as personal potency in participation. An individual feels personal power when his capacities to feel, to reason, and to do are allowed to operate. Power is only felt in relation to other people or to things.

Capacities to feel, think, and to act are related to other constitutional capacities. The capacity for movement is based upon one's body build; a small, wiry, overactive child feels differently about certain events than a fat, large, underactive child does. The capacity for perception is based upon innate temperament and the ways in which other people have responded to it; an energetic, quick-tempered child will feel, reason, and act differently than a quiet, placid child will. These differences will not only be based upon innate temperament but also upon how parents and other important people in their lives have looked upon their expression of temperament. These capacities are also related to the developmental level which the individual has reached; an adult has many more tools to choose from in establishing relations with people than a 3-year-old child has. At each era of his development an individual feels power when new tools (new ways of dealing with life situations) are recognized, and their purpose and use is respected, allowed, understood, and guided by others.

Everyone needs to feel power in some form. Speculate for a moment on what can be done without power—think of being without the power to feel warm or angry, power to reason through one's intentions or to comply with the orders of others, power to act (wisely and otherwise) or to refuse to act.

If power is not experienced, the feeling of powerlessness takes over. But this is a disorganizing feeling and the anxiety that underlies feelings of inadequacy, incompetence, powerlessness, cannot be experienced indefinitely. Power to act, think, or feel for oneself can be translated into various distortions— power over others to manipulate or to exploit them; power to follow others and thus gain strength by allying oneself with stronger individuals. Power to make others do things is an important aspect of advertising, public relations, and managerial services. The power to persuade is very different from the power of eliciting understanding, out of which flows the desire to do what is called for in a situation.

RATIONAL AND IRRATIONAL POWER. Rational power can be defined as power to do—to express honestly and directly what one feels, to say openly and forthrightly what one thinks, to act and to participate according to one's actual feelings and thoughts. Non-rational power is experienced as not doing —structuring one's behavior in ways that cover or hide one's actual feelings or thoughts.

Rational power is expressed through active participation in seeking, asking, struggling, finding out, and in working to get acceptance or validation for ideas, plans, and so forth. It may be difficult to accept expressions of hostility or rebellion on the part of adults as expressions of rational power. But, in children, the relation of expressions of hostility to personal integrity is perhaps more readily recognized than it is in adults. For example, a teacher constantly asks a group of exuberant children to be quiet. That is, she imposes actions related to quiet upon children who honestly feel exuberant. To retain the teacher's approval, these children need to deny their feelings by complying with her demands. If they were to express what they actually felt naturally and spontaneously, or if they harnessed their energy and used it to find out what the new demands in the situation were, they would be expressing rational power. But their compliance becomes non-rational expression of power—these children have the power to be liked for not doing what their own feelings dictate.

It is a serious hazard to the mental health of children when such demands for distortion of perception and feelings are constantly made and when opportunity to understand the basis for such demands is not available. It leads to disparity between feelings, thoughts, and actions such as one sees in schizophrenic processes. Disharmony or splitting between "felt relations," reasoned intentions, and concomitant actions is an outstanding feature of the schizophrenic process and should concern psychiatric nurses.

DEFENSIVE USAGE. The use of non-rational power is a defense against anxiety and against feelings of powerlessness. It would be well to consider what there is in psychiatric ward situations that disempowers us, makes us feel anxious, inadequate, ineffectual, or insecure. Until we identify these problems and understand the various factors in them, we cannot decide what we want to do to change the situation. How is non-rational power expressed by nurses in some of their relationships with psychiatric patients? Is the "busy-work" of nurses—clerical work, housekeeping, manipulative routines—done largely as a way of avoiding close contact and active struggle with the nursing problems which patients present? Why have we delegated contacts with patients to non-professional personnel and hung onto the office work connected with the management of a psychiatric ward? Have we rejected—unwittingly, perhaps—what we do not want to do?

Nurses say that their intention and choice is to have active and close relations with patients. They have not made this choice in psychiatry—there are 9000 nurses to care for 600,000 psychiatric patients or 54.6 percent of all the hospitalized patients. *What is there in nurse-patient relations in psychiatry that leads to feelings of powerlessness against which defensive practices are instituted?* This is our problem. Psychiatric nurses need to understand this problem and all its interrelated factors. Then, when we understand what is going on now, we can determine what we want to do.

Nurses need to become aware of the ways that interaction among nursing personnel and psychiatric patients renders the patient powerless and how the patient then rallies his non-rational power operations as defenses against the anxiety generated in his relations with nurses. Several studies have been reported which point up some of the outcomes when patients feel powerless. Incontinence has been shown to be one of the defensive responses which a patient will use when he feels devaluated or powerless (3). It has also been shown that there are many aspects of patients' needs which practicing nurses are not aware of—a fact which is particularly important in psychiatric nursing (4). Another study highlights three themes—deprivation, indulgence, and indifference—as characteristic of interpersonal relations (5). Perhaps a logical fourth might be mutual learning. How are these themes—deprivation, indulgence, indifference, and learning—expressed in nursing situations and how are they connected with the need for personal power which nurses, patients, doctors, attendants, and the public all have?

Are there differences in the way nurses feel and use power in their relations with particular patients—those diagnosed schizophrenic, paranoic, manic-depressive, and so on? Does the age of the patient make a difference? Are there differences based upon prognosis?

Everyone needs to feel power in some form and in some degree. It enters into every interpersonal relation and every situation; it determines the products of interaction. It cuts across descriptive-diagnostic psychiatry and is a theme to be taken into account in every institution as well as every face-to-face relationship. How is power experienced? How is it expressed? What are its outcomes to the psychiatric patient? Discussing these questions may help us to understand what goes on in psychiatric situations in which we attempt to work creatively and productively.

REFERENCES

1. Ruesch, Jurgen and Bateson, Gregory. *Communication: The Social Matrix of Psychiatry*, New York, W. W. Norton, 1951.
2. Tudor, Gwen E. A sociopsychiatric nursing approach to intervention in a problem of mutual withdrawal on a mental hospital ward. *Psychiatry* 15:193-217, May 1952.
3. Schwartz, M. S. and Stanton, A. H. Social psychological study of incontinence. *Psychiatry*. 13:399-416, Nov. 1950.
4. Schwartz, Charlotte G., Schwartz, M. S. and Stanton, A. H. Study of need-fulfillment on a mental hospital ward. *Psychiatry*. 14:223-242, May 1951.
5. Lasswell, Harold. Person, personality, group and culture. Contained in *A Study of Interpersonal Relations*. Ed. by Patrick Mullahy. New York, Hermitage Press, 1949, pp. 309-364.

22

Themes in
Nursing Situations—Safety

Hildegard E. Peplau*

This is the second in a series of articles describing themes that recur in nurses' relationships with their patients. Safety is one of these themes.

An important trend in the continuing development of psychiatry is the thematic phase—concern with the recurring themes or focal problems in the patient's past and present relationships with people.

When we talk about themes we are referring to qualitative judgments or abstractions that characterize an event and help us to recall and to understand what went on during the event. When we are aware of what went on—or is going on—in an interaction with a psychiatric patient, we are able to make useful inferences which may lead us to change our ways of interacting with the patient and thus establish a more therapeutic relationship with him.

Consider, for example, the theme of power. Everyone needs to feel power in some way. If the nurses' use of power in a ward situation strips the patient of his power and makes him feel powerless, what will he do to defend himself against this feeling? How will his defense operations affect his recovery process? If, on the other hand, the nurse recognizes power as the theme of the interaction, the situation can be controlled—she can change her part in the interaction and foster a more therapeutic relationship with the patient.

---

*From *American Journal of Nursing*, Vol. 53, No. 11 (November, 1953).

Miss Peplau (Pottstown, Pa., Hospital School of Nursing; B.A. Bennington College; M.A., Ed.D., Teacher's College, Columbia) is associate professor of nursing and director of the graduate program in advanced psychiatric nursing at Rutgers University College of Nursing.

SAFETY

Safety is another outstanding theme in psychiatric nursing practice, one which bears strong influence on our work. We need to recognize whether this influence is mainly constrictive or constructive in our relationships with patients. We need to know how this theme can be used constructively in a psychotherapeutic nurse-patient experience.

For whom does the theme of safety operate, primarily? The patient, the nurse, the doctor, the other workers, the public? What practices are related to safety in psychiatric situations? Are these practices sound in the light of therapeutic intentions? Are they sound in relation to the actual need for safety?

We can distinguish satisfaction and security as two goals toward which human behavior is oriented. Satisfaction has to do with going after and getting what we really want; it is therefore based upon knowing and understanding what is actually wanted. Security has to do with feeling safe—with seeking something in order to avoid getting something else that we do not want. We seek success to avoid being a failure; we seek prestige to avoid being unnoticed; we seek money to avoid being poor.

A certain amount of security—or safety—is essential for survival. You really cannot eat unless you have enough money to pay for food; you really cannot feel related to people unless they notice you and you in turn notice them and join with them in activities of one sort or another. But security is not an either-or proposition; it is relative. When we talk about the need for safety or security, we are talking about relative safety—the amount of safety needed for human psychological and physiological survival.

In psychiatric nursing practice, we see patients who focus almost exclusively upon security. Their ways of relating to people—whether by direct aggression, withdrawal, compliance, or whatever—are calculated to ensure safety more than to bring personal satisfaction. Yet, deep down, everyone has wants, desires, wishes, hopes, and can eventually formulate what it is that will bring his satisfaction. Many patients who are diagnosed as schizophrenic—if not all of them—are no longer able to identify and to express what they want. Their language, their total bodily involvement in a situation, expresses their need to feel safe, to keep from revealing themselves further to themselves or to others, to preclude the threatening results of their earlier efforts to relate to people.

Everything the schizophrenic patient says and does is calculated to ensure safety for him in the current situation. His withdrawal and seclusiveness are security operations—ways of avoiding contacts with people who, he expects, may disrespect, hurt, or even destroy him. A person's expectations and preconceptions about people are based on the feelings he has had in his relationships with people who were significant earlier in his life. To the psychiatric patient, nursing personnel symbolize, or are illusory reminders of, these earlier figures. In his relationships with nurses, therefore, safety is a dominant theme.

Coupled with this need of the patient to protect himself is another safety operation which markedly affects psychiatric care—the public's need to know that it is safe from any intrusion by psychiatric patients. There is tremendous fear in this culture that the "insane" will harm some one; consequently, there is the need to feel protected against this potential harm. Protection for the public is achieved by building hospitals that emphasize security—places that people know have the means for holding patients in such a way as to ensure that the public will not be harmed by the patients. In fact, most of the emphasis in building psychiatric hospitals has been upon safety for the public—rather than on organizing the brick and stone in the way that best provides a place for sound treatment of patients.

Just as the patient seeks safety and the public seeks to ensure its own safety, professional workers also focus upon safety for themselves. In textbooks on psychiatric nursing, we find recommended procedures to protect the nurse from injury—placing herself so that she cannot be attacked from the back while she is talking with a patient, for instance. These procedures are expected to help the nurse feel secure enough so that her talks with the patient can be functionally effective. But, very often, the effect of these precautions is to get the nurse so involved with her own safety that she is not aware of what actually is going on in her interaction with the patient. Work that is focused primarily on escape from possible danger is bound to be different from work that is focused on fulfillment of therapeutic intentions.

We can see then that in a psychiatric situation, everyone involved—patients, professional persons, the public—seems to share the common theme, safety. But does this shared focus on safety actually aid and abet the recovery process? Does it help nurses and patients to learn, grow, change, and mature as they interact? Educators and psychiatrists have decried our cultural emphasis upon security. They say that maybe we are helping our children to become so secure and to value security so highly that they cannot live in this insecure, anxiety-ridden world. What might this radical change in our way of looking at security mean?

Is it possible that the exclusive focus on safety and security by everyone relating to the patient actually leads to a stalemate—that it becomes an obstacle rather than an aid to progress? What ulterior effects does it have on psychiatric nursing care? Does it distract us from paying attention to satisfactions, and keep us from developing practices that help patients to achieve satisfactions? Do we miss growth cues and possibilities because of this exclusive focus on safety?

Newspaper stories about recent prison riots frequently refer to security as the main concern of penal institutions. This attitude is in contrast to thinking of a prison as a social hospital for the rehabilitation of individuals who are guilty of not conforming to the existing, socially sanctioned mores. Here, also, the focus upon security detracts from attention to the rehabilitative aspects of imprisonment. Perhaps the public is not ready to see the prison function as anything except a place for punishment, although we know that punishment does nothing to correct the distorted interpersonal processes of which prisoners are capable—in fact they are often made worse by imprisonment. Nurses should study the parallels—with particular reference to the theme of safety—in prison situations and psychiatric institutions.

In all nursing there is an element of safety—"the need to give safe, efficient care" is a cliché which expresses an idea that every nurse subscribes to in some degree—but professional work calls for more than this. Professional work is distinguished from vocational employment in that a professional person can and does take calculated risks. That is, the professional person goes beyond what is merely safe, and experiments so that new and more productive practices can be evolved.

An example of this in medical practice is the Blalock operation for "blue babies." Dr. Blalock took many risks as he tried out and perfected the techniques that are now used to save the lives of many babies. In doing this he made judgments which were based upon his view of the problem and his understanding of the principles involved. He risked the scorn of those who condemned him for not allowing the babies to die of "natural causes," and even the disapproval of some of his peers. All these factors are involved in experimenting and devising something new. What about the nurses in an experimental situation? Many nurses feel that no one should take chances with a patient's life. Yet we take chances and make grave errors by default. By not knowing better practices to use in psychiatric nursing, we offer services of questionable safety—if the patient's psychological safety is considered to be an element in his recovery. Only by trying out new practices and studying what happens can one understand the extent to which the patient's full functioning can be restored. To take the chance is the first step in evolving sound and productive practices.

Let us recall what the word "error" meant to us when we were students in basic nursing schools. To most of us the word was anathema—an error was something that must not be made under any circumstances. It is almost impossible to get a graduate nurse to admit having made an error in practice or in judgment. Nurses are not supposed to make mistakes. It is hard to say what dire consequences would result from admitting such human faults. Yet, at the same time, we don't think of ourselves as "perfect" people, above and beyond human error. We ought to think about this inconsistency and begin to permit ourselves, openly, to take risks and to acknowledge that we are human enough to make mistakes. We might then be able to examine and profit from mistakes. Nurses make many mistakes that they are not aware of and take risks in interpersonal relations all the time—saying something that might hurt a patient or provoke his anxiety or anger. We must become aware of our errors and begin to make experiments in nursing practice.

In psychiatric nursing, taking risks may mean breaking the existing pattern of "safe custodial care." It may involve incurring the disapproval of other workers; daring to suggest new ways of nursing practice to the medical director and the nursing service director; and persisting in one's efforts despite the disapproval of one's peers and also of those in authority.

Most existing nursing practices afford a considerable amount of certainty, safety, security—they keep patients in line, they keep patients clean, they keep wards quiet, they keep order. But are cleanliness, quiet, and order crucial elements in the patient's recovery process? Could it be that noise, disorder, and dirt are tools that a patient needs if he is to express his feelings and free himself from restraint that was imposed on him earlier?

Authorities indicate that self-examination, learning, and therapy do not occur in an orderly, step-by-step fashion. Broad phases can be identified for each of these processes. Insight occurs when all the elements of a problem are grasped in a total concept, but even these elements do not become apparent in an easy, orderly fashion. Many are recognized only after they have been acted out in a situation that brings them to the individual's attention in a way that makes their real meaning clear to him.

The patient who wants to remain unbathed, to be noisy or disorderly, may be using these practices, which are usually disapproved, to test the strength of the nurse's respect for him as a person. Do we make it plain to him that he is the object of our respect, that we are concerned primarily with him, not with the cleanliness, quiet, and order of his unit? What does a nurse feel, think, and do in the processes of bathing, feeding, dressing, and socializing with a patient, to show her respect for him?

Shouldn't certain of the standardized routines which meet the nurses', doctors', and public's need for safety be relaxed in order to meet the patient's need for safety? Shouldn't nurses spend less time learning to establish such routines to assure safety and more time developing the ability to carry out psychiatric nursing functions?

The central functions of psychiatric nursing are: (1) to observe—and take part in while observing—the patient's interactions; (2) to make inferences by identifying the themes, making judgments and forming hypotheses from the data she has observed; (3) to experiment with ways of intervening in the nurse-patient situation that will effect changes which are favorable to patients.[1] These functions are carried out within the broad limits of existing hospital policies which, desirably, are determined interprofessionally according to the soundest therapeutic intentions of members of a professional team. Where such teams do not exist, nurses have a role in seeking to have them established or to have a voice in determining policies that influence nursing practices. Nurses cannot afford to sit back and wait until others notice the importance of this principle. We must ask for, struggle for, demonstrate the right to have, and be willing to work to have a voice in determining policies that affect nursing care.

In carrying out her function as a participant-observer the nurse must be able to take part in the patient's continuing struggle to locate, clarify, and solve his problems. To do this, the nurse needs to examine herself, to understand the meaning of her own actions, and how her feelings enter into them. She needs to have a sound method for finding out what is going on, for seeking to know, in contrast to knowing. She must be able to see the patient's responses in relation to something—to others in a situation, in a culture, in a period in time—rather than in isolation. Thus, the nurse becomes a participant—a party to the interaction and an observer of it at the same time—rather than a mere spectator of the peculiarities of others.

---

[1]For a more comprehensive discussion of functions see Claire Mintzer Fagin's report, *A Study of Desirable Functions and Qualifications for Psychiatric Nurses.* New York, National League for Nursing, 1953.

There is far less certainty, safety, and security in the role of participant-observer than in the role of spectator-observer. The comfortable safety of hard and fast rules must give way to the relative security of the inquiring method—through which the professional nurse can secure the data she needs; from this data, she infers meanings and makes judgments about what is going on. Positive, useful, professional nursing practices evolve from these inferences—practices which make the nurse's intervention in the patient's problem situation both therapeutic and satisfying.

23

Utilizing Themes in Nursing Situations

Hildegard E. Peplau*

How can nurses recognize the themes which characterize productive participation and use them in making their interactions with patients therapeutic experiences?

Interaction is a process that we read a great deal about in psychiatric literature today. The contributions of Lewin and the *Gestalt* theorists have led to a shift in emphasis in the meaning of this concept. Lewin referred to the field as the whole framework within which an individual operates and interacts with other forces at work in a situation. A situation is viewed as a field of interacting forces which can be studied in their relations with other forces and not as a sum total of separate parts. Einstein calls these forces *pushes* and *pulls* and has said that the world is more a question of these pushes and pulls than it is of atoms.

INTERACTION WITH PSYCHIATRIC PATIENTS

Psychiatric nurses have always claimed that one of their functions is to help develop a therapeutic environment in which the patient can move toward recovery. This function requires that nurses be aware of what is meant by "therapeutic environment" and by "recovery." The nurse's awareness of the pushes and pulls going on in a situation in which she is a participant with patients is a major aspect of this function.

*From *American Journal of Nursing*, Vol. 54, No. 3 (March, 1954).

Miss Peplau (Pottstown, Pa., Hospital School of Nursing; B.A. Bennington College; M.A., Ed.D., Teacher's College, Columbia) is associate professor of nursing and director of the graduate program in advanced psychiatric nursing at Rutgers University College of Nursing.

A situation develops its unique characteristics from the interactions that occur. Nurses can learn how to find out who and what interacts in a particular situation so that a broad pattern of the themes of interaction can be identified.

It would be easy to answer the question of who interacts by confining the discussion to nurses and patients. But this assumption would be correct only if we considered interaction as a matter of actual contact and communication between real people. According to Harry Stack Sullivan's definition of psychiatry, however, the term interpersonal relations—or interaction—refers to "what goes on between people all but one of whom may be completely illusory" (1). The question of who interacts, therefore, involves not only the people who are actually present in a situation but also the figures who are projected into the situation. This is perhaps most clearly seen when a patient is hallucinating, that is, expressing an inner experience about people as though these figures were present in an external situation. Patients who relate to nurses as if they were figures out of the past, or nurses who relate to patients who are strangers to them as if they were familiar persons, distort interpersonal interaction. The complex task of observing and recognizing what goes on in an interaction is, therefore, made even more difficult. It would seem, then, that an initial step in developing a therapeutic environment would be for the nurse to become aware of how she feels about and views the patient and then to inquire into how the situation looks to the patient.

When we consider the question of what interacts, we are certainly not talking about literal rubbing of elbows. What then do we mean when we speak of the pushes and pulls or the forces that interact?

A long time ago Kant and others began referring to three aspects of human behavior: the cognitive, affective, and conative aspects. With the emergence of field and interpersonal theory came the recognition that these three facets of an individual's behavior must be considered, not each alone, but rather in relation to other aspects.

Cognitive refers to our perception of roles and events—that is, it describes the way in which an object (a person or thing) is viewed. How the nurse views the patient, how the patient sees the nurse, and how the nurse and patient each view themselves—these four views constantly interact. In one small sampling of observations, we found that compatability, not identical views, is essential for movement in a relationship (2). For example, if the nurse sees herself as an authority and the patient as a child, and if at the same time the patient sees the nurse as a sibling and himself as an authority, marked incompatability stalemates any constructive movement in the situation.

Affective refers to our feelings about an event. Since "felt" relations precede intellectual operations in an infant it is conceivable that this aspect of an interpersonal interaction occurs first in a person's general development, and that cognitive and conative aspects follow. Feelings are communicated knowingly and unknowingly. When we know and can state what we feel about a patient, our awareness may lead to our being able to control this aspect of interaction. But when we do not know what we actually feel, or when there is great disparity between what we say we feel and what is actually going on in us, psychobiologically, the latter is most likely to be communicated. This points up our need to recognize the variety of feelings of which we are capable—anger, guilt, hatred, warmth, tenderness, and the like.

We know that many psychiatric patients—if not all—are hypersensitive. Their previous experiences with people have alerted them to expect particular feelings to arise in an interpersonal situation—from others and in themselves. In addition, they use selective perception in viewing all that actually does happen. In other words, the patient decides—unwittingly, for the most part—what the nurse's feelings toward him will be and then selects what he *expects* to find from all that she does; so does the nurse. What each perceives about the other's feelings, on a selective basis, is what interacts.

Conative refers to the meanings, evaluations, or appraisals made in an interpersonal event. The patient's perceptions, feelings, and meanings interlock and interact with those of the nurse.

A recent article reaffirms this structural basis for studying interpersonal relations:

. . . two interacting persons must be conceived to be objects to each other in two primary respects, and in a third respect which is in a sense derived from the first two. These are (1) cognitive perception and conceptualization, the answer to the question of what the object is, and (2) cathexis—attachment or aversion, the answer to the question of what the object means in an emotional sense. The third mode by which a person orients himself to an object is by evaluation—the integration of cognitive and cathectic meanings of the object to form a system, including the stability of such a system over time. It may be maintained that no stable relation between two or more objects is possible without all three of these modes of orientation being present for both parties to the relationship.

Consideration of the conditions on which such a stable, mutually oriented system of interaction depends leads to the conclusion that on the human level this mutuality of interaction must be mediated and stabilized by a *common culture*—that is, by a commonly shared system of symbols, the meanings of which are understood on both sides with an approximation to agreement (3).

This description of a system for viewing an interaction—recognizing the object, sensing what it means, and evaluating these judgments—also points to a need for psychiatric nurses to identify the steps through which commonly shared symbols of communication can be expressed more and more directly among nurses and psychiatric patients. Nurses need to be able to observe behavior and to desymbolize it— to find out what the behavior says and what it asks for that the patient cannot communicate directly, verbally. Another concept ought to be considered in relation to this commonly shared culture.

. . . only where there is difference between two persons in contact is it possible for those persons to achieve a new understanding, a new awareness of the previously unconscious premises which underlie their own habits of communication . . . [each] is driven to some awareness of his own and of the [other's] premises. And even with the help of difference and contrast the task will still be difficult (4).

Issues, disagreements, differences in views and feelings are here postulated as the basis for change. If this proposition is correct, then psychiatric nurses also have the task of locating statements in ward situations or in nurse-patient interactions that overstabilize relations and then delay, disrupt, and disallow movement in the patient's recovery process.

STALEMATES

Some of us have been wondering for a long time whether the theme of hopelessness—in our culture, in the medical and nursing professions, among auxiliary personnel, and among patients—is one stalemate that interferes with progress. Is there tacit sharing of this unconscious premise about psychiatric work to such an extent that movement is possible only for a few patients who do not share the "hopelessness" of those around them? Are patients, nurses, attendants, and others caught in a closed circle of hopelessness? Does not this theme emerge from the data on interactions? Do we dare to observe and to find out how many people in supposedly therapeutic situations feel deep down inside themselves that psychiatric patients cannot be cured?

Too often I have heard statements like this: We must do something for these 600,000 patients . . . People think that nothing can be done, but in psychiatry we have learned a great deal . . . We have new and effective treatments . . . Only we have to get cases earlier . . . In fact, prevention is more important than treatment . . . The truth of the matter is that even recovered patients have relapses . . . There is so little we can actually do.

To me such a statement points up how a person went all the way around the closed circle of hopelessness to defend what was felt in the first place.

Themes in interaction, when we are aware of them, help us to determine how to intervene in stalemated situations. A study done by Gwen Tudor showed how the theme of mutual withdrawal stymied the patient, doctor, and nurse. Treatment was practically at a standstill until the nurse became aware of this all-pervasive theme, and then ways of intervening were devised.

Another interpersonal study showed respect and disrespect as the outstanding themes of an interaction. The nurse genuinely felt and communicated respect to a patient who felt and communicated only disrespect. As interaction proceeded, quite favorable changes—judged according to the criteria of social acceptability—took place in the patient. But, all the while, there were pushes and pulls going on between the nurse and the patient. The patient continued to test out—expecting, seeking, indeed courting disrespect from the nurse. One day, the nurse—anxious for one reason or another and not entirely aware of it—showed disrespect. The patient then courted, sought, practically asked for respect, but the nurse—understandably, from the documenting data—missed these subtle cues. In a few days, the patient's panic, instead of the nurse's awareness, gained ascendence in this situation and the patient was sent to the ward for disturbed patients. This error—along with hindsight gained from reviewing the interpersonal data—was the beginning of real learning for the nurse who has since rectified relations with this patient. It behooves us to recognize the therapeutic role of nurses and to realize that this role depends on observation and awareness leading to productive participation.

PARTICIPATION IN PATIENTS' LIVING

Participation is a word we often see in psychiatric literature. We read about active and passive participation, or negative and positive, or productive and nonproductive participation.

Participation in living in a society is an important aspect of an individual's life history—throughout infancy, childhood, and adulthood.

Participation in living always involves communication which can occur on many levels: (1) biochemical; (2) psychobiological (3) interpersonal; (4) intergroup; (5) international or intercultural. The body's biochemical structures constantly undergo changes which are demanded by the functions they are called upon to perform. Psychosomatic research reveals ample evidence that such a structure as the stomach can change as it is called upon to function as an instrument for expressing feelings, rather than primarily to receive and dispose of nutritive materials.

Participation in living means being related to others; this requires that others know how we view them, what we feel about them, and what they mean to us. It would be ideal if all such interchanges could be direct, forthright, and carried out verbally, but since this is not possible, for many reasons, distortions in participation and communication occur. "Organ language" is one way to say something and to ask for what is needed from others; consequently, in order to understand this kind of participation it is essential that nurses understand the language of illness, as well as the dynamics and generic roots of disease processes.

Highly distorted and disguised communications occur in our current song hits, comics, movies, dreams, and in the language used by patients who are diagnosed as schizophrenic. The nurse needs to be able to desymbolize these and to abstract the central themes thus communicated. Many song hits communicate a need for unconditional love—mother love rather than mature, collaborative relations. Many of the comics have been dealing lately with the theme of dishonesty among parents and in our culture, as if to desensitize children as they become aware of this problem. The movie, *Death of a Salesman*, also deals with the theme. Themes which can be inferred from these cultural communications often point up social pathology which is also expressed as part of individual pathology. The themes in what a patient tells us directly or indirectly communicate his concerns and needs.

Participation occurs wittingly and unwittingly; that is, it can be guided by intentions of which we are aware or by unconscious motivations that lie outside our awareness. Only when we are aware of what is going on does a situation become amenable to control. Panic in a theater fire demonstrates this principle dramatically; a positive example is an instance in which a nurse's keen observation and intervention keep a patient from committing suicide.

Conditioning and learning occur in situations in which we participate. What is actually learned depends upon how the various individuals in the situation participate and how this participation is experienced by everyone concerned—that is, how it is viewed and felt and what effect it has. Nurses have this paramount task: to become aware of how they experience the participation of patients in ward situations and to find out how patients experience their participation.

BRINGING ABOUT FAVORABLE CHANGE. Patients generally relate to nurses according to their earlier life experiences. Selective perception—a well documented psychobiological principle—means simply that we see and hear what our previous experiences have made it possible for us to perceive. In new situations changes can occur—if reason operates effectively, if we can safely know what we actually feel, and if new ways to participate are actually available. The case of the patient diagnosed as schizophrenic offers us striking examples of this. Deprivation and indifference which he has experienced in lieu of mother love leads to gross mistrust of the affectionate, tender interest of others. The schizophrenic patient cannot foresee the possibility of our accepting him. He cannot participate, as we would like him to, in accepting the relationship which we offer him. Yet, at the same time, there is his unrecognized longing for the unconditional acceptance of which he has been deprived.

A patient's participation is always based upon his concept of self—how he views himself—and this has been derived from appraisals others have made of him earlier in life. The schizophrenic patient sees himself as a person to be derogated, ignored, deprived. When the psychiatric nurse can understand this—and can see it in relation to the unique context of the patient's life history—then she can begin to plan her intervention. She sees that her role is consistently to demonstrate respect, acceptance, and willingness to struggle—at the patient's rate of movement and according to his temperament—with the patient's nursing problem until both are clear about it.

The greatest hope of bringing about favorable change in the patient's behavior in nursing situations—through the use of interpersonal relations—lies in the nurse's observation and awareness of what goes on. When she can recognize how she participates, when she can find out how she affects patients, then she knows what changes, if any, she needs to make in her own behavior.

Any change in one's view of self—for nurse or patient—involves experiencing anxiety. This is a concept that we should understand thoroughly. Every psychiatric nurse should own a copy of Rollo May's *The Meaning of Anxiety* and should study it for comparison with the inferences she makes about what she observes and for guides to developing methods of productive intervention.

GROWTH AND LEARNING EXPERIENCES

Changes in one's view of self signify growth and understanding. How we view ourselves is directly related to the modes or patterns of participation that we use recurrently. These patterns are also related to our need for getting approval and avoiding disapproval, and in this way are connected with power and security operations.

The maturing adult becomes increasingly better able to get away from merely seeking approval and avoiding disapproval; he becomes able to take the risks involved in experimenting with new experiences in learning. One such new experience is the psychotherapeutic aspect of nursing practice—helping the patient to recognize and understand those problems which the nurse can help him with. There is urgent need for nurses to shed some of their expendable busywork and take on this professional function. More and more doctors are saying that this is a part of our job.

What is involved in the nurse's participation in therapy? Perhaps we should review some of the interlocking factors involved:

1. Nurses need to observe and thus to locate the nursing problem. The problem is a thematic inference which underlies and is expressed in symptomatic communication.
2. They must be aware of the factors in the problem and recognize how the factors are interrelated; these judgments are based upon inferences and themes abstracted from observed data.
3. Their intervention must be based upon their observations and the inferences which they have made and are aware of.
4. They must recognize the developmental level reached by the patient and how it can vary at different times.
5. They must recognize cues which indicate the patient's growth, and respond to them as they occur.
6. They must recognize themes that are inherent in patients' interactions with other patients: (a) in the "inner circle" grouping of patients; (b) in the casual formal groupings, as at meal times; or (c) in the large, informal ward group. Nurses may intervene in any of these interactions.

None of these are special "office" experiences in the usual sense of psychotherapy; rather they are aspects of the nurse's participation in life on the psychiatric ward. If the activities which are unique to nursing practice—bathing, feeding, toileting, dressing, socializing—can be viewed as instruments for developing and implementing participation that becomes more and more productive, then perhaps new and more rewarding "mothering" can be offered to patients. Making these daily events count as learning experiences is a nursing task. We must see the situation as a whole and respond to whole concepts of what goes on rather than fractionalize nursing practice on the basis of data concerning one particular problem.

Nursing participation can be viewed as one way of *not* repeating, *not* perpetuating, *not* reinforcing cultural experiences that have already done damage. This requires not only that we understand the prevailing expectations and preconceptions of the culture—both today and at significant periods in the patient's early life—but also that we attempt to understand how the patient has experienced them. Relating constructively to patients requires constructive attack on all minor problems as and when they emerge. This can be done to some degree in the time which nurses customarily spend with patients but it requires that the nurse be able to conceptualize processes rather than products and themes rather than details.

REFERENCES

1. Sullivan, Harry S. *The Interpersonal Theory of Psychiatry*. Edited by Helen S. Perry and Mary L. Gawel. New York, W. W. Norton and Co., 1953.
2. Roth, Dorothy I. Role call—a study of roles in nurse-patient relations. *Nursing Research* 1:41-42, Oct. 1952.
3. Parsons, Talcott. The superego and the theory of social systems. *Psychiatry* 15:15-25, Feb. 1952.
4. Ruesch, Jurgen and Bateson, Gregory. *Communication: the Social Matrix of Psychiatry*. New York, W. W. Norton and Co., 1951, p. 229.
5. Tudor, Gwen E. A sociopsychiatric nursing approach to intervention in a problem of mutual withdrawal on a mental hospital ward. *Psychiatry* 15:193-217, May 1952.

24

Psychotherapeutic
Nursing

Claire M. Fagin*

Unlike many other therapists—social workers, psychologists, psychiatrists—the nurse functions in many ways, sometimes moving from individual to group to milieu therapy several times within the same day, continuing, as well, to pay attention to patients' physical needs. To do this successfully, the nurse needs to understand herself and her reactions, her patients and their needs, the nature of her practice, and the philosophy within which she functions. This author believes that emotional illness can be "influenced, interrupted, or altered by what nurses do to and with patients."

Psychotherapeutic nursing consists of those acts, those interventions through which nurses help patients use new or healthy patterns in consistent and continuous ways. To do this the nurse moves on three avenues of approach: through the milieu, that is, through manipulating the organization of the social system in the patient setting; through her one-to-one relationship with the patient; and through her interactions with groups of patients.

The nurse may work in all of these ways simultaneously or in one way exclusively. For example, she may have a one-to-one interview with a patient in a structured setting where she is aware of the social system which affects the patient but is not a part of it. Or the one-to-one relationship may occur

*Reprinted from *American Journal of Nursing*, Vol. 67, No. 2, February 1967, pp. 298-304, by permission of the author and The American Journal of Nursing Company. Copyright February 1967, The American Journal of Nursing Company.

Dr. Fagin received a B. S. degree with a major in nursing from Wagner College, Staten Island, N.Y., and M. A. from Teachers College, Columbia University, New York, N.Y., and a Ph.D. from New York University. She is director of the Graduate Programs in Psychiatric Mental Health Nursing at New York University.

within the context of a milieu—home, hospital, or institution of any kind—which the nurse may attempt to change.

The place of treatment need not be the hospital. It could be the home, the community center, the storefront. And within this frame of reference, it is not only the patient who is deemed sick; his family also, as a social system, is seen as functioning in a pathologic way. There is, in other words, an integration constructed within this family unit which serves to elicit and continue disturbing behavior on the part of the patient.

The nurse's intervention with groups of patients also has a specific configuration. Even though she may work with groups of patients in the same structured way as other therapists, she also works with groups of patients and plans intervention with groups on the ward or in the home where the setting is far less structured. It is in these less structured areas that our theoretic frame of reference regarding nursing therapy is not well developed. In the more structured aspects of individual and group interviews, nurses can borrow and adapt from the approaches of other professional workers. However, in our manipulations of the more typical nursing roles, we are less scientific even though we have much pragmatic evidence. But, this neither has been shared nor researched.

For example, seven dimensions of nursing practice may be identified:

Time spent with patients. Nursing personnel live with their patients within the hospital for an entire tour of duty. If we think of the concept of anxiety, it is obvious that one cannot live with anxiety for extended periods—neither patients for their twenty-four-hour day nor nurses for their eight. Nursing personnel must, therefore, be able to intervene in anxiety-producing situations wherever these occur—in the hospital, in the home, or in the clinic.

The spatial area. Nursing personnel have to be able to participate effectively in areas as varied as bedroom, bath, dining room, living room, or recreation area. This is in sharp contrast to the psychiatrist or social worker, whose spatial area generally is structured.

Variety of patients. The nurse must relate simultaneously with many individuals who have varying degrees of health and illness with multiple and possibly conflicting needs.

Care for the whole patient. The nurse's ability in relation to patients' physical as well as emotional care needs can be extremely useful in her psychotherapeutic efforts. It can also pose a problem, however, of too great intimacy for the patient and a lack of clarity of role for the nurse. Again, this is in sharp contrast to the psychiatrist or the social worker whose roles tend to remain more or less constant.

Rapid adjustments. Throughout her working day, the nurse moves frequently from relating to individual patients to relating to groups of patients. Her effectiveness is determined by her ability to make rapid adjustments to these changes in situations and to creatively utilize and influence the interactions. In other words, the movement from individual therapy to group therapy and vice versa should not be seen as an interference with the relationships but as a learning experience in the daily life of the patients.

Care for patients as a group. Frequently nurses are involved with groups of patients. Group interactions are inherently complex, especially in terms of the meaning of relationships and communications between nurse and patients, patient and patients, and nurse and family.

On-the-spot decision making. The nurse has to make moment-to-moment decisions, compromises, improvisations, and take risks for prolonged periods of time.

Although each nurse may add to this list on the basis of her own experience, considering these seven dimensions has been useful in thinking through nursing roles and relationships.[1]

To achieve therapeutic effectiveness, the first step the nurse must take is to look at the preconceptions she brings to the situation. What is of particular concern is her concept of illness which, overtly and covertly, influences her philosophy of nursing and her approach to therapy. The nurse must understand the meaning of illness in our society and, more particularly, the meaning of mental illness.

Action for Mental Health, the report of the Joint Commission on Mental Illness and Health, noted sharply that attitudes about mental illness were obstacles to therapeutic efforts. They found an underlying attitude of rejection and disapproval of mental illness and the mentally ill which frequently engendered more rather than less estrangement of the sick person (1). The patient, too, holds these attitudes and, therefore, he tends to reject himself for some of the same reasons that others do: fear of his acts, his destructive impulses, his anger, and his helplessness. Lack of awareness of our own feelings about mental illness and the mentally ill covertly influences our behavior. This is true, of course, of preconceptions in general.

By way of illustration, let's take the preconception some people have of nurses. Occasionally, it is said that nurses are authoritarian and coldhearted. The nurse who is not authoritarian may provoke anxiety in patients who think this. Such a patient comes to the nurse expecting that she will give him answers and tell him what to do. If, instead, the nurse is warm and spontaneous and tries to make decisions *with* the patient instead of *for* the patient, his preconceptions may clash with reality. But if this nurse also notes the cues to the patient's anxiety and tries to understand and clarify with the patient what is going on, there is possibility for growth.

The nurse's concepts and attitudes also are relevant. For example, the nurse working with a specific cultural group needs to examine her preconceptions about this group, test them with reality, and then attempt changes if her findings so dictate.

The recognition and subsequent alteration of one's preconceptions are essential modes of behavior in any area in which the nurse finds herself. And unless she is clear on the degree to which her preconceptions are accurate and on how they influence her thinking, she cannot begin to be therapeutically effective in any relationship: one-to-one, group, or milieu. Morris Schwartz points out:

There has been increasing acceptance of the idea that non-organic mental illness is not a disease entity lodged within the patient. Rather, it is seen as a pattern of difficulty that the person manifests in relating to himself and others. This pattern

---

[1]This list is based on but is not identical with that developed through collaborative efforts with Gwen Tudor Will and Agnes Middleton.

of difficulty is seen not only as a product of what a patient "is" but of what he does and what others think about him and do to, and with, him. This line of thinking further maintains that, if the patient's difficulties are to be alleviated—his thinking and behavior changed—not only must the patient do something about himself but personnel who are part of his daily social environment must develop attitudes and behavior toward him that best fit his needs and are most appropriate for his current and changing condition. (2)

This concept leads to the view that is within the behavior, within the interpersonal relations which develop between staff and patient, that the patient can learn and grow and, therefore, get well. Such a concept can determine a philosophy of psychotherapeutic nursing that is essentially interpersonal. It is, for example, no longer believed that a therapeutic hour each day, alone, helps the patient get well but, rather, that one or many persons in many situations with the patient can bring about therapeutic results. Patients, and their families as well, are seen as active participants in treatment.

Quite simply, one might say that a patient comes into contact with psychiatric personnel because he is having difficulty in living; specifically, difficulty in living with other people. One of the purposes of nursing intervention, then, is to provide experiences in living which will enable the patient to establish relationships that are less anxiety provoking and more comfortable, making possible other less threatening, less forbidding relationships.

METHODOLOGY

The obvious question then is, "How does the nurse do this?" First of all she *observes and collects data*. Part of this data is theory: information about personality development, interpersonal interaction, the concept of anxiety, and how social systems operate (3). She acquires this knowledge from the literature and from her own observations and research.

In addition to theory, the data include specific observations about the patient: his verbal and nonverbal communications; that is, his words, actions, expressions, and gestures. The extent to which the patient uses gestures rather than verbal communication, for example, will indicate something about the level of personality development at which he is operating.

In addition to these observations, the nurse needs to look at her own words, actions, and gestures and, even more important, at her thoughts and feelings for the clues they give. Thoughts and feelings of patients are not always obvious yet they often are the first clues that something is amiss with patients, the group, or the social setting. They may, on the other hand, tell us that things are going well and that the situation is comfortable.

Harry Stack Sullivan said that two overall goals in interpersonal relations were satisfaction and security (4). These two broad categories are helpful in grouping patients' needs. Satisfaction, for example, is produced when needs that are primarily biologic are met; security when needs that are primarily interpersonal are fulfilled. Both of these categories are of concern in nursing since a patient's problems often are entwined with frustrations in both biologic and interpersonal areas. A patient on a special diet who is always hungry may feel a lack of physiologic satisfaction but, since food plays a significant role in our interpersonal context from birth to death, he also may have his need for security breached. Or a man seriously mutilated in an accident may be more troubled by the change in his self-image than with his severe pain.

Needs which have to do with maintenance of the self, that is, who we are and what we are, are included in the category of security needs. For example, such needs as the feeling of respect for oneself, for approval, prestige, love, friendship, recognition, power, and so forth, obviously deal with personal security. When these needs are unmet or, in other words, when there is a threat to the self-esteem, a feeling of anxiety may be experienced. All of us are familiar, in one degree or another, with the discomfort of anxiety, as well as with the desire to avoid such discomfort. The wish to avoid anxiety gives rise to patterns of behavior that will meet needs or, at least, preserve the self with a minimum of discomfort.

Anxiety is essentially an emergency emotion that warns the individual that something is likely to interfere with the self-concept. This emotion can be generated interpersonally by co-workers, patients, family, or others in the situation, or it may be generated by something in the present situation which unconsciously reminds the individual of a painful experience in the past.

People have different ways of seeking relief from the feeling of helplessness that arises with anxiety. Some persons may become more dependent and submissive, clearly demonstrating the helplessness that they feel. Others may respond with defiance or stubbornness, or they may become demanding. Each response that a person makes is apt to bring a response from others which may reinforce the way the person feels or alter it.

Most people have experienced anxiety from being with a very anxious person. But this reaction often is not realized until a later time. This process —one person's anxiety being communicated to another person—may become circular if there is no awareness of the anxiety and no understanding of it. Self-observation, therefore, is crucial in being therapeutic.

The second function is to *make inferences* from the data gathered. Here the nurse looks at the data and tries to relate her own observations of the situation to the theory and also to past situations she and others have observed. She makes an attempt to decode and infer meaning from the communications, and to look at the whole: herself and the patient, the nonverbal and the verbal communications, and at the theory.

Third, the nurse *structures her interventions according to her inferences.* These three—collecting data, making inferences, and structuring nursing interventions—may occur on a rapid moment-to-moment basis or over a long period of time. The nurse working with a patient thinks about what is happening and plans her interventions accordingly. But she also thinks about the relationship of today's activities with those of the week before and the weeks to follow; she thinks of the continuous process, the themes that emerge, the unique patterns, the recurring patterns.

Fourth, she also *evaluates.* The correctness or incorrectness of particular interventions or of inferences she draws about the patient's responses, the feeling tone of the group, progress, regression, obvious or subtle changes, or even no change are looked at in this process. Evaluation is a separate function, yet it also is a part of the nurse's other therapeutic functions.

The nurse cannot practice psychotherapeutic nursing unless she is able to take these four steps independently as well as interdependently. Unless she can use her own intellectual abilities, she will function only in rote fashion and not consistently and continuously in terms of the specific situation in which she is interacting with the patient.

For example, if the principle is accepted that behavior is reciprocal—that is, what we do with patients influences their responses—the nurse can alter her behavior on the basis of what she knows about the situation. But this may elicit any of a variety of responses from the patient since no set response to a particular behavior can be predicted. In determining a correct and useful response to make to the patient, the nurse uses the skills with which understanding is built—observing, listening, studying, decoding, inferring, acting, and evaluating. Patients' needs, however, are often expressed in obscure and confusing ways, and any conflict between the nurses' and the patients' interpretation of what is being communicated must be resolved if there is to be understanding of the problems the patients are facing.

So far this paper has focused on the ideas which are relevant to the three avenues of approach in psychotherapeutic nursing intervention—the one-to-one relationship, group relationships, and the milieu. The remainder of the paper will identify some specific techniques that can be used in each of these three areas.

INDIVIDUAL THERAPY

A useful beginning in individual, or one-to-one therapy is to look at how the patient might see the nurse. Every patient will have ideas about the nurse and her job because of the cultural stereotype. But each nurse needs to examine this stereotype for herself. If the patient has had pleasant experiences with nurses, he might see the nurse as somone who cares for or helps people, who goes out of her way to do something for someone. This concept of doing something for someone may be of positive value with patients who are dependent, yet unable to express their dependency in a way that will get them constructive help. Such a patient may find it difficult to seek help or to express his needs for help. The nurse, on the other hand, can go to the patient. Some writers describe this approach to patients as positive aggression (5). That is, the nurse goes after the patient and meets the patient on his own terms. The one-to-one relationship, thus, may be started in an unstructured way and continued on an appointment basis when both nurse and patient so choose. The nurse by virtue of role is in a position to seek out the patient and to see him in a variety of places rather than waiting for him to come to her.

Another aspect of nursing that is essential with many patients is the nurse's ease in physical caring and doing for others. In this instance, the mother-surrogate role, spelled out by Peplau has particular relevance (6). In tending the patient physically, the nurse demonstrates how much she cares but the anxiety and disapproval which the patient's mother may have conveyed to him in her caring is absent. Caring activities are vehicles for deepening the relationship; the nurse may find it is when she is giving physical care that the patient will discuss his real concerns. But the patient who has difficulty in what he views as intimacy with another person will have increased anxiety if the nurse is not clear about the differences between her professional and her social roles, and about her own needs. The nurse may have a need to be liked and accepted by patients. The clearer she is on how this need affects her behavior the more useful she will be. By consciously manipulating her own behavior she can help the patient find himself through the acceptance, learnings, and subsequent satisfactions of their relationship.

When the nurse is helping a patient express and resolve his dependency needs, it is essential that she be alert to minute changes in his responses. She addresses herself to the healthy aspects of the patient. As she watches, listens, and infers meaning, she is able to sense when he has made some movement which she then uses in helping him to gradually assume more responsibility for himself and lessen his need to continue his mentally ill behavior. If the nurse does not notice the change in behavior, she will continue to deal with the patient as if it had not occurred, and thus make it more difficult for him to sustain the improvement. A small change in behavior may be a big step for the patient, and if the nurse fails to sense it, the patient may become greatly discouraged.

The very subtle cues which may come from the patient, particularly in terms of any movement toward a higher level of functioning, are extremely important. Even a small amount of understanding will reinforce his healthy behavior and help him feel that he is not completely "crazy." Understanding the patient's communication makes the whole process of illness more rational and brings about a sharing experience which for the patient may be a unique event. Each experience of this kind gives him hope that other experiences like this can happen to him, that he isn't so different from others, that he can be understood.

One difficult aspect of the one-to-one relationship is the silent listening and observing that is necessary. This skill is not easy to acquire because the nurse often feels unsucessful if she hasn't been able to get the patient to talk to her. But if she recognizes the importance of the nonverbal cues and develops her ability to observe them, she will uncover signs she previously would have ignored.

One essential aspect of therapy is reflection on the meaning of what the nurse sees or hears, reflection that encourages the patient to expand on it further. The nurse who jumps in to say something, or says the first thing that comes to her mind, will shut off the patient's flow of self-expression. If she can sustain her own tension and anxiety and respond thoughtfully to the patient's comments, she will often learn more about the patient's particular modes of behavior. She may find out what he is looking for in other people; themes or consistencies may become obvious; knowledge may be obtained, for example, about a phase of his development. Is he operating for the most part at an infantile level? If so, what might be done to help him move to the next level of development?

The one-to-one relationship allows the nurse to structure her interventions to include experiences geared toward helping the patient accomplish a particular developmental task. But, one-to-one therapy is not always feasible nor always desirable. Some patients respond better to group therapy, and for some nurses group work is their métier.

WORKING WITH GROUPS

Obviously, the important aspect in groups is the reaction of personalities on one another. There is stimulation and contagion of emotion from one patient to another, and correlation of one person's problems with those of others

—of help particularly to those patients who find it hard to verbalize their difficulties.

Another value of a group experience for a patient may be a realization that his problems are not unique. This realization tends to dispel his guilt and sometimes even lessens the weight of his problem. In the group, the individual obtains support not only from the therapist but from other patients as well. A problem the nurse needs to keep aware of is that of competition among patients for attention from the therapist and for status in the group.

Sensitivity to the needs and tensions in the group is very important. A common error is to focus more on individual rather than on group interaction. Another is to fail to recognize the unofficial patient leader and channel his leadership into healthy rather than destructive patterns.

A therapist working with groups learns to verbalize the underlying feelings of the group only when they are near the surface and only when many group members share them. In other words, the feelings should be easily perceived. In general, probing questions are ruled out, both in individual and in group therapy. Patients will discuss the topics of importance to them when they are ready to do so. The responsibility to make choices and to institute change belongs to them.

Group therapy draws only part of its methodology, dynamics, and techniques from psychiatry; sources of knowledge about the particular ways in which groups operate, cultural and class values and configurations, and concepts of role come from sociology, social psychology, and anthropology. Such ideas as role complementarity and role set have relevance in individual therapy, but these ideas are even more significant in situations where there are multiple "others" to assume roles in relation to particular problem situations.

Although group interviews deal predominately with current problems—following the patients' leads—the therapist develops a sensitivity to group themes, individual incongruities, topics around which the group clusters, silences, and the direction which patients are taking. She notes whether silences occur around specific topics or whether there are situational changes. Continued silence by some patients may mean that they are too embarrassed or too ashamed for the group discussion. Their usual patterns of withdrawal might be reinforced by the discussion. Sensitivity to this behavior would lead the nurse to help plan subsequent individual approaches.

This paper, focusing on psychotherapeutic function, is not meant to imply any view of the nurse as omnipotent. Although she may work independently, there are, of course, times when she collaborates with members of other disciplines. However, when and how she collaborates is a subject for another paper.

THE MILIEU

In the third avenue of approach—the milieu—the nurse has the authority as well as the responsibility for creative action. Many authors believe that the milieu is the most important treatment modality for psychiatric patients. In the first place, psychiatric patients often are not able to express themselves in a traditional interview, and often are not able to talk easily about many aspects of their lives. Second, improvements in the milieu reach a greater number of patients than do other therapies. Third, and probably most important, the patient lives in a situation 24 hours a day, 7 days a week; the benefits of a few scheduled therapy hours often can be undone, or at least not capitalized upon, by the social setting.

In examining and creating a therapeutic milieu, a philosophy of psychotherapeutic nursing must first be developed and then implemented in the situation. For example, admission routines are a good place to start. Frequently, the way a patient is treated on admission reinforces his negative feelings about himself and about hospitals. The procedure often is depersonalized, the patient's belongings are removed, and few explanations are given. Good practice would be to see that he has everything he needs, and to introduce him, regardless of his behavior, to patients and personnel he is going to live with in his immediate area.

For example, a graduate student told about seeing, on her first day on a psychiatric ward, a tall, thin, well-groomed young man pacing the long hall. Occasionally, he would pause, look into the living room, nurses' station, or music room, but would never enter. The student introduced herself to him; he told her his name was Bob. Presently, another patient joined them, remarked upon her Boston accent, and spent a few moments in conversation. Soon Bob resumed his pacing. At lunchtime, the student asked one of the nurses to tell her about Bob. The nurse replied, "Who knows him? He has been here for three weeks but doesn't say very much and just seems to wander about the ward. He's a chronic schizophrenic."

Three days later, when the student returned to the ward, she was told that Bob was becoming catatonic, had been posturing, was not able to swallow, and consequently had not eaten. He had been given sodium amytal and had been sleeping most of the afternoon. Following this report she saw him lying on the bed, unshaven and unkempt. She brought him a tray for supper and when she awakened him to eat, she noticed that he appeared dazed, frightened, and had tremors. In order to alleviate some of his fears, she forewarned him about all of her actions and told him that she would help him eat and remain with him. To her surprise, he ate all the food on the tray, but did not speak. Following supper, he stood up. The student asked him if he would like to walk in the hall; he responded by turning toward the door. He was unsteady, so she offered to hold his arm. They walked into the hall and the first words he said were, "Have you been to Boston lately?" Obviously, he remembered her.

She spent most of the evening pacing the hall with him. His verbalization was autistic for the most part. At one point, he told her he was frightened and he took her hand in his as they paced. An undergraduate nursing student relieved her for dinner and coffee break. Bob went to bed at 10:00 p.m. after the graduate student had told him she would return in two days. The night staff discussed Bob and his feelings of depersonalization as evidenced by some of his activities. When the student returned two days later, she found that Bob had been eating and that members of the staff, especially the nursing students, were taking turns pacing with him in the hall. When the graduate student began walking with Bob again, he was walking with a shuffling gait but shortly changed to a normal gait. At times, he was confused, but he told her about his brothers and sisters, and some of his interests. He was initiating conversation, not merely responding to the nurse's questions.

163

The staff nurse assigned to the patient was amazed at the change in his behavior and said, "His medication must finally be working." But the student said she thought the interpersonal attention he had been receiving might well be related to the change, pointing out that at the beginning of the week he was alone most of the time and no one had seemed to know anything about him (7).

This example illustrates a patient's awareness of events at times when he does not seem to know what is going on, the overlapping nature of the one-to-one and milieu approaches, and the contagious effect of one person's behavior on another. In this case, it was the nursing student who picked up the behavior of the graduate student. Sometimes, a nurse's behavior will be reflected by patients on the unit who, when they see how a patient is treated, may also begin to behave toward the patient in similar ways. In fact, patients, like other people, are influenced as much by the nurse's behavior as by what she says.

In implementing a psychotherapeutic philosophy, another area to examine is that of communications. Are there opportunities for staff and patients to meet formally and informally? And for personnel to share information, both verbal and written? Is the ward routine so arranged that nurses can devote time to listening to patients and to each other? Does the setting allow for exploiting life issues? For example, is it possible for interviews to be held when necessary and when indicated rather than only at prescribed hours during the day?

The direction of communication and the way decisions are made is another index of the philosophy of care. If the patient is to benefit from the milieu, he must participate in it so that his behavior actually influences what is going on. The same principle holds for the optimum functioning of all levels of nursing personnel. Personnel who are involved in decision making have an investment in the policies they have helped to frame.

Program, policies, and routines should insure that the patient is protected from traumatic handling by any personnel associated with the unit. In addition, there must be gratification divorced from consideration of whether the patient deserves it or not. Patients need gratification as part of their treatment; they don't win it on the basis of good behavior. Tolerance of symptoms and leeway for regression is necessary within the treatment environment, but protective interference by the staff at the moment when it is necessary to protect the patient from his own guilt, anxiety, or depression, or to protect other patients, is also a part of effective milieu therapy.

A patient may not be able to handle a permissive environment, especially at the beginning of hospitalization. Acceptance of him, his problems, and his symptoms may make him anxious. In this instance, patients and personnel need to recognize the difference between acceptance of symptoms and indifference or permissive enjoyment of problem behavior. Accepting a patient does not mean approval of everything he does. Approval of negative feelings may, in fact, be a hindrance rather than a help. The patient group, itself, will indicate over and over to individual patients the concept of permissiveness and acceptance that really exists. And the patient will sense this from the nurse's responses to him and from what he observes of her acceptance of other patients.

A treatment milieu also has rules or limits—rules for social and for physical behavior that are really necessary, rules that are clearly understood and carefully observed. First of all, dangerous, aggressive behavior against self and others obviously cannot be permitted. Some forms of obscene language and some forms of acting out also may be too seductive under certain circumstances. Judiciously planned, rules, limits, or routines will help to increase a patient's sense of security.

Routines should be part of the design, however, rather than a challenge to patients to behave in ways which would then call out reward, punishment, acceptance, or rejection on the part of the personnel. Whatever the rules, let them be few, explicit, and understood by staff as well as by patients. Nothing is more attractive to patients than testing limits, especially with new staff.

Creative manipulation of the milieu is an exciting aspect of psychotherapeutic nursing. It suggests an infinite variety of work roles with personnel and patients, and poses a fruitful arena for nursing research.

SUMMARY

The role of the nurse as a therapeutic agent has been identified, using three overlapping avenues of approach—the one-to-one relationship, the group relationship, and the milieu. The philosophic frame of reference has been that the patient has become ill as a result of the experience he has had in living. His illness then can be influenced, interrupted, or altered by what other people do, to and with him. Behind a patient's rejecting behavior is potential for warmth and responsive behavior. This potential can be reached through persistence in offering the patient a responsive and respectful relationship.

REFERENCES

1. Joint Commission on Mental Illness and Health. *Action for Mental Health.* Final report. New York, Basic Books, 1961.
2. Schwartz, M. S., and Shockley, Emmy L. *Nurse and the Mental Patient.* Science Editions, John Wiley and Sons, New York, 1966, (Paperback) Introduction.
3. Fagin, Claire M. *Study of Desirable Functions and Qualifications for Psychiatric Nurses.* New York, National League for Nursing, 1953. (Mimeographed)
4. Sullivan, H. S. *Conceptions of Modern Psychiatry.* Washington, D. C., William Alanson White Psychiatric Foundation, 1947, p. 6.
5. Bruce, Sylvia J. Adolescence; delinquent and distressed. *Nurs. Outlook* 8:499-501, Sept. 1960.
6. Peplau, Hildegarde E. Principles of psychiatric nursing. In *American Handbook of Psychiatry,* ed. by Arietis Silvano. New York, Basic Books, 1959, Vol. 2, pp. 1840-1856.
7. Davidites, Rose Marie. (Unpublished paper)

25

With Suicidal Patients
Caring For
Is Caring About

Sister Theophane Umscheid*

"No other way out but suicide." This thought may not always
be verbalized, but it is generally expressed. It is the expression
that the nurse must see. And if she sees, she can help, not
with light-hearted cheering up, but with sensitive listening,
understanding, respecting, and caring. It is through this use
of self that she is more likely to reach the patient—the person
who feels helpless, hopeless, and deserted.

Most people have experienced depression, to a greater or lesser degree,
at some time or other in their lives. They have known, to some extent, the
feelings of sadness, worthlessness, hopelessness, and emptiness which characterize it psychologically. Chief among the physiologic symptoms are gastro-
intestinal and sleep disturbances, and decrease in muscle tone. Slumped shoulders, a slowing gait, drooping facies, burping, decreasing interest in work and
in personal appearance, and lack of communication are physical signs.

The wise nurse knows there is no pat list of techniques to use in helping
someone in the anguish of depression, but she will be able to develop skill
in offering support to the depressed person while he works through his feelings if she understands what is happening.

*Reprinted from *American Journal of Nursing*, Vol. 67, No. 6, June 1967,
pp. 1230-1232, by permission of the author and The American Journal of Nursing
Company. Copyright June 1967, The American Journal of Nursing Company.

Sister Theophane (St. Joseph Hospital School of Nursing, Concordia, Kan.;
A.B., Marymount College, Salina, Kan.; M.S.N.E., Catholic University, Washington, D. C.) is mental health coordinator and professor of nursing at Marymount
College in Salina. Her specialty is psychiatric nursing and she has had many years
of experience in caring for patients, in teaching, and in administration. This paper
is based on material she presented at programs sponsored by KSNA, KLN, and
the Educational Division of Kansas Institutions.

Hopelessness is probably the most distressing of all symptoms. The person feels muzzled, hemmed-in, and utterly incapable. These feelings are so devastating that if relief does not come, suicidal tendencies are inevitable. Lincoln's biographer wrote that the plague of hopelessness nearly drove Lincoln to the Potomac River. In describing one of his blackest moments, Lincoln wrote to his law partner:

I am now the most miserable man living. If what I feel were equally distributed to the whole human family, there would not be one cheerful face on earth. Whether I shall ever be better I cannot tell. I awfully forbode I shall not. To remain as I am is quite impossible. I must die to be better, it appears to me. (1)

And in the same tone, Edgar Allen Poe once wrote to a friend:

My feelings at this moment are pitiable indeed. I have struggled against the influence of this melancholy but am miserable in spite of the vast improvement of my circumstances. I am wretched and I know not why. Console me if you can. But let it be quickly or it will be too late. Write me immediately. Convince me that life is worth while. Oh, the bliss of putting one's self to sleep, never to wake. (2)

There are other examples of apparently successful people whose periods of depression were intense. One whose cry for help did not suffice to prevent the "traitor from within" from accomplishing his deed of betrayal was James Forrestal. A few hours before Mr. Forrestal leaped to his death, he exclaimed hopefully to his brother, "I'll be all right. We'll pull out of this." But at the very time he made this remark, he was in the process of copying the following quotation from Sophocles:

When Reason's day sets rayless—joyless quenched in cold decay,
Better to die, and sleep—
The never-waking sleep, than linger on,
And dare to live,
    When the soul's life (the spirit) is gone. . . . (3)

No one—Forrestal's brother nor the hospital personnel—saw anything amiss in his concern with this particular poetry. But after Forrestal pushed the window aside and leaped, the pencil, the pad, and the book of Greek poetry lay ghostlike on the table telling a story of despair.

It is not so important that the nurse understand the motives for suicide as it is for her to understand the helplessness and hopelessness of the suffering person. However, a reference to Meerloo's discussion on suicide is enlightening. Meerloo points out that the suicidal attempts are *communications,* communications which may go something like this:

Look what you've done to me; now you've killed me.
I'll die and then they will be sorry.
I can't kill you (hostility) so I'll kill myself.
I can't *stand* this any longer.
It is more than I can take.
They'll be glad when I'm out of their way. (4)

In any case, whatever the communication, suicide is a cry for help. The greater the nurse's comprehension of human behavior, the greater will be her perception of clues to depression, and she will then recognize the potential for suicide in all persons who are depressed and anxious.

The novel, drama, and biography can sharpen the nurse's observation and feeling skills. Look into the life of Van Gogh, and see where he was driven. Live for awhile with the author of the "Missouri Waltz," "When Day is Done," and hundreds of other beautiful ballads and find why the songs on the lips of James Royce Shannon were not able to put a song in his heart. View and discuss such films as *Death of a Salesman, David and Lisa,* and *La Strada,* to develop sensitivity to the utter helplessness and hopelessness of the depressed person who is plagued with suicidal thoughts. The nurse cannot remain cold, indifferent, and unfeeling. The cry for help must be answered.

The responsible nurse will give that help—provide protection against self-destruction and reduce environmental hazards. And she will try to understand the relationship between anger and depression. The angry child can kick and scream, but the angry adult in our culture must repress his emotions. If he does this repeatedly, the anger often is expressed in self-destructive behavior. It takes time to work through the anger and depression which accompany suicidal tendencies. While the patient is working through his problems and is gaining insights, the nurse can offer support against the impulse of self-punishment.

Basic needs must be met before we can ever hope to meet more complex needs. The nurse, therefore, first supplies nourishment and other physical care. She uses measures to induce rest and sleep. And, at the same time, she tries to bolster the patient's self-confidence and self-esteem. When he feels worthless and of no value, she seeks out tasks for him which are therapeutic such as doing something useful for others. If the patient himself chooses such seemingly degrading tasks as emptying ash trays, scrubbing wastebaskets, and the like, she permits them, remembering that to him they may be symbolic of "cleaning away his bad self." Appelbaum suggests that more could be done in a systematic and conscious way to undermine the patients' suicidal premise through encouraging decision and responsibility at every level of integration possible for him: letting him decide what to eat for dinner, whether or not to watch a television program, what attire to wear for the day, and so forth (5). But, there is danger in this form of approach. The demands on the patient must not be out of proportion to his capabilities at the moment; otherwise, his feelings of hopelessness may be intensified. Confrontation, therefore, may be harmful unless it is used with great skill. In general, most authorities believe that patients should not be required to make any but the most simple decisions until the depression is somewhat elevated.

Diversional activities may also help to reduce the self-centeredness that accompanies potential suicide. The activity must be carefully selected for each individual. *Learning to know the patient* is the key to finding the most effective type of diversional therapy.

Verbal and nonverbal communication skills are important. Many a suicide has been prevented because the patient knew that the nurse was interested in him. He had hope when he sensed that there was at least one person who cared about him. The need to be accepted, respected, and appreciated is human. A nurse's acceptance and respect do get through to even the most deeply depressed person, but the communicating person must be sincere. If a person is to perceive that I care for him, that I respect him, that I have faith in him, I must be genuine; I must *really* care; I must respect; and I must trust.

I could elaborate on the value of drugs—the tranquilizers and the anti-depressants—in the treatment of depression and the alleviation of suicidal tendencies. And I have mentioned nothing about specific environmental safety measures. This is intentional because I know that these are stressed in all inservice programs. However, there is one area that is not stressed and does need mentioning—the successful suicide or unsuccessful nursing intervention. What then?

A patient hangs himself, or throws himself down an elevator shaft, or jumps from the eighth-story window. What happens? Listen, and you may hear:

1. Mr. Schmidt, the patient in the next room, recalls that Jack gave him the bacon from his breakfast tray this morning, saying, "Here you can have this. I won't be eating any more bacon." "Of course, it's my fault," muses Mr. Schmidt, "I should have known. If I had told the nurse, the suicide may have been prevented."

2. Jack's mother relates, "Over the weekend I noticed that Jack was very careless about his personal appearance. I should have told the nurses because this was unusual for Jack. He has always been so particular about his clothing."

3. Mrs. Kelley, the night nurse, forgot to report to the day nurse that Jack slept poorly last night, but she tries to justify herself saying, "But it isn't unusual. Jack often prowls around at night."

4. Mr. Drummond, the occupational therapy supervisor, admits that Jack didn't appear for his morning assignment but, "I didn't think much about it because Jack is often late."

5. The nursing student becomes panicky. "It's my fault. I should have known. Jack told me this very morning how he had felt—worse than ever before."

And so there is self-blame, guilt feelings, and anxiety accompanying the tragedy in retrospect.

This is a time for talking. There must be group sessions for the patients with effective, therapeutic leadership. Dialogue and verbalization are essential. The atmosphere must be free and permissive. Patients need to express their thoughts and feelings—not just once, but often. These sessions should be continued until there is no evidence of further need.

And what about the personnel? Equally important, and simultaneously with the patients' discussions, there is great need for personnel to give vent to their feelings of guilt and self-blame, and to their ideas of negligence. Through being able to ventilate and to listen, members of the staff can be supportive to each other. It is during such times of great stress that people realize how much they really need and can help each other.

There really are no formulas for dealing with depression and suicide. However, Hofling states that there are three general therapeutic aims in handling depressed patients: provide protection from self-destruction until the patient is able to assume this responsibility for himself; help him to express his feelings of aggression and hostility constructively and outwardly rather than destructively turning them inward on himself; and help him achieve a more realistic and positive concept of himself so that his feelings of self-esteem, self-respect, and acceptance by others and his feelings of belonging are enhanced (6).

Nurses can build and plan for the specific nursing care needs of patients on these therapeutic aims. But each patient's specific conflicts and highly individualized needs must be kept in mind. Perhaps the most important factor in helping a suicidal patient is skill in maintaining a therapeutic relationship. The nurse lends support and protection through her sincere interest, warmth of personality, and understanding until the patient is able to manage his self-destructive urges. The genuineness of the nurse does not consist of external manifestations alone; it comes from an inner realness, a humanness revealed in a consistent flow of strength, concern, and protection.

If I were to suggest some general principles for nursing intervention in suicide proneness, they would be:

1. Know yourself—your strength, your weaknesses, your feelings, your beliefs. Know what you feel and why you feel as you do. Know how you feel about people who want to destroy themselves—people who are weak. If you have feelings and thoughts that are nonaccepting, you will surely communicate them.
2. Know your patients. Make it your business to understand them. It is not always easy to get through the wall around the patient that holds the nurse out, but the nurse should never cease trying.
3. See each patient as an individual with dignity and worth. Learn to accept him as he is, love him, and respect him. Weakness is not easily respected, but the nurse who has truly lived knows how thin is the line between weakness and fear.
4. Plan his activities to meet *his* individual needs. And, if possible, allow him to share this planning without making demands that are too great.
5. Use every free moment to communicate with patients. Patients must know that you care. Listen. Walls are not easily penetrated; gates do not open readily; it takes a great deal of *just being there,* being there at the right moment, being there when resistance cries out for help through understanding.
6. Be genuine. The patient knows if what you say is compatible with what you think and feel. A nurse cannot think and feel nonacceptance and, at the same time, communicate acceptance. She cannot dislike and at the same time make the patient believe that she cares.

This kind of care is exhausting. It drains. But this is the nurse's job. This is what psychiatric nursing is like.

REFERENCES

1. Allen, G. N. and Ellis, E. R. *Traitor Within; Our Suicide Problem.* New York, Doubleday and Co., 1961.
2. *Ibid.*
3. Meaker, M. J. *Sudden Endings.* New York, Doubleday and Co., 1964.
4. Meerloo, J. A. M. *Suicide and Mass Suicide.* New York, Grune and Stratton, 1962.
5. Appelbaum, S. A. The problem-solving aspect of suicide. *J. Project. Techn.* 27:259-268, Sept. 1963.

6. Hofling, C. K., and Leininger, Madeleine M. *Basic Psychiatric Concepts in Nursing*. Philadelphia, Pa., J. B. Lippincott Co., 1960.

BIBLIOGRAPHY

Bidder, George. Are drugs the answer in mental depression? *Amer. J. Nurs.* 61:60-63, Oct. 1961.

Hillman, James. *Suicide and the Soul*. New York, Harper and Row, 1965.

Manfreda, Marguerite L. *Psychiatric Nursing*. 7th ed. Philadelphia, Pa., F. A. Davis Co., 1964.

Matheney, Ruth V., and Topalis, Mary. *Psychiatric Nursing*. 4th ed. St. Louis, Mo., C. V. Mosby Co., 1965.

Mereness, Dorothy, and Karnosh, L. J. *Essentials of Psychiatric Nursing*. 6th ed. St. Louis, Mo., C. V. Mosby Co., 1962.

Murphy, K. B. Do they really want to die? *Today's Health* 43:48-49, 66, Apr. 1965.

Neylan, Margaret P. The depressed patient. *Amer. J. Nurs.* 61:77-78, July 1961.

Shneidman, E. S., and Farberow, N. L. *Clues to Suicide*. New York, McGraw-Hill Book Co., 1957.

St. John-Stevas, Norman. *The Right to Life*. New York, Holt, Rinehart and Winston, 1964.

Thomas, Betty J. Clues to patients' behavior. *Amer. J. Nurs.* 63:100-102, July 1963.

Vipond, Eleanor. A time for talking. *Amer. J. Nurs.* 63:111, July 1963.

26

Nurse-Doctor-Patient Relationships in Psychiatry

Melvin Sabshin*

> *We cannot deny that certain tensions arise in these relationships. By far the most important reason for recognizing and relieving them is the welfare of the patient himself.*

Traditionally, the doctor and the nurse have been pictured as an efficient team, working for the benefit of the sick patient. By and large, this is the case, but often complex strains between them lie just beneath the surface.

Recent trends in psychiatry and psychiatric nursing have led to a new look at the doctor-nurse-patient relationship. Some of these trends have been:

1. The growing predominance of therapeutic optimism in all types of psychiatric hospitals with diminished emphasis on custodial care alone.
2. The increased emphasis on milieu, or environmental, therapy and on the need for well-trained psychiatrists and psychiatric nurses to participate in such a program.
3. The rapidly increasing number of new psychiatric sections of general hospitals.
4. The increased utilization of psychotherapy on psychotic patients.

All of these trends are still in the developmental stage and the next several decades should see continued advances. The progress, however, has

---

*From *American Journal of Nursing*, Vol. 11, No. 5 (May, 1963).

Dr. Sabshin is assistant director of the Institute for Psychosomatic and Psychiatric Research and Training at Michael Reese Hospital in Chicago. He is a member of the Committee on Psychiatric Nursing of the Group for the Advancement of Psychiatry.

This paper was prepared in collaboration with two nurses at the institute: Helen Ruch, assistant director, in charge of psychiatric nursing, and Dorothy Sabolsice, day supervisor.

brought latent tension between doctors and nurses to the surface. Psychiatric patients are sensitive barometers of doctor-nurse relationships, and when tensions exist, patients tend to respond with problems of their own.

PROBLEMS INVOLVING PSYCHOTHERAPY

The increased use of psychotherapy on institutionalized psychiatric patients is one of the most important and promising current aspects of psychiatric therapy. It has the potentiality to allow patients to work through their problems and make their readjustment to the community more meaningful and successful. It follows the best traditions of medical therapy in going beyond symptomatic relief. It may seem somewhat paradoxical that such a promising development should stir up problems, but there are signs that this is happening.

The difficulties center on two fronts. First, the development of milieu therapy is also proceeding rapidly at the present time and, frequently, problems occur in attempts to integrate psychotherapy and milieu therapy. The second problem evolves from the increasing use of psychotherapy in settings where somatotherapies have been the traditional clinical treatment.

Part of the problem is an emotional one. Psychiatrists and psychiatric nurses tend to identify with certain forms of therapy and be opposed to others. The problems that stem from these identifications are among the most persistent and difficult ones to solve.

In attempting to integrate psychotherapy and milieu therapy, one basic problem that arises can be characterized as "the therapeutic hour versus the other 23 hours." The psychotherapist, focusing on what is going on between himself and the patient, often is not really interested in what is happening the rest of the day on the ward. He strongly believes that he is applying the *specific* treatment in his sessions with the patient. In this sense he feels like the surgeon who has removed an appendix as the specific curative measure for a specific illness. The surgeon's attitude is that if his postoperative orders are followed by the nursing personnel, things will go well. Most surgeons make little comment about postoperative care until something goes wrong. Strongly psychotherapeutically oriented psychiatrists often follow exactly the same procedure. They will complain about the staff if something goes wrong with a patient's treatment, but otherwise have little contact with nursing personnel.

Indeed, many psychiatrists oppose an active milieu program in which nursing, occupational and recreational therapy, and social work are part of the treatment plan. The most frequent complaint, usually voiced informally, is "everyone wants to be a therapist." I know of one psychiatrist who will not bring a patient to a psychiatric hospital with an active milieu therapy program, preferring places where there is less contact with personnel. He feels that in these circumstances the psychotherapy clearly emerges as the most important factor in the patient's life.

ISOLATION OF THE PROCESS. Many of us, however, question whether this isolation of the psychotherapeutic process is beneficial to the patient. We also question whether the model of the specific treatment for a specific illness, as in surgery, is correct for treating psychiatric patients. Distortions may occur in the therapeutic process itself unless the therapist has at least minimal awareness of what is going on the rest of the day on the unit.

Caudill has given an excellent illustration of this type of distortion (1). At one psychiatric hospital all the patients on the unit were in intensive psychotherapy. When the phonograph broke down, the patients started to talk with their doctors about their reactions to this occurrence. The set remained broken for weeks, and the patients continued to discuss it in their therapeutic sessions. The therapists, each focusing on his individual patient, began to interpret the unconscious meaning of music and how it related to other problems. When the set was repaired, however, the patients ceased talking about it and the therapists made no comments about the fact that music was no longer discussed.

Of course, the individual meaning of music has many ramifications and exploring them can be very useful, but this phonograph had many other meanings. It was often the gathering place for much meaningful group interaction on the unit. The failure to have the set repaired quickly had many implications, also. The nursing personnel were keenly aware of the situation on the unit, but they had little knowledge of what was going on in the therapeutic sessions. The doctors had little knowledge of the social implications of the phonograph. The fundamental breakdown was in the communication between the doctors and the nurses, but the doctors' relative disinterest in what was happening on the ward contributed significantly to the problem. The patients might have benefited if the therapists' interpretations had integrated the meaning of music with the specific set of circumstances.

Here is another example of the problems that develop from a concept of psychotherapy as isolated from the total ward situation. A psychotherapist worked intensively with a young, inhibited, depressed patient. It became clear in the therapeutic sessions that a nuclear problem in this case involved repression of hostility. The physician encouraged the patient to be free to express angry feelings at him during the therapeutic hours and also tacitly encouraged the expression of anger elsewhere. The patient experienced pleasure in his new ability to be more spontaneous and his behavior changed remarkably. However, he became manipulating, demanding, and somewhat destructive.

Unfortunately this change occurred at a time when the unit was already in a turmoil with a number of very difficult patients, taxing the nursing personnel to their limit. The physician had discussed this patient's case only superficially with the nursing personnel, and they had very little understanding of his new behavior patterns. These seemed to them the proverbial straw that breaks the camel's back, and the nurses responded with tension and barely suppressed anger to his new aggressivity. The patient sensed this and regressed to a state of increased guilt and depression.

In this case, the therapist acted as a "lone wolf" and induced changes which boomeranged against his patient. He acted as if the nursing personnel should always be ready to accept and tolerate any type of behavior. His concept of a psychiatric nurse was of an all-giving and all-understanding mother. In this sense psychiatrists are often like some of the people who write books on raising children. It is easy to advocate warmth, love, and unlimited toleration from a distance, but in everyday life human beings are not all-giving and all-understanding, nor should this be expected of them. The doctor sees his patient and then leaves the psychiatric unit. The nurse must live with the patient for eight hours and retain responsibility for his care over this longer time span. These very different roles lead to widely different perspectives.

Another point illustrated in this case is the necessity of understanding the current situation on the psychiatric unit. With this patient it would have been possible to encourage spontaneity and also explain the reality of the situation on the unit. Hospital treatment in which such reality is not taken into account creates tension between the doctors and the nurses, and this affects the therapeutic process.

THE PERMISSIVE-RESTRICTIVE CONFLICT. Closely related to this is a chronic difficulty which can be called the "permissive-restrictive problem." Psychiatrists often complain that psychiatric nurses are rigid, compulsive, and restrictive, that they do everything "by the rule book." Nurses in turn complain that psychiatrists are often permissive and lax, endangering their patients' security by allowing too many privileges. A favorite quote from psychiatric nurses is "I hope those psychiatrists don't raise their children without setting limits." The problem, of course, is very complex. One basic difficulty involves the psychiatrist's idea about the role of the psychiatric nurse. Many psychotherapeutically oriented psychiatrists act as if the only thing that the nurse does is spend time with his patient.

This leads to the much discussed question: what is the role of a good psychiatric nurse? I have noted, in reading statements on this subject, how often writers will list a single attribute as the main function of the nurse. Psychiatrists, especially, are apt to say simply, "The psychiatric nurse should be able to understand and tolerate psychotic behavior" or "She should be a giving mother."

There are, of course, a wide variety of alternative patterns which different nurses can utilize in functioning quite successfully in their role. This is true of members of any medical professional group. Some nurses work best in rather intensive relationships with patients while others function much better in group situations.

A colleague of mine once read another psychiatrist's prescription to the nurses, which stated that they should consistently treat this patient with warmth and tender loving care. My colleague remarked tersely, "What if they don't love the patient?" He was saying, in effect, that this type of psychiatric order often is unrealistic. Nurses differ greatly in personality. Some psychiatric nurses function best as leaders or administrators. Others need the opportunity to carry out various combinations of managerial and therapeutic functions.

The role of the nurse is much broader, and yet much more poorly defined, than that of the psychiatrist. When the psychiatrist focuses on psychotherapy, his place is even more clearly demarcated. He has spent many years training for psychotherapeutic work. The role of the psychiatric nurse, however, may include not only working intensively with patients, but also managerial duties, administering medications, playing mother and big sister, being a teacher, and so on. Attempts are being made now to define these functions more sharply. For example, the psychiatric nursing committee of the Group for the Advancement of Psychiatry has attempted to clarify aspects of the psychiatric nurse's role (2). My impression is that, at the present time, any definition of the psychiatric nurse's role should involve recognition of her many different types and areas of functions. Too much emphasis on any one function seems premature and unwise.

THE "NURSE-PATIENT SYNDROME." One type of difficulty can be found in what Stanton and Schwartz have called the "nurse-patient syndrome" (3). In this situation a nurse takes special interest in a particular patient on a psychiatric unit. She spends increasing amounts of time with this patient and begins to pay less attention to her other duties. Other nursing personnel begin to react negatively to this development and criticize her, either overtly or secretly. She becomes defensive and soon makes errors of judgment because of her need to justify her role with the patient. Tension increases and the patient often suffers because hostility is displaced to him. A common result of this type of difficulty is the resignation of the nurse.

I have observed that this type of behavior is often encouraged by a psychiatrist. Thus, the chain of events may start because a nurse likes a special doctor, and wishes to do something extra for a patient of his. On the other hand, a nurse may become unusually involved with a patient because of hostile or competitive feelings with the therapist. One of the key errors in this situation is the omission of other ward duties. The nurse must have good working relationships with other nurses if she is to be able to help the patient, and psychiatrists often forget this. The example highlights the point that the nurse must be more than a therapist and has many *group* functions.

DIFFERENCES IN THERAPEUTIC PHILOSOPHY. Many of the changes in the use of somatotherapies are giving rise to problems in doctor-nurse relationships. At some hospitals there is considerable difference of opinion regarding the indications for the new tranquilizing drugs. Occasionally nurses feel that the psychiatrist is too slow in ordering daytime sedation. Or the reverse may occur, and nursing personnel may show considerable resistance to the use of shock and drug therapy.

Another important problem in doctor-nurse-patient interaction relates most closely to the remarkable expansion of psychiatric sections of general hospitals, and involves status and hierarchy. Hamburg has pointed out that in most general hospitals the social structure tends to be quite authoritarian (4). The physicians are at the top of the hierarchical pyramid and nurses are considerably lower. Decisions made at the top are expected to be carried out by those in the lower echelons, who have had no part in making them. Patients are considered very passive individuals without any role in policy-making. The psychiatric section of the general hospital usually follows the same routines and pattern of social relationships as the rest of the hospital. The kind of psychiatric treatment possible under such an arrangement is certainly open to question.

PROBLEMS INVOLVING STATUS. It is paradoxical that the people at the lower end of the echelon have the closest and most sustained contact with the patient. There is danger that they may act out on their patients the tensions they feel regarding the authoritarian structure. Of course, status barriers exist in all psychiatric hospitals, not just in psychiatric sections of general hospitals. Stainbrook has illustrated this by showing that at psychiatric clinical conferences high-ranking doctors speak the most, residents less, nurses still less, and so on down to aides who hardly talk at all (5). There are definite inhibitions against crossing status barriers freely and speaking one's mind in the formal setting. What is said informally is another matter.

In hospitals which emphasize milieu therapy, there is a tendency to cut across these lines and allow all levels of staff and patients to participate in decision-making. In psychiatric sections of general hospitals, it is much more difficult to alter the status barriers, which are often deeply ingrained in the medical and surgical sections. This frequently presents a dilemma to the mature psychiatric nurse. She wants to be respectful towards the physician, but she also wants to take an active part in the therapeutic program. In addition, she wants the physician's attitude to communicate that he has genuine respect for her as an individual and as a professional person. Psychiatric nursing education makes her aware of the fact that her own conscious and unconscious reactions to rigid lines and lack of respect for her can affect her work with patients.

These problems are by no means unique to the psychiatric unit. In recent years it has become more obvious that doctor-nurse tensions can affect the medical and surgical care of patients. Nursing personnel may displace emotional reactions towards patients if the social structure of the hospital permits no other outlet. Patients hospitalized for medical and surgical illnesses may be given a minimum of information. Frightened and lonely, they may complain that the hospital atmosphere is cold and impersonal.

There has been a growing tendency to broaden decision-making in general hospitals and promote the participation of more personnel. One technique has been to create committees in which there can be free discussion of problems. The results indicate that this type of expression makes for a more effectively administered hospital.

The way clinical conferences are conducted is often a good indication of the types of social relationships in the hospital. At one extreme are clinical conferences from which everyone is excluded except the doctors. In these situations the hierarchy is strongly maintained. At the other extreme are nursing care conferences in which all personnel join in the discussion of a patient's care. There are many variations between these extremes.

Psychiatrists often claim that they are too busy to spend time discussing their cases with nursing personnel. Yet a few moments of discussion may save a great deal of time in the long run. For example, one therapist discussed his vacation plans in some detail with the nursing personnel. He indicated the ways in which the patient would become anxious and suggested techniques that could be used in each situation.

The threatened resident. Problems frequently arise between nurses and new psychiatric residents. The resident often feels inadequate and realizes that he knows much less than the experienced psychiatric nurse. A conflict arises between his desire to learn and the need to follow the hierarchy system which implies that "doctors know more than nurses in all situations." He becomes very defensive and has to pretend to know things that he may not really understand. One of his defenses may be to use complex terminology which he has learned from his psychiatric reading. Another defense frequently used by young psychiatrists is making interpretations about the behavior of the nurses.

Experienced psychiatric nurses are aware of this reaction and have adjusted to it over the years. As the psychiatric resident advances in experience, he usually becomes more relaxed and doesn't have to use such methods of coping with the situation. Unfortunately, however, even some senior psychiatrists occasionally use these techniques in relating to nurses. Psychiatry is still in an exploratory stage, and relative ignorance tends to put the psychiatrist in a position where he often finds it difficult to admit that he does not know the answer to questions. This realization is a frightening experience for nurses, too, and many have to deny its reality. For others, the mistakes of the psychiatrists become an area upon which to displace a great deal of hostility.

SOME POSSIBLE SOLUTIONS

Thus far, we have been pointing out problems, giving only brief mention to possible solutions. Now I would like to focus more sharply on some suggested solutions. Most of the following discussion is based on the ideas of Hamburg (4).

The solutions involve the following three major areas: 1) techniques of recognizing tension points in doctor-nurse-patient interaction; 2) roles of the doctor, nurse, and patient in matters concerning hospital policy-making; 3) implications for hospital administration.

At the present time it is inevitable that some tension will arise in doctor-nurse-patient interaction. At one psychiatric hospital it was claimed that the interpersonal interaction was excellent, but there was a remarkably high turnover of psychiatric nurses. In that hospital there was a great deal of informal complaining about hospital policy, but there were no channels to express the complaints constructively.

Nurses and doctors often use informal channels of communication to discuss problems. Many hospital administrators rely on the "hospital scuttlebutt" for information. Relying on informal communication alone is dangerous, however, since information gets distorted in these channels and useful action is often impossible in such situations.

There should be *consistent* communication channels within the hospital structure so that problems can be aired. These channels must extend to every group within the hospital—and this includes patients. Such factors as the size of the hospital and type of patient treated alter the form that the communication process takes. Obviously there will be differences between a state mental hospital with 7500 beds and a 10-bed single unit in a general hospital. Nevertheless, certain common principles can be applied.

A key factor in this process is the attitude of the people in high administrative positions. They must give genuine encouragement to the open expression of difficulties and tensions. Their inability really to listen to criticism will block the process entirely and will lead merely to a downward flow of orders through the communication channel.

More subtle difficulties arise with the administrator who needs to have his personnel admire him consistently. He creates a feeling that he will be personally hurt if everyone is not happy. Tensions cannot be aired in such an atmosphere either.

OPEN CHANNELS OF COMMUNICATION. Among the things that have been done at some hospitals, including ours, to maintain a consistent flow of useful information are these:

1. The patients meet as a group on every unit each week to discuss ward problems. These meetings are conducted by the unit resident, but the head nurse and the nursing supervisor attend also.

2. Staff psychotherapists, including residents, and private attending psychiatrists are encouraged to relay information from their patients regarding the functioning of the hospital to members of the administration. Thus information relevant to hospital policy, obtained in therapeutic sessions, can be channelled into constructive use.

3. Psychiatric residents have been assigned as "unit physicians" with the coordination of various treatment efforts as their prime function. The resident serves as the key communication link between the private attending psychiatrist and the nursing personnel. He works closely with both groups and is familiar with the day-to-day situation on the unit. The nurses at our hospital report that this has been very helpful to them. One of them commented that by being in the situation, the resident has a better understanding of problems which exist there. He can be there to listen to the problems of personnel and give support. He also serves as another person who can contact the attending physician in the event the nurse is not successful.

We strongly suggest that a resident be assigned to each hospital unit; if no residents are available an attempt should be made to find an adequate substitute.

4. Having an administrative person to coordinate the functions on a number of units is also helpful. This must be someone sensitive to problems who allows free expression of difficulties. At our hospital the coordinator has weekly meetings with the staff on each unit, during which the focus is on difficult management problems. Intrastaff difficulties can frequently rise to the surface and be acted upon at such meetings. A common area for discussion is the integration of the treatment needs for a particular patient and the welfare of the unit as a whole. For example, if three manic patients are on a small unit at the same time, it may be necessary to sedate them heavily because of the effect of their behavior on other patients, as well as on the staff. With only one manic patient, more individual attention is often possible and less heavy sedation may be required.

5. The nursing administrators and the psychiatric administrators should meet regularly. Here again emphasis should be on sensitivity to problem areas so that they can be acted on before they reach crisis proportions.

Communication and the recognition of tension points have little meaning unless they are followed by reasonable solutions. The most constructive methods to achieve such solutions involve broadening participation in decision-making processes. There are some decisions which can be made on the ward level. Others involve larger sections of the hospital, while some decisions involve the entire hospital's relation to the community.

WIDER PARTICIPATION IN DECISION MAKING. Wider participation on all levels of decision making raises staff morale and tends to decrease tension and feelings of noninvolvement. The extent of the patients' role varies at different hospitals. Some, like the Boston Psychopathic Hospital, have organized patient government (6). At others the patients are active participants without a structured patient government. Still others see the patients as passive nonparticipants.

At our hospital we have organized a "hospital policy committee." This is an interdisciplinary committee on which every group of full-time staff members dealing with patients is represented—nurses, aides, resident psychiatrists, attending psychiatrists, social workers, occupational therapists, and dietitians. This committee, meeting biweekly with one of the members of the administration as chairman, makes most of the major policy decisions for the psychiatric section. It deals with problems that involve more than one unit or more than one discipline. Its decisions are subject to review by the hospital director, but are rarely changed by him. Except for a few permanent representatives, members of this committee serve six months and are then replaced by others of their own group. In this way there is widespread participation.

Some of the issues discussed by the hospital policy committee have been: 1) the admission procedure; 2) the security policy on the hospital units; 3) criteria for placement of patients on the various hospital units; 4) plans for a new unit; 5) policies concerning the ordering of sedation for patients. After the committee makes recommendations on a particular issue, it also attempts to follow through on them, using the appropriate channels.

IMPLICATIONS FOR HOSPITAL ADMINISTRATION. In considering these implications, we must recognize first that we don't know all the answers in the field of hospital psychiatry, although there are some promising developments on the horizon. Smugness and dogmatism have little place in our field. The medical and nursing professions are both grappling with serious problems in regard to role definition. They are also re-evaluating the goals of therapy in psychiatry. There are, and there will continue to be, complex tensions in this period of working out better techniques to treat the patient.

It is important for hospital administration to be cognizant of these problems and to help provide an atmosphere where they can be discussed reasonably and with mutual respect.

With this kind of openness it will be possible over the coming years to make a better evaluation of psychotherapy, milieu therapy, and the somatotherapies in the treatment of the hospitalized patient. It will also be possible for the new trends to advance with minimum tension between doctors and nurses.

REFERENCES

1. Caudill, W., and others. Social structure and interaction processes on a psychiatric ward. Am. J. Orthopsychiat. 22:314-334, April 1952.
2. Group for Advancement of Psychiatry, Committee on Psychiatric Nursing. Therapeutic Use of the Self. (Report No. 33) Topeka, Kan., Group for Advancement of Psychiatry, 1955.

3. Stanton, A. H., and Schwartz, M. S. *The Mental Hospital.* New York, Basic Books, 1954.
4. Hamburg, D. A. *Therapeutic Aspects of Communication, Decision Making and Administrative Policy.* Presented at the Conference on Socio-Environmental Aspects of Treatment of Patients in Mental Hospitals, sponsored by the U.S. Public Health Service and the Harvard Medical School at Boston, Mass., Dec. 1955.
5. Stainbrook, Edward. Human action in the social system of the psychiatric hospital. In *Better Social Services for Mentally Ill Patients,* edited by Ruth I. Knee. New York, American Association of Psychiatric Social Workers, 1955, pp. 19-26.
6. Hyde, R. W., and Solomon, H. C. Patient government: a new form of group therapy. *Digest Neurol. and Psychiat.* 18:207-218, April 1950.

Section 4

Developing the Nurse's Therapeutic Roles

27

Reassurance

Dorothy E. Gregg*

We see the phrase, "Reassure the patient," in every nursing procedure. What does it really mean?

A nurse walked into a patient's room and found her looking very forlorn and upset. This was their conversation.

Nurse: Oh, come now, Mrs. Carson, nothing could be that bad! You look like you have lost your last friend!

Patient: The doctor just told me that it will be impossible for me to get well if I don't have the operation. I'm so mixed up—I wish I knew what to do.

Nurse: There is only one thing to do, and that is to have the surgery! You haven't a thing to worry about. You have the best surgeon in town. He has done hundreds of operations just like yours.

Patient: You don't understand—I have confidence in my doctor's skill—it's—well—.

Nurse: Most people are a little scared when they think about having an operation. Remember when you had your first baby several years ago while I was working on OB? You had the longest and hardest labor of anyone on the ward, and I never heard a whimper out of you! I was so proud of you! You were the best patient in the whole hospital! After what you went through, this operation should be a picnic, and this time you'll be completely unconscious from the anesthetic. You won't feel a thing.

During this conversation the nurse probably was sincere in her desire to reassure the patient, but she was not aware of what constitutes reassurance.

---

*From *American Journal of Nursing*, Vol. 55, No. 2 (February, 1955).

Miss Gregg (B.S., University of Colorado School of Nursing; M.A., Teachers College, Columbia) is coordinator of psychiatric nursing and mental hygiene at the University of Colorado School of Nursing.

She may not even discover that she has failed, but she will probably wonder why the patient talked more freely to someone else than she did to her. If we attempt to see how the patient felt in this conversation, maybe we can make some guesses about what she experienced.

Mrs. Carson's reaction to the nurse's first comment might have been: *I feel very upset, and she can see that I am upset. Why does she say, "nothing could be that bad?" How could she possibly know? And losing friends has nothing to do with how I feel. This is worse than losing friends—what a silly remark!*

Such clichés frequently are used socially to reduce the danger of an unwanted "scene" and to preserve social equanimity. What happens most often is that they reduce the importance of the other person's feelings. In this situation they failed to convey to the patient that the nurse understood the concern that she has perceived in the patient. Webster defines reassurance as a "restoration of confidence." There was little in this opening to the conversation that restored Mrs. Carson's confidence.

The patient's feelings about the nurse's second comment might have been: *I tried to tell her that I was mixed up. It is hard for me to explain to another person how I feel, and she didn't even let me finish! Maybe she doesn't care how I feel. Now she thinks I am frightened about the operation. I guess she wouldn't know what it's like to be afraid of something bigger than an operation! She tells me there is only one thing to do—if life were only that simple! Why does she have to tell me what to do? I didn't ask for that! What does she mean—"I haven't anything to worry about"? I wonder what she would do if she had my little boy? She doesn't even know what I'm worried about! Maybe that's it—maybe she doesn't want to know—maybe she is afraid to know. I guess I really shouldn't bother other people with this. No one could possibly understand how I feel. What is this about the surgeon? Does she think my doctor isn't good enough? Why else would she be so eager to tell me he is good? I have confidence in him—well—I think I have—.*

This is one possible outcome of jumping ahead of a patient's expression of her feelings and guessing at what she is trying to say. The guess can easily be wrong and, furthermore, it conveys that the patient is not important enough to the nurse for her to care what the patient has to say. A second error in the nurse's approach was that she immediately started telling the patient what to do. This action was based on the assumption that the patient couldn't make a decision for herself and that she wished the nurse to make it for her. Erroneously, the nurse believed that she was helping the patient when she told her what to do.

In addition, in an attempt to allay unknown fears, she made another guess that the patient was not sure of her doctor's skill, and in so doing, she was in danger of creating doubt. If the nurse is fortunate, the patient may be able to perceive that the nurse is anxious and has made a false assumption regarding her own fears, but there is the possibility that an anxiety-ridden patient may not be capable of such perception at the moment, so she takes the cue from the nurse to worry about her surgeon's skill.

Regarding the nurse's third response, the patient may have felt: *She didn't let me finish—she must think I am stupid because I can't talk without stumbling over my words. There she goes on about the operation again. She just can't understand! There is just no point in talking with her! What is this about the way I behaved at the birth of my baby? If she only knew—I was so scared I couldn't whimper—but she was proud of me! That very baby is my biggest problem! What is she saying? Does she mean good patients don't cry? I guess I'm supposed to be brave and silent, and here I am telling her about being so mixed up! Is she afraid I'll make a scene? Oh, what's the use? How could anyone understand about John? She says I won't feel a thing—maybe I won't—maybe I really won't!*

Twice the patient tried to express to the nurse how she felt and as she hesitated and searched for words, the nurse became anxious and guessed at her problem, thereby cutting off the patient's chance to talk about what was bothering her. The nurse further expressed her own anxiety when she un-wittingly told the patient how she expected her to behave by holding her past performance up to her as an example of behaving as a "good" patient should. She also conveyed disrespect for the patient in her present disturbance by telling her that the coming episode would be "a picnic." The implication was that she blamed the patient for her present distressed behavior. It is rarely comforting to an anxiety-ridden person to be told that she will be unconscious, for in her apprehension, she may look upon this as simply another situation in which she will be "out of control."

Later in the day, another nurse entered the same patient's room to prepare her for the night. Mrs. Carson smiled a greeting, but initiated no further conversation. She seemed preoccupied, and her face was tearstained. The nurse began to rub her back.

Nurse: It seems hard for you to relax tonight. You must have had a difficult day.

Patient: Yes.

(silence)

Nurse: Would you like to tell me about it?

Patient: It would seem silly to you. It's so hard to explain—. If I thought I could make it home, I would leave—. No one understands.

Nurse: I would like to try to understand if it will help you.

Patient: They say I have to have an operation, and I'm so scared and mixed up. They think it's the operation that scares me, but—oh, well—I don't know how you could understand. I'm such a mess!

(silence)

Nurse: It's hard to talk about it.

Patient: Yes—if I weren't around maybe he could get someone who would really help John. I just don't have the patience any more—maybe I never did! (pause)

Nurse: Could you tell me who John is, and who could get someone else?

Patient: John is my oldest child. He has cerebral palsy. He is a sweet little boy but he needs so much care, and you have to be so patient with him, and I'm just not. Since I've been sick we haven't been able to send him to his special school. My medical bills stand in the way of his chances to get help, and when he is home all the time—well—I guess I get impatient with his troubles, and I'm always scolding when I know he can't help it. My husband has the burden of both of us. He is so kind to the boy, and so patient with me. They would both be better off without me. I shouldn't have the operation.

Nurse: Are you saying that you may not live if you don't have the operation and that this would be better for John and your husband?

Patient: The doctor said I can't expect to live long without surgery. (thoughtful silence) I guess I really am silly—that would be kind of like suicide, wouldn't it? (crying) Now you know how mixed up I am! I guess I am a little crazy—worrying about John and the money and everything. (sobbing)

Nurse: (hands patient a handkerchief): It's such a tough problem that you would just like to escape from it.

Patient: Yes, but I don't really want to die. I can't really say that my husband would be better off if I died. He would be all alone with our little boy. What a coward I am! What would he do all alone? And Johnny—he needs me even if I'm not much of a mother. If I just knew what to do! If I could just be patient like other mothers!

Nurse: All mothers get angry and impatient with their children sometimes.

Patient: I do get angry at the other children, but I don't feel so bad when I jump on them.

Nurse: It's more difficult with John, because he has special problems.

Patient: Yes. I feel so helpless with John. I guess if I knew how to work with him better I wouldn't be so impatient.

Nurse: There is a specially trained person on our staff who works with children with cerebral palsy. She might be helpful to you and John, and if you feel you would like to talk with her, it can be arranged.

Patient: Yes, I would. I used to talk with John's teacher, and that helped a lot, but since he hasn't been in school I haven't seen her. We must get him back in school soon. We will have to borrow money for the operation; that is why his schooling has to wait. I wish there were some way to pay for both at the same time.

Nurse: There are also people on our staff who are trained to help with financial problems. Maybe one of them could help you make a payment plan for your operation so it would not be such a burden to you.

Patient: Could my husband and I both talk to them before I have the operation? I would want him to see the person with me.

In this conversation, the nurse recognized the patient's distress, as the nurse in the first episode did. Contrary to the way her colleague responded, however, she did not derogate the patient by making light of her feelings. She made an opening for the patient to communicate her distress, which the discouraged patient fenced off by a simple "Yes."

The nurse's next question, "Would you like to tell me about it?" opened further the opportunity for the patient to speak. To be helpful, this question would have to reflect the nurse's sincere interest and warmth for the patient. If it were a curious probe without real interest in understanding the patient better, the patient would probably be able to detect it as such. This is only one of several similar kinds of openings. For example, one might use, "Tell me what happened," or further identification of feelings might be attempted to encourage expression, such as, "It must have been pretty upsetting." The nurse observed that the patient had a need to talk with someone, but at this point she needed a little help to feel that the nurse would actually accept her.

Next, the nurse attempted to convey to the patient that she wanted to try to understand her, even though the patient thought that it was impossible. The patient gave three clues to the fact that it would be difficult for her to feel accepted enough to talk about her problem: (1) she expected nurses to think that her distress was silly; (2) she said that her feelings were hard to explain; and (3) she wished to escape the whole issue by going home. The nurse made the inference that the patient's confidence might begin to be restored if she could be assisted to work out her problem for herself. The nurse's second inference was that the patient might experience further distress, perhaps to the point of devastation, if she were allowed to escape from working with her difficulties.

The patient's first step in having a successful experience in problem-solving is to feel accepted and understood, so she can feel free to talk about all the facets of her problems in order to view them clearly in making her decisions. The nurse created a feeling of acceptance by what she said and did as she listened to her. By listening with sincere interest, by identifying the feelings that the patient was expressing and by seeking clarification when meanings were not clear to her, the nurse conveyed that she was trying to understand.

The nurse's statement, "It is hard to talk about it," was an attempt to identify and accept the patient's feeling of half-wanting and half-notwanting to talk "it" over, and to show that she accepted the turmoil that the patient felt.

As the patient started to work with her problem, she made opening statements that were not quite clear. When the nurse sought clarification by asking, "Could you tell me who John is. . . ?" she accomplished two things. First she conveyed that she was really interested in knowing exactly what was being said, and secondly, she helped the patient communicate more clearly. Issues sometimes can be perceived more adequately as they are described to another person. If the factors involved in a problem are clear, accurate identification of the problem is possible.

The nurse's question, "Are you saying that you may not live. . . ?" was also a clarification maneuver, using a slightly different method. The nurse picked up something the patient said and tried to help her re-examine it to see if she really meant what she was saying. There are a variety of clarification-seeking responses that might have been used. For instance, "What do you mean?" or "Why shouldn't you have the operation?"

When one uses any "helping measure" there is the possibility that he is using it to serve his own purpose rather than that of the person he is helping. If the nurse uses a clarification maneuver to help the patient look at her meanings more clearly and use her own resources to reformulate her concepts, the patient experiences a feeling of confidence that comes when a problem is successfully resolved. However, if the nurse uses the clarification maneuver to achieve a sense of power in manipulating the patient and thus to raise her own feeling of prestige, her patient may feel foolish for approaching her difficulties as she did. She will not be reassured about her own strength, but she may feel more helpless and inadequate than she did before, and become more anxious and less able to solve her problems rationally.

Within an accepting relationship, a patient is able to take the next step in problem-solving. Mrs. Carson took a second look at what her death would mean. As she realized somewhat more clearly what she had been thinking, she became self-condemnatory. She expressed her feeling through crying and by saying that she was "mixed up" and "crazy." The nurse's behavior conveyed that it is all right for her to feel and act upset. She sympathetically realized with her that hers was a difficult situation. This acceptance made it possible for the patient to explore and express her feelings further, and perhaps to uncover more facets of the problem.

The nurse made several responses that identified the patient's feelings. This helped the patient look at the feeling herself and identify what she actually felt. Secondly, they helped her realize that the nurse saw the feelings too, and did not dislike her or blame her for having them. Thirdly, the nurse identified feelings that Mrs. Carson had in common with other mothers which helped her realize that she was not an unusual, bizarre, or bad person. In other words, these responses conveyed to the patient that the nurse could accept what she was saying and understand what she was feeling. This made it possible for the patient to look at her feelings more realistically and to express some of her other feelings that were difficult for her to accept.

The nurse would be of little value to her patient if her role stopped here. The purpose of exploring and examining feelings is to help the patient see how they relate to her problem and to make it possible for her to identify her problem. Mrs. Carson identified her problem as being an indaquate mother to a child with special needs. As she was helped to express and clarify her feelings, she replaced her nonrational thinking of death as a solution with a more constructive approach. She began to consider making plans for the care of her child with the assistance of someone else, and she began to take steps to work out her financial problems.

Talking things over is helpful only if new insights are gained, insights that were not present when the situation was being mulled over alone. The nurse uses techniques in her interpersonal relationship that convey acceptance, ask for clarification, and identify feelings and issues to help her patient get all of the parts of a problem examined. This examination includes a survey of the facets that make up the problem, identification of the problem, the choice of possible solutions, and the recognition of factors that are involved in possible outcomes. Whether a problem is great or small, the nurse's role is not to make choices for the patient, but to help him arrive at a solution after considering all the factors involved.

To return to Webster's definition that reassurance is "a restoration of confidence," a patient experiences this restoration when his "mixed-up" and indecisive feelings disappear and his thinking becomes clearer. He can then discard the nonrational solutions made in panic and begin to work toward a realistic outcome.

Frequently the patient will need the aid of specially trained persons to deal with certain problems or facets of problems. The nurse needs to know who is available on the health team and in what ways other services can be useful to patients. She also needs to interpret these services skillfully to the patient. Concrete help, such as finding a resource person to help with a financial problem, is not always a part of the reassuring process. Also, one cannot assume that simply referring a patient to a source of aid suffices as a reassuring experience, for it does not replace the necessary emotional reassurance.

Essentially, then, the technique of giving is very difficult to separate from the total interpersonal process of the nurse-patient relationship. In the examples we have cited of nurses' conversations with patients, we have suggested that patients feel reassured when they are helped to use their own skills to work with problems that seem overwhelming at the outset. Patients probably feel reassured when someone is willing to listen and to value them as persons, accepting what they say without condemning them for expressing what they feel. As a part of this, there is probably a feeling of reassurance when a patient feels that the nurse's actions, feelings, and words indicate her respect for him.

There are other elements in the problem of reassuring people that command our attention. There are times when a person is so anxious that reasonable problem-solving is not possible at the moment. Reassurance for this person requires a different approach. In moments of great apprehension it is usually comforting not to be left alone. A child is comforted by the calm presence of his mother when he runs to her terrified, and finds that the terror is not duplicated in her. As the mother comforts the child by holding him and saying she will not allow him to be hurt, his terror is reduced, and eventually he begins to talk about the experience that frightened him; thus the problem-solving process begins. This is similar to many situations with adult patients. During labor or just before electrotherapy or surgery, for example, the adult experiences reassurance by having someone with him whom he knows and trusts. The reassuring person may be a member of the patient's family, a friend, or a churchman; in the hospital, this person is often one of the members of the health team—most frequently, the nurse.

Correcting a false expectation or a misconception by giving correct information can be a reassuring measure if the patient has an opportunity to discuss the issue adequately with someone he trusts. A patient's apparent efforts to seek information are not always an attempt to get the facts, however. For example, when a patient who is about to have an electrotherapy treatment asks the nurse, "How many patients die from this?" he is usually not seeking a factual answer. More likely, this is a "front" question that tests to see if the nurse will respond with understanding. Behind this "front" the patient may be feeling, "I'm afraid I am going to die, and I need to tell you how afraid I am!" If the nurse responds with a factual answer, she conveys that she does not understand his underlying fear, and the patient will usually refrain from pushing the matter further. She has not given the patient the opportunity to express his feeling, and what she expected to be reassuring has become a blocking measure. On the other hand, when information is needed but is withheld, a situation is produced that is far from reassuring. A patient experiences reassurance when he is given authentic information, by someone he trusts, when he needs it.

Reassurance is also experienced when a limit that is reasonable is set with fairness. There are always a few necessary limitations on one's behavior, at any age and in any situation. In illness, patients are sometimes unable to set their own limits without help. It is reassuring to a psychiatric patient when a nurse enforces a limit that prevents him from damaging himself or others. It is reassuring to a patient when the nurse sets some necessary limitations on the behavior of those around him as, for example, when she observes that visitors are disturbing to him, and tactfully helps them terminate their visit. It is also reassuring to a patient to be oriented to the limitations and the expectations of the hospital setting.

A patient is reassured by his trust in those who are in the "helping" role—trust in both their interpersonal and functional abilities. The patient observes the nurse's competence in administering technical procedures and hygienic measures, and when he perceives that these are done well, he is reassured. He is aware of the clinical and administrative judgments that concern him directly and indirectly. When he feels that competent people are making these judgments, he is reassured. Verbal reassurance cannot substitute for functional competence, nor for sincerity and warmth of feeling toward people.

It is not uncommon to hear professional people attempting to reassure patients with the social "bromides," such as, "Everything is going to be all right" and "There is no reason to worry." These are of little value to a person in trouble. They are false reassurance because they lack a rational operating principle and do not provide the opportunity for the person to experience reassurance. The urgings to "cheer up" or "buck up" are equally useless to the person in distress. Another kind of false reassurance, the frank falsification or lie, can be quite devastating when the patient discovers the falsehood.

A common misconception is that it helps to change the subject when a patient starts to talk about something that is disturbing, either to himself or to the listener. This maneuver only prevents the patient from working a problem through, and it betrays the listener's lack of acceptance. A similar measure is to stay away from, or leave, patients who are upset, in order to avoid a "scene." In this situation, the patient experiences isolation and loneliness; he is rarely reassured.

Reassurance involves all of nursing. It is an element of every procedure and every personal contact with patients. Its effectiveness depends on a basic philosophy of respect for another person. Reassurance is experienced by a patient when he finds that he is respected and understood by the nurse who assists him to recognize and develop his own resources and thereby restore his confidence in himself.

[In preparing this paper, Miss Gregg consulted Ewald W. Busse, M.D., Chairman, Department of Psychiatry, Duke University School of Medicine, and Betty Van Huben, Instructor in Psychiatric Nursing, University of Colorado School of Nursing; she acknowledges their help.]

28

The Psychiatric Nurse's Role

Dorothy E. Gregg*

The work of the psychiatric nurse is to help create an environment in which the patient will have an opportunity to develop new behavior patterns, to examine his beliefs with a new perspective, and to work on his problems with new capacities.

The work of the psychiatric nurse is to help create an environment in which the patient will have an opportunity to develop new behavior patterns that will enable him to make a more mature adjustment to life. This change in behavior is a growth process in which the patient learns through his experiences with others to examine his beliefs with a new perspective and to work with his problems with new capacities.

If we assume that recovery from mental illness is essentially a growth process, then the kinds of experience through which growth may take place must be provided in the ward life of the hospitalized patient. Skilled persons within the patient's environment must be able to detect the kinds of experiences he needs and to create them in ways that he can use them with his capacity to function at the moment. We assume that the accomplishment of each task opens the possibility that a more advanced task can be met (1). Through this process, the patient gradually accomplishes the tasks that allow him to mature.

These learning experiences take place within the patient's relationships with people, and therefore our focus is on the interpersonal relationships in his environment. We are interested in the interaction between people and how interpersonal relationships can be used to extend the therapeutic process to the patient's life in the ward. The goal is to help him work through his

---

*From *American Journal of Nursing*, Vol. 54, No. 7 (July, 1954).

problems by providing learning experiences that give him new tools and a new perspective with which to meet them.

This orientation is different from another kind of ward environment in which the emphasis is on helping the patient conform to accepted social behavior by keeping him occupied with activities and routines that are planned to keep him in touch with the familiar patterns of daily living. The goal in this orientation is to try to make reality more desirable than illness with the hope that he will choose the former. This type of environment has value, but it is somewhat limited.

There is a third kind of ward environment in which the patient is merely confined for a course of psychiatric treatment or for custodial care. The goal here seems to be to provide a protected living area for the patient.

THERAPEUTIC ENVIRONMENT

Our concern is with the first kind of ward in which the environment is a part of the therapeutic program. In the therapeutic ward, first, the patient is allowed to express conflict; second, the staff tries to understand him and his problems; and third, there is an opportunity for interpersonal relationships in which the patient may test his beliefs and possibly change some of them through experiential learning.

If the hospital ward is to be a place in which the patient can express conflict, it must be free from unnecessary limitations, inhibiting routines, and attitudes that prevent freedom of expression. The interpersonal environment should offer the patient the experience of being accepted and respected as a person in his own right, with the freedom to talk out his problems and act out his conflicts—within the limits of safety and group living—without censure or sanction. Such an environment allows him to communicate his feelings, to examine his thoughts and actions, and to make choices and test out solutions to his problems. As communication is established with the patient, some understandings are possible, his needs can be recognized, and provisions to help him meet them can begin to be made.

GROUP PLANNING. Group planning by the psychiatric team is required to create a therapeutic environment and to work out a consistent approach that is in accord with the psychiatrist's goals in therapy. Close working relationships should be developed among all of the psychiatric workers who are in contact with the patient. Group participation serves several purposes: (a) workers have the opportunity to share observations and compare notes on the patient's responses to various situations; (b) cues to the patient's patterns of behavior and kinds of responses to people can be picked up from these shared observations that are useful in ascertaining the patient's needs; (c) the group can formulate ways to help meet the patient's needs and plan the learning experiences he might require for emotional growth; and (d) the workers can plan how their interpersonal relationships might be used to structure these experiences.

The group has another important function. Group meetings offer an opportunity for each member of the staff to discuss his relationship with the patient and possibly to gain insight into some of the interaction between himself and the patient that may be taking place outside of his awareness. Inferences can be made from these discussions on how the relationship is used by the patient and by the team member, and how the behavior of the team member might be changed or modified to effect a change in the patient's behavior. This kind of group work requires mutual respect and acceptance, and freedom to express feelings and ideas within the group.

Group planning might be developed in a variety of ways; the method chosen would depend on the type of ward unit in which the group works. The team membership also would vary according to the kinds of personnel working in the ward unit, and the kind of teamwork that is planned. Psychiatrists, nurses, social workers, psychologists, psychiatric aides, occupational and recreational therapists, and others who work with the patient might all be members of the team.

A system of interlocking teams may be useful. People who are working closely with the patient would be on the first team and would plan the therapeutic program. Members of this team would join allied teams to communicate information to and from personnel working in other divisions or on other shifts. In large units, it might be expedient to have ward group conferences for all workers, and to have the planning for small groups of patients or individual patients centered in small teams operating within the large group. If interlocking groups are used, it is important to have free communication between them.

There are many problems in establishing a group approach of this kind. It is not easy for people with different orientations and different kinds of training and competencies to work closely together. There has been much enthusiasm lately about the team approach, but it is hard to raise our concept of the team beyond the horse and buggy stage in which every team has a driver. Truly collaborative teamwork is difficult to achieve, but if we can approximate it on the psychiatric ward, we have a valuable therapeutic tool with which to shape changes in the social patterns of ward life. As a team develops, it is also a positive educational device for those taking part in it. It can be used as an inservice teaching group to help members who need further training.

THE NURSES'S ROLE. If the ward is to become a place in which the patient experiences therapeutic learning, the psychiatric nurse must have interpersonal skills that enable her to work with the patient in these learning experiences. In many units, the nurse is now expected to be mainly an observer who records and verbally reports her observations to the psychiatrist and others. She is expected to provide a safe living area for the patient and to give him things to do that help him socialize. Her focus is to encourage the patient to drop his symptoms and adopt the accepted patterns of behavior through conforming to the social patterns of the ward.

In fostering a change that involves experiential learning rather than mere conforming, the nurse's goal changes. She assures a more active role of interaction with the patient. Hildegard Peplau outlines the nurse's function as that of a participant-observer who makes inferences from her observations and who intervenes in behavior patterns (1). As the nurse works with the patient she questions: What is the patient saying with his behavior? What is he trying to communicate to me? What are his needs? How do my responses affect his behavior? What kinds of experiences with people does he need? How can I use my interpersonal relationship with him to help him learn? How can experiences in the ward life be used to help him?

With this approach, the nurse is still an observer and she still communicates her observations to other members of the therapeutic team, but she also uses her observations and makes judgments in determining how to help the patient use his relationship with her to foster emotional growth. Some of the judgments affecting her relationship with the patient may be made collaboratively with other team members, and some she makes alone. For example, she may observe that a patient repeatedly creates situations in which people will reject him. To change this pattern of behavior, he must repeatedly experience acceptance and inclusion by others. As a group, the psychiatric team may discuss ways in which team members may intervene in this behavior pattern through their individual contacts with the patient and how they may construct group situations in which he can feel accepted. The nurse must be able to recognize when the patient is creating such a situation with her, and she must decide how to respond to prevent him from feeling the rejection that he expects. She should also be able to detect how the patient reinforces this pattern with other patients, and she should learn ways to intervene in this behavior in group situations.

As a participant in an interpersonal relationship with a patient, the nurse observes not only the patient's behavior, but also her own, and she studies responses and learns to use the interpersonal experience constructively. Naturally, there are limitations in her ability to be aware of her behavior and to make inferences about what is going on in the relationship. Therefore, a collaborative relationship with the therapist and other team members is essential to the nurse. In her communication with others, she has the opportunity to clarify her role, validate her judgments and experiences, and use the group's formulations more effectively.

The nurse's functions in intervention include interrupting behavior patterns by her own response to the patient. For example, the patient who feels unworthy and disrespected may need the experience of learning personal worth. The nurse may convey a feeling of respect and an impression of his personal value as she carries out nursing procedures, such as dressing, feeding, or bathing. Through her manner, as well as through verbal communication in these contacts, she can provide the patient with the experience of being accepted. Many similar patterns of behavior may be changed when the patient repeatedly experiences a different kind of relationship than his beliefs have led him to expect. As psychiatric problems are worked with in the doctor-patient relationship, the therapist can plan with the nurse intervention techniques consistent with his therapeutic goals.

The nurse's role in intervention also involves setting necessary limits with the patient, and helping him to work within these limits. She must learn the skills of handling individual differences in groups so that each patient's needs are met. She learns to intervene in interaction between two patients in such a way that they may be able to talk out and accept each other's differences without either feeling that one has been favored over the other. She often becomes the strategic person who helps to coordinate team relationships and to clarify interrelationships of the various people in the ward society with the patient.

Defenses in problem situations. The nurse becomes more acutely aware of patterns or themes in behavior that interfere with relationships as she works with the problems that are involved in establishing therapeutic interpersonal relationships. These patterns often become social forces that affect both patient and staff, and, in the course of planning a therapeutic ward environment, many of them require intervention or modification. One such pattern is the tendency to move away from situations that are uncomfortable. This is seen in a nurse's withdrawal from patients who are withdrawn when unresponsiveness makes her anxious (2). Avoidance of the patient whose behavior is erotic, bizarre, hostile, or overdependent is also common.

Milton Sapirstein says that we use three defenses against anxiety—we run away, we battle it out, or we go for help (3). If the nurse does not have the skills to handle an interpersonal problem, running away is one of the defenses readily available on the psychiatric ward. She may avoid the withdrawn patient and still feel useful because she spends her time with the more responsive patients, or she may find other useful tasks such as arranging the medicine closet or doing the book work. Some of the complicated procedures and routines of psychiatric wards seem to have been created out of a need to withdraw from patients. This defense may be used not only by nurses, but by any member of the psychiatric team.

The second defense—to approach the problem situation—presupposes that the person has certain skills, that she has some understanding of the meaning of the behavior she observes, and that she has learned ways to communicate with the patient. If such skills are lacking or if the attempt is unsuccessful, the approach may become hostile. Since overt hostility is rarely accepted, the nurse may make covert expressions of hostility without recognizing that she is hostile.

The third defense—to go for help—might be useful if constructive help were available. If assistance is not available when it is sought or if the help obtained is consistently not useful, attitudes of indifference or hopelessness may result.

These patterns of behavior alert us to the nurse's need to acquire techniques for handling interpersonal problems with the patient before changes in patterns of withdrawal, hostility, or indifference can be expected. If we find ways to decrease the "detail work" of nursing to give the nurse more time with her patients, and yet fail to teach her the skills she needs, the anxiety that is created in her because she does not know what to do only increases her need to use a variety of unprofitable defenses.

Another pattern of behavior or theme that may interfere with a therapeutic environment is control. This theme may promote inflexible regulations and rigid routines which seriously inhibit the freedom to express conflict. If the nurse has the notion that she must always have the situation under control, she sets limits on the patient's behavior if it is unmeaningful or upsetting to her; and thus interferes with her opportunity to learn what he is trying to communicate. For example, the patient who becomes disturbed may be immediately secluded or transferred to a ward for disturbed patients, without having an opportunity to talk about what is upsetting him, because his behavior interferes with the nurse's control of the situation.

In the carefully controlled setting, a pattern of efficient routine is often adopted. The expediency with which bathing, feeding, dressing, and other tasks may be done becomes more important than the patient who is involved in the procedure; his needs and feelings may be disregarded in the process, and the opportunity to use these tasks in communicating with him is lost. For example, on one ward, the admission routine included a shampoo. The shampoo was given to one patient even though she had spent the morning having her hair done.

An atmosphere of hurriedness may be a part of the nurse's concept of efficiency, and this interferes with the establishment of satisfactory interpersonal relationships with patients. The importance of being busy is so well ingrained in nursing that student nurses feel uncomfortable when they are just talking with patients during the first part of their psychiatric affiliation. In one well-staffed ward that I visited recently, patients prefixed every request with "Nurse, I know you are busy, but . . ." The nurses were far from busy, but the impressions of busyness had been effectively established.

The theme of control is manifested also in the behavior of the nurse who always operates in an information-giving role. This interferes with her ability to listen and accept, and her patient may be denied the understanding he needs and the chance to communicate his feelings. This pattern stereotypes the nurse as "the informer," and the patient as "the uninformed." The role may be adopted by the nurse who needs to feel important, with the consequence that the patient is made to feel unimportant. The connotation that the patient does not understand and cannot understand may develop with this trend. The result is that attempts at conversation are reduced, or conversation may be carried on in the patient's presence, but without including him.

The theme of control is also reinforced when there is a pattern of set expectations on the part of the staff regarding the patient's behavior and a demand that he conform to these expectations. One operation in this pattern is the stereotyping of the patient's behavior by the staff. When the patient moves out of his stereotype, the staff becomes anxious and places restrictions upon him. Take, for example, the patient who has attempted suicide and whose every move may be taken to be a suicidal gesture. He is rigidly restricted in his activities far beyond the point of reasonable protection. Another stereotype is that an excited patient cannot communicate, so the opportunity for him to communicate with others is not provided. A common belief is that a "good" patient is a quiet patient and all behavior outside this stereotype must be restricted.

Real understanding of patients is not possible if the staff operates within set expectations of behavior. Patients learn to take on the fixed, expected behavior pattern to gain approval or to be left alone, or they learn to cross the limits of their stereotype so that they will be noticed. Thus a patient may stay disturbed because it is expected, or because it is the only way he gets attention.

In some situations a patient needs merely to conform to our concept of proper adjustment to the ward life to be considered well enough to go home. This may be seen in wards where the emphasis is on short-term treatment. In one such unit which I visited, I was interested to see that there was very little "acting-out" behavior and very few verbal expressions of conflict from patients. They knew that if they were not able to show improvement within two weeks they would be committed to the state hospital, and they seemed to concentrate all their effort on gaining control and hiding their symptoms in order to be well-behaved patients. When so little time is allowed for working with complex problems, conformity seems to be the only chance for survival.

Some administrative policies develop from the theme of conformity. The methods of working with patients may be so predetermined that sensitive nurses who are aware of their patients' needs are unable to work effectively within the seriously limiting circumstances. For example, disapproval of dependence may be so great that dependence cannot be allowed even when it is therapeutic. Disapproval for neglecting to carry out a ward routine may be so marked that personnel will forfeit the patient's welfare. For example, a very anxious patient was forcefully stripped of her own clothing and dressed in hospital attire upon admission to a hospital. Nurses were aware that this was extremely disturbing to her, but the hospital policy was followed and the patient's feelings were ignored.

Patterns of conformity are usually enforced by fear of punishment or disapproval for the violation of limits. A nurse who expects blame or punishment from her teammates or the administration if something goes wrong in her interpersonal relationship with a patient will find it quite difficult to accept behavior that makes her feel that she has lost control. Thus, one of the basic premises of the therapeutic ward—freedom of expression—cannot be attained. It is difficult for the nurse to be accepting of patients when she does not experience acceptance in her working relationships, and to be permissive with patients when she works in a rigidly regulated setting. In one instance, a head nurse who was able to develop a permissive environment in a ward of a rigidly regimented hospital was regarded by the administrator as poor and inefficient, and was derogated by other head nurses.

The need to cling to these themes of control and conformity may be partially reduced when the nurse learns new techniques for meeting problems and has different kinds of experiences with patients as she tries out these techniques in clinical situations. For example, as she learns communication skills through which she can relate to disturbed patients, the impression that disturbed people cannot and do not want to communicate with others may be changed.

We have considered here only a few of the many themes in the ward life that concern us in creating a therapeutic environment; most of these themes present multifaceted problems as we seek methods to change them. We have been concerned with ways in which these themes influence the patient-nurse relationship, but they affect other team members similarly.

There are many sources from which these themes develop—cultural patterns, community patterns, the patterns of professional training, of hospital life, and individual patterns. To change well-established social patterns is a laborious process; however, it seems possible that of the most effective tools for instigating social change in the ward environment is the psychiatric team whose members are constantly working with social forces in their interpersonal relationships with patients. As a part of the social group in the ward life of the patient, the team member is capable of increasing or reducing the influence of prevailing ward themes.

SUMMARY

The psychiatric nurse's role, then, is to help extend the therapeutic process into the ward environment by creating nurse-patient relationships that promote emotional growth and that are consistent with the therapeutic plan of the doctor-patient relationship. She functions in interpersonal relationships with individuals and with groups of patients, and she collaborates with others to plan learning experiences and to discover and modify the social patterns or themes that influence the ward life of the patient.

REFERENCES

1. Peplau, Hildegard, Lectures and discussions at Teachers College, Columbia University, Division of Nursing Education.
2. Tudor, Gwen E. A sociopsychiatric nursing approach to intervention in a problem of mutual withdrawal on a mental hospital ward. *Psychiatry* 15:193-217, May 1952.
3. Sapirstein, Milton R. *Emotional Security*. New York, Crown Publications, 1948.
4. Ruesch, Jurgen and Bateson, Gregory. *Communication: The Social Matrix of Psychiatry*. New York, W. W. Norton and Co., 1951.
5. Busse, Ewald W., Director, Department of Psychosomatic Medicine, University of Colorado School of Medicine. Personal communication.
6. Van Huben, Betty J., Instructor in Psychiatric Nursing, University of Colorado School of Nursing. Personal communication.

29

A Day Hospital
for Psychiatric Patients

Anne Hargreaves, Patricia Warsaw,
and Edith P. Lewis*

Traditional methods of caring for psychiatric patients are being challenged by this newer concept of care, which stresses treatment of the patient within family and community relationships.

It is becoming less and less possible to speak of Boston's Massachusetts Mental Health Center as a hospital with a given "bed" capacity. As Dr. Milton Greenblatt, director of research and laboratories there, puts it: "We have facilities to care for something like 200 patients—but, actually, we have only about 100 beds. The rest of our patients are cared for on a day basis and go home to their own beds at night."

At the Center, an average of about 40 to 50 patients are cared for in what might be called the Day Hospital proper: a separate but integral unit of this psychiatric hospital. And about an equal number of persons receive day care on the inpatient services: that is, they spend the day with the patients who are in the hospital on a 24-hour basis, but return to their own homes at night.

Again quoting Dr. Greenblatt: "We are looking forward to a relative numerical dominance of day patients over full-time hospitalized cases. How far this process can be extended depends on future developments, particularly the education and cooperation of staff, relatives, and the community. What-

*From *American Journal of Nursing*, Vol. 62, No. 9 (September, 1962).
Collaborating in the preparation of this article were Anne Hargreaves (Boston City; B.S., M.S., Boston University) assistant professor of nursing at Boston University who developed and directed the student program described in the paper; Patricia Warsaw (Peter Bent Brigham) head nurse at Massachusetts Mental Health Center's Day Hospital; and Edith P. Lewis, contributing editor for the *Journal*.

ever the ultimate success, the day hospital idea has struck a severe blow to the 'bricks and plaster' answer to mental illness problems—that is, the construction of ever more full-time custodial type institutions to care for mental cases." (1)

It could be added that the day hospital concept of care has also struck a severe blow to the traditional practice of psychiatric nursing and is creating a new and dynamic concept of the nurse's role in psychiatric care.

The idea for a day hospital at the Massachusetts Mental Health Center began to germinate about 10 years ago when it was noted that a number of discharged patients were returning to the hospital almost daily—apparently simply to pass the time or to take refuge from the difficulties of life at home or in the community. They would sit in the lounge chairs in the lobby, greeting old friends among patients and staff as they passed through, occasionally joining in available recreational activities. Some interaction took place among themselves but their attempts at socialization were for the most part feeble and fumbling.

Obviously, some step was missing in the discharge of these individuals; some needs were not being met. Consequently, exploration was started to find out what brought these former patients back to the hospital so often—sometimes just to visit, sometimes for readmission—and to ascertain what more helpful service could be provided to aid in the transition to community life.

A somewhat tentative day program was inaugurated for this group, with the investigating social worker serving as staff person. A small room near the lobby—originally a cloak room—became the official "center." There the patients could check in and out, hang up their coats and hats, meet for group or individual discussions with the social worker, or take refuge when they were overwhelmed in the course of the day. An activity program was also provided for the group, dovetailing with ongoing social and recreational activities in the hospital. Eventually, students from the Boston University School of Nursing were assigned to this rudimentary day care program as part of their educational experience in psychiatric nursing. Along with their psychiatric nursing instructor from the university, they helped develop a program of meaningful therapeutic activity for this "unattached" group.

In its early years at the Massachusetts Mental Health Center, the day care idea, although soon a living program, was nevertheless a rather diffuse and loosely organized one. Patients came not by referral but on their own initiative. There were no set criteria for admission to the program; in fact, there was no clear-cut program. Medical responsibility for the patients was not clearly defined and nurse participation was limited to the activities of the psychiatric nursing faculty members from Boston University and her students.

Even under these limited circumstances, however, the day care program continued to demonstrate its usefulness as one way of caring for psychiatric patients. By the end of 1956, the Day Hospital was established as an official, functioning unit within the institution, with a large area equivalent to a ward setting given over to it. Psychiatrists were assigned to the unit and, in 1957, the first full-time professional nurse was added to the staff. Now, in 1962, the Day Hospital is a going concern, caring for 40 to 50 patients at any given time.

THE DAY HOSPITAL IN ACTION

The patient population runs the gamut from semi-acute, bordering on acute, to severely incapacitated chronic patients. The most common diagnoses are depression and schizophrenia. Within our present state of knowledge, drug addicts and patients with alcoholism or severe character disorders do not seem to benefit from this type of care.

At first, most of the Day Hospital patients were received from the in-patient services, the Day Hospital thus serving a primarily transitional function in returning these patients to full community living. Even in the beginning, however, from a quarter to a third of the patients were admitted to the Day Hospital without preceding inpatient hospitalization. Now, since the recent establishment of day care on the hospital's inpatient services, too, practically all of the patients in the Day Hospital proper are admitted directly from the community on referral from physicians, community agencies, or outpatient and clinical services. On the whole, any patient who seems likely to benefit from therapy and who, along with his family, is willing to enter into a co-operative approach with the staff is considered suitable for admission.

The hospital day begins officially at 9:00 A.M. but the patients start arriving from 8:30 on. Occasionally, they drive their own cars to the hospital. Most often, they come by public transportation or are brought by a family member.

The Day Hospital operates from 9:00 to 4:00, Monday through Friday, but schedules are adjusted to the individual patient. Some arrive late or leave early, depending on transportation problems or family considerations. Some don't come every day. But each patient has his own schedule and is expected to adhere to it. If he doesn't put in an appearance at the given time and nothing has been heard from him, then the nurse phones his home—not to upbraid or discipline him, but to find out what the problem is and what can be done to help with it.

The Day Hospital is a self-contained unit within the larger hospital. A large living room is divided by halfway lattices into a number of smaller areas: a place to sit, read, or talk; a ping-pong and active games area; and a spot with a refrigerator and hot plate for coffee and snacks. Card tables, games, a piano, a sewing machine, and a radio are in frequent use. No television, though. This is considered too likely to foster withdrawal and isolation, but for special events—the World Series, for instance, a presidential inauguration, our first manned space flight—a television set is borrowed temporarily.

Adjacent to the large activity area are a number of smaller rooms: a sort of treatment or examining room with a small cot, which serves various purposes; a room with a record player for quiet listening or reading; offices for the psychiatrist, social worker, and other staff members; and a large, centrally located nursing office.

The latter bears little resemblance to the nursing office typical of the custodial type of institution: no locked doors, no shatterproof glass, no aspect whatsoever of an observation post in enemy territory. Instead it is a large, almost cluttered, somewhat shabby room, furnished with a desk, a few comfortable chairs, some straight ones, and plenty of "leaning" areas. A bulletin board on one wall contains not only official notices but also a random collection of cartoons culled from magazines and newspapers and poking fun at psychiatry. Patients as well as staff bring these in and they seem to be as much enjoyed by the one group as the other.

Aside from a medicine cabinet high on one wall, nothing is locked in this room and the door is rarely, if ever, closed. Patients, nurses, other staff members—in fact, anyone who has any business on the ward at all—wander freely in and out. At a given moment, a nurse may be giving a patient a medication in one corner; in another, an earnest conference is taking place between psychiatrist and social worker; and in still another, two patients are having a goodnatured argument while waiting for the head nurse to hang up the phone and attend to them.

The atmosphere, not only in the nursing office, but throughout the entire Day Hospital, is definitely informal. Everyone wears street clothes and the visitor would be hard put to distinguish staff from patient, mostly because of the deceptively casual, give-and-take relationships that obtain between personnel and patients.

Neither the atmosphere nor the relationships, however, are as casual as they may seem. In almost every interaction between nurse and patient, for instance, the nurse's ear is tuned for deeper implications, evidence of feelings and motivations, clues to problems and behavior.

In this calculatedly "open" environment, with no one arbitrarily dictating behavior or activities, the staff assumes—and makes clear in one way, or another to the patients—that the latter are expected to act like responsible human beings. Realistic standards are set in matters of general behavior, dress, feeding, and toileting. When in the nursing office, patients are expected to respect the private conversations of others, to stay away from desk drawers, charts, and the like, and to make themselves scarce when requested. Rarely do they overstep their boundaries; they meet the expectations that are implicitly set before them.

THE THERAPEUTIC GOALS. The philosophy of treatment in the Day Hospital, very generally stated, emphasizes four factors: psychotherapy, in individual or group settings or both; full use of the therapeutic milieu, with stress on meaningful staff-patient interrelationships; resocialization, as the patient is encouraged to take part in both the social and occupational activities of normal living; and a concerted effort to return the patient to full community living as soon as possible. Three months is the approximate period of hospitalization for Day Hospital patients.

Against the background of these general principles, the Day Hospital provides a place to which the patient can take his anxieties, people for him to relate to, and an opportunity for him to learn to understand his difficulties. The therapeutic plan is carefully modeled to meet each patient's individual needs, and is broad enough to include the family, as well as the patient. Chemotherapy may also form part of the treatment and, in an occasional instance, convulsive shock therapy may be used.

Within the first few days of his admission, the patient's own doctor, nurse, and social worker meet with him and his family in an attempt to tailor a plan of care that will be most useful to all concerned. The same team—as well as other members of the staff who have become concerned with the patient—expedites this plan of care in cooperation with others, and reviews and re-evaluates it at frequent intervals in both formal and informal conferences.

The boundaries between the various disciplines represented on the Day Hospital staff tend to be fluid. Very roughly speaking, it might be said that the doctor is concerned with individual psychotherapy, the social worker with patient-family problems, and the nurse with maintaining a sociotherapeutic atmosphere and relationships. No one is yet prepared to spell out specifically, however, each one's "role," since the team approach is an integral part of the program.

Each staff member more or less works out his own relationship with the patient in line with the total therapeutic goal. There is free and frequent communication among all the personnel, a constant pooling and exchange of information, and cooperative planning as to approaches and attitudes.

THE PATIENT'S DAY. The patient's day is not very formally structured. (Old line psychiatric nurses will remember the frequent calls: "Time for O.T., ladies" or "Time to go outdoors," and so on.) Each patient, however, is expected to spend at least two hours daily (this time increases as the patient improves) at some sort of work therapy: serving in the coffee or gift shop; typing in one of the offices; or lending a hand with the gardening in the greenhouse.

One of the most explicit objectives of this form of therapy is to build "work tolerance." The program is considered especially valuable, encouraging as it does a sense of responsibility, of participation in the normal workaday world of the well, of relationships with others, and of sharing in an activity of use to others.

In the course of the day, the patient will also have conferences, formal or informal, with doctor, social worker, or nurse. He will take part in the recreational activities on the ward or in other parts of the hospital. A small school with certified teachers is maintained for school-age patients, and they attend this regularly.

There may also be organized trips to a nearby bowling alley or to parks, museums, and other places of interest in the city. On occasion, the patient may prefer to sit quietly and read or listen to the radio. During the course of most days, too, he will spend some time with the nursing student who has been especially assigned to his case. Together they will explore feelings and attitudes as the student works on developing with the patient a relationship of true therapeutic significance.

Films are shown from time to time and there are also organized classes in such varied subjects as the modern dance, cooking, current events, or the Bible. Some of these classes are held in the Day Hospital itself. Others include patients from the other hospital services, and may be conducted by occupational therapists, volunteers, or other hospital personnel, and may be held almost anywhere in the hospital. Generally speaking, however, it is the nurse who carries the major responsibility for group activities, although she brings in others—occupational therapists, theologians, volunteers—as needed.

Group meetings are held at scheduled times during the week, sometimes for the entire Day Hospital population, sometimes for a smaller segment of the group. Patients are expected to attend these sessions—one of the few structured elements in their day.

The group discussion leader may be the resident psychiatrist, a social worker, or one of the nurses. Each one of these, although drawing on the accepted principles of group dynamics, develops his own style of leadership and determines his own purpose. This means that both the content and form of the group sessions will depend to a considerable degree on the person leading the group.

THE NURSING STAFF. The nursing service of a 5-day-a-week day hospital has one great and unique advantage over conventional 24-hour nursing services: the same staff is there each day. For the nurses, this means the elimination of one more problem in communication—passing on the day's information to the evening and then to the night staff. It means, too, that the nurses are on the scene during the patient's entire hospitalization, informed through their own presence of both problems and progress. A final and obvious advantage, of course, is that this system makes it possible to have more nurses available for day care.

For the patient, this setup not only cuts down on the number of people with whom he must establish relationships but, more importantly, assures him continuity of care, with a feeling of consistency in relationships. What may be important to him, for instance, is not just receiving a certain pill two or three times a day, but who gives it to him, her approach, and what the whole business of being medicated may signify to him. With the same nurse responsible for the same activities each day, a sense of stability and security is introduced into the patient's anxious world.

The professional nursing staff, which has grown steadily in numbers since the Day Hospital was first established, now numbers four: the head nurse, who has been with the unit since 1957, and three staff nurses. Stress for the staff in the early days was very great. Repeatedly they were asked to clarify the role of the nurse in the Day Hospital: how did it differ from social work? Was there a place for the nurse at all? The anxiety was great and often the nurses tended to fall back on traditional functions: ordering supplies, checking blood pressures, dispensing medications, and coordinating activities.

Today, however, there is no doubt that the nurse *is* a significant member of the staff of the day hospital, even though the nurses most intimately concerned are still exploring the full and exact potential of their contribution. As a social scientist who studied the day care program remarks, "The Day Hospital nurse engages in activities which are quite different from the traditional nurse's activities. Her work is much more oriented toward the patient's emotional life and toward his activity and participation in the unit." (2)

The head nurse, of course, in collaboration with the medical and social work staff, is the over-all administrator of the unit, and coordinator of its activities. She is also a vital central link in the necessarily complex communication network. Finally, she is always available to talk with patients who may be having difficulties and to discuss with them problems arising from environmental stresses or intrapsychic conflicts.

Each of the three staff nurses has a specific area of responsibilty. One is responsible for the social and recreational activities of the patients, both within and without the ward setting; another is in charge of medications and any physical treatments that may be indicated; and the third plans and supervises the patient's work program.

Each of these areas has its own special significance for the nurse-patient relationship that develops, as well as its own special problems. Take medications, for instance, which might seem to be the routine affair it usually is in a general hospital of checking cards, preparing medicines, and making a quick trip through the ward to dispense them. Not in the Day Hospital, however.

To begin with, the patients are expected to come to the nursing office at specified times to receive their medications: this is their responsibility. They may be consistently early or consistently late—or they may "forget" to come at all. They may watch carefully, almost suspiciously, to be sure they receive the "right" pills from the "right" bottle, or be completely indifferent to the process; they may report each possible side effect with anxiety, or ignore obvious ones completely; they may see medication time as an opportunity to socialize or discuss problems, or as something to be gotten over with as soon as possible.

Whatever their attitude or reaction, it is of concern to the medication nurse. It tells her something about their problems, and she recognizes that *her* reaction to *their* reactions may have as much significance as the medication itself. As soon as the nurse thinks it is feasible, incidentally, the patient is given a week's supply of his medication and expected to take care of it himself—this, to free him from dependence and to encourage self-reliance.

The fact that each nurse has her own special area of responsibility should not be interpreted as a return to the old "functional" approach to nursing. It means, rather, that each nurse has a specific contribution to make to the total therapeutic program, and a specific role to play in which she develops real expertness. This system also provides for consistency in nurse-patient relationships, with the patient learning to whom he should turn and for what within this small community. Furthermore, each nurse of course develops relationships with all the patients—inside and outside her own particular area of responsiblity—and she pools her observations and experiences with those of the rest of the staff.

Boston University School of Nursing undergraduate students have an eight-week clinical experience in psychiatric nursing in the Day Hospital during their senior year. In collaboration with the head nurse, their own instructor provides for a meaningful learning experience for them. Each nursing student is assigned to a doctor and social worker who join forces with her to make up a team which works with individual patients.

Often uneasy at first, the student soon grows in understanding of herself, the patient, and team interaction as she explores the developing relationship with "her" patients. Some patients she works with from admission through to discharge, participating in orientation, diagnostic and treatment plan formulation, and termination. In all, she contributes substantially to the total therapeutic plan.

Medical and social work students, in addition to nursing students, are also assigned to the Day Hospital. The entire student group brings to the unit youth, enthusiasm, and scientific curiosity which seem to have a wholesome and stimulating effect on the patients and staff. Through their presence, spontaneity, questions, and turnover, these students add even more flexibility and movement to an already dynamic environment.

CRISIS SITUATIONS. Suicidal risk, of course, is always a concern of any institution or personnel caring for psychiatric patients. Its handling at the Day Hospital remains largely an area of judgment and of maintaining good communication with the patient and his family.

Occasionally, for this and other reasons, it becomes necessary to consider whether a particular patient at a particular time might not better be transferred to full-time hospitalization, at least for a while. Making the decision is again a matter of clinical judgment.

The patient or family may indicate, either verbally or in other ways, when this step seems indicated. The patient may seem overwhelmed in situations of daily living or may be temporarily "out of control." Sometimes his reactions or behavior constitute almost a direct request for someone to "take over," and the nurse's, doctor's, or social worker's ear soon becomes tuned to this unspoken plea.

What is important, when around-the-clock hospitalization for a period is decided upon, is that the situation be considered in the nature of a temporary upheaval, with a goal of returning the patient as rapidly as possible to the Day Hospital setting. In the meantime, while he is on full hospitalization, the Day Hospital staff still maintains contact with him so that ongoing medical and nursing relationships can be preserved.

DAY CARE ON INPATIENT SERVICES. One of the outgrowths of the Day Hospital's demonstrated success in caring for patients who would once have been admitted for around-the-clock care has been the extension of day care to selected patients within the hospital's inservice population. Almost as soon as a patient is admitted to the Massachusetts Mental Health Center these days, consideration is given to the possibility of day care. Physician, nurse, and social worker discuss this with the patient and his family and, as soon as it seems therapeutically and socially feasible, day care is started.

This means that, on a given inpatient service, certain patients are in residence only during the day, returning to their own homes at night. (This situation is occasionally reversed. There have been instances where a patient holding a full-time job spends only his evenings and nights at the hospital, his therapeutic hours being arranged accordingly.) During his time at the hospital, the patient shares in all the activities—social, recreational, and therapeutic—of the full-time group.

Still another example of the flexibility of approach at the Massachusetts Mental Health Center is the fact that sometimes the family comes to the hospital instead of the patient returning to the family. One young mother on day care arrived at the hospital each day with her six-month-old baby. The sight of this baby placidly asleep in a playpen in an old-time seclusion room provides a sharp contrast between the old and the new in psychiatric care.

IMPLICATIONS FOR THE FUTURE

Until recently, hospitalization to most people has meant spending 24 hours a day under the direct care of the hospital staff when ill, and then being discharged home when well. With the rising costs of hospitalization, however, alternatives in care are developing—the system of progressive patient care in general hospitals, for instance, or the extension of home nursing care plans. Perhaps one of the most significant contributions to the present trend has been the increasing awareness of the fact that hospitalization, for both physical and mental illness, may create as many problems as it tries to resolve.

The traditional mental hospital system, with its borrowed medical-surgical orientation, fosters isolation, dependency, and a lack of self-direction. The mentally ill person's relationships with people, especially with his family, have broken down, and only in the setting of family and community relationships can effective therapy take place.

One of the most vexing problems in psychiatric therapy has been the loss of contact between patient and family; at first, this is unwittingly fostered by enforced separation, but eventually grows into lack of emotional investment as the months and years accumulate. It often becomes virtually impossible for the patient to return to the community after contact with home breaks down.

The advent of day care for psychiatric patients gets around many of these difficulties. It permits—in fact, almost insists—that the sick person continue his relationships with family and community. It provides an opportunity for psychiatric and nursing care to be truly therapeutic, integrated into a framework of more or less normal family and community living.

Also lending support to the day care idea is the fact that more and more individuals are seekings psychiatric help and at an earlier stage of illness than they once did. The public is becoming better informed about the importance of prevention and early recognition and treatment of mental illness, and the stigma once associated with psychiatric disorders is gradually disappearing.

Day hospitals—and, in some places, night hospitals—plus the development of psychiatric clinics and units in general hospitals make it more and more possible for these individuals to receive the help they need in a meaningful therapeutic setting and without too much disruption of their personal, family, and community relationships.

The patient in turmoil needing full-time hospitalization during an acute phase will probably be with us for some time to come. So, in all likelihood, will be the patient who needs temporary asylum from a very disturbed relationship with his family and community. The feeling at the Massachusetts Mental Health Center is, however, that as the medical and nursing staff become more comfortable with the trend toward noninstitutionalized care and more skilled in administering it, increasing numbers of patients can be cared for on a day care basis.

REFERENCES

1. Kramer, B. M. *Day Hospital; A Study of Partial Hospitalization in Psychiatry.* Boston, Massachusetts Mental Health Center, 1960, Preface, pp. iii-iv. (Mimeographed)
2. Ibid, Chap. 3, pp. 9-10.

30

The Psychiatric Nurse
as Sociotherapist

Joyce Samhammer Hays*

A primary function is to help the patient take advantage of the therapeutic possibilities on a psychiatric ward. A technique is described which the nurse can use for studying the ward social structure and the patient's interaction with others.

In the past two decades there has been considerable progress in the practice of hospital psychiatry. We no longer read of "snake pits" or of wards of neglected, denuding patients. Now we hear of the "open" hospital, of day care units, foster home care, halfway houses, and patient government (1). Paralleling this progress, there has been a corresponding evolution in the role of the psychiatric nurse. As psychiatry passed from a lengthy custodial stage through a somatic treatment period to its present rehabilitative phase, the functions of the nurse have changed to keep pace with the goals and aims of hospitalization.

CUSTODIAL PHASE . . . CONTROL,
CLEANLINESS, CONFORMITY

During the custodial phase, the aim of hospitalization was primarily the protection of society. Hospital personnel sought similar protection from the patient. Nurses and attendants spent much of their time "supervising" and

*From *American Journal of Nursing*, Vol. 62, No. 6 (June, 1962).

Mrs. Hays (Philadelphia General Hospital School of Nursing; B.S., M.S., University of Pennsylvania) has taught at the Veterans Administration Hospital in Coatesville, Pa., and in the school of nursing at the University of Pennsylvania. Since 1960, she has been consultant in psychiatric nursing at the Veterans Administration Hospital in Northport, New York.

"observing" patients for behavioral expressions of pathology. They provided a clean, safe, secure environment devoted to avoiding escapes, controlling assaultiveness, and preventing suicides. In this context, a "good" patient was one who could be described as "quiet" and "cooperative." Individual initiative in any form was discouraged, while conformity was rewarded with approval. Large and frequent doses of sedation, restraints, and seclusion were used for those who did not readily comply. The nurse's role was much like that of a jailer, complete with an unwieldy ring of keys.

SOMATIC TREATMENT PHASE . . . SHOCK, SURGERY, PSYCHIC DRUGS

As physical methods of treatment became widespread, the nurse assumed a new role, a primarily technical one. She learned to assist with insulin and electric shock treatments, to care for patients after lobotomy, and, finally, to administer massive doses of the new tranquilizers. In addition, she became enlightened about the different diagnoses and her nursing care was dispensed in terms of the kind of "label" attached to the patient, much as her general hospital counterpart managed appendectomies and thyroidectomies.

A great rush of "total push" and activity programs came in during this phase. Nursing personnel sought to "activate" patients, keeping them on the move rather than sitting in the endless rows of chairs and benches.

The new drugs were seen as being only slightly short of miraculous and quickly displaced the majority of other somatic treatments. Consequently, nurses devoted long periods to pouring, administering, and charting, as soon almost every patient was given one drug or another—tranquilizers for the active patients, energizers for the inactive ones. In many settings, the role of pill-dispenser continues as the nurse's paramount reason for existence.

REHABILITATIVE PHASE . . . RE-EDUCATION, REMOTIVATION, RESOCIALIZATION

Currently, there is a new emphasis. In progressive mental hospitals, the patient is viewed as an individual and as a social being. Mere custodial care has had little therapeutic value. Even the drastic physical methods have not produced lasting results in the majority of patients. The new drugs have made patients more amenable to further therapy which, on the whole, has not been available. Now there has come the realization that hospitalization must also be "education."

We have discovered that patients are people who have not learned to live comfortably with others and, hence, are in need of experience in social living. The hospital ward is no longer a place for the patient merely to stay between "treatments," but rather ward living itself is recognized as being treatment. Patients are no longer expected to spend their entire lifetime or even a large part of it locked away from society. The expectation is for early return to community life after therapeutic experiences in a sort of "model community." Consequently, the nurse's role is altered drastically. No longer is she a keeper of the keys or even primarily a technician. A new role is emerging—that of "sociotherapist."

If a major goal of treatment is to have patients learn to live successfully with others and if ward living itself is to have therapeutic value, then the nurse's role becomes increasingly important. For it is nursing personnel who provide the 24-hour supervision of the patient's living. And it is nursing personnel who, in effect, *live with* the patient group. Hence, it will be up to nurses, aides, and attendants to utilize the everyday experiences of the patients' ward living—eating, rising and retiring, meeting personal hygiene needs, working, talking, and playing together—as therapy. To understand this role of "sociotherapist" more fully, consider the functions it comprises.

CREATING A FAMILYLIKE ENVIRONMENT. To create a familylike environment means more than hanging pictures on the walls and curtains on the windows. Just as a good home is first a place where there is love and respect for each member, so must the ward become a setting where there is consideration for each person and his needs, where there is acceptance, understanding, and opportunity for emotional growth. The physical trappings can add to, but not make, a desirable ward environment any more than they can make a good home.

Furthermore, each patient must be allowed a voice in ward affairs, and the nurse's voice must be valued not as that of a figure of irrational authority—always "right" because she is the nurse—but for its real value, for its contribution to ward living. Her authority, then, is based on competence, not on power over others.

Perhaps this concept is best epitomized in the "therapeutic community" which Dr. Maxwell Jones established at Belmont Hospital in England (2). Responsibilities for ward living must rest on all members—patients as well as personnel. Every patient is capable of accepting some responsibility, although it may take a great deal of cooperative effort to discover just what tasks are appropriate and then to alter these duties as capabilities change.

A step toward creating a familylike environment is the elimination of unnecessary regimentation—for example, lines of patients waiting for medications, for meals, for walks. Many status symbols might also be removed—the starched white uniforms, the different manner of address for professional personnel as contrasted with that for patients or attendants.

If patients are to be prepared for living outside the hospital, life inside must parallel such living wherever possible. Patients can eat together in a manner which promotes socialization, rather than just fulfilling their nutritional needs. And personnel who are observing during the meal can sit with patients rather than stand and stare at them. The administration of medications can provide a therapeutic contact with patients rather than be the impersonal act of "pill-passing" which it often becomes. There is need to examine *every* activity of the day or night—showering, shaving, eating, sleeping, working, playing—in the light of its potential therapeutic value.

No activity or incident is too small or unimportant. Let us consider a common experience: an attendant enters a dayroom to find several patients arguing about which television channel to watch. What might he do? (1) He could be very authoritarian and declare, "We'll put it on channel 6." (2) He could suggest, "Let's take a vote and watch what the majority want." This would be a proposal of a more democratic nature. (3) He might say,

"It looks as though we're faced with a problem. How should we handle it?" Such a confrontation would place the responsibility for solution on the group where it rightly belongs. Thus, a dispute could become a learning experience.

Creating such an environment demands continuing cooperation and communication between personnel and patients—in a word, teamwork. Time must be set aside for daily ward meetings—planning and evaluation sessions—in which there is representation from the patient group and from all levels of the ward's nursing personnel. Here, there would be discussion of problems of group living and problems of individuals as they affect group harmony—aimed not at placing blame, but at finding workable solutions.

In addition, ward units should be administratively as small as possible. If two nurses are assigned to a building of 100 patients, it would be preferable to have two groups of 50—with one nurse responsible for each of the groups—than to have both nurses care for all the patients. (This would be true even if it were necessary for each nurse to cover both units on the other's days off duty.) Similarly, if there were eight attendants assigned to this building, care would be best personalized if each attendant were responsible for 12 or 13 patients (3). Such divisions of responsibility would allow each patient to be known well individually and to feel that there was some member of the staff to whom he could turn for understanding and help.

Studying the ward social structure. If healthy socialization is to be promoted, it is necessary first to study the ward social structure already in exist-

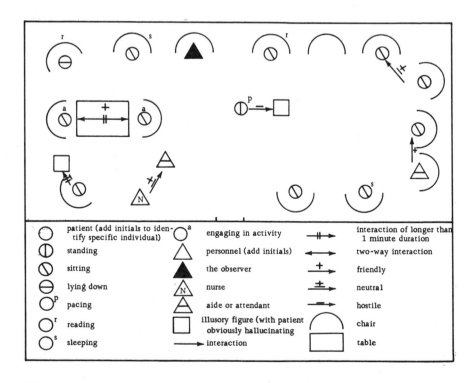

ence. Who are the leaders among the patients, the members of already existing groups, the isolates, the fringe members? Where does most of the socialization occur? In the dining room, the dayroom, outdoors, in the occupational
therapy shop? What activities and what persons promote friendly interaction
and which deter it? With which patients do the personnel spend most time
and effort?

A simple technique for answering these questions and others is diagram-
ming ward interaction (see figure). Any variety of symbols can be used.

One diagram of this sort, made at one particular time has, of course,
little significance. Only when many diagrams have been made at different
times of day, on different days, and in different places over a period of time,
can conclusions having validity be drawn.

A tool such as the interaction diagram can readily be used by all levels
of nursing personnel. As its use continues and the findings it reveals are
discussed by the personnel, they become acutely aware of those patients who
need the most help in interacting with others. Patients who have the greatest
problems in interacting, either because they withdraw or relate in a hostile
fashion, can be selected for more intensive individual nurse-patient relationship. Personnel who are found to avoid relating to patients or to relate non-
therapeutically can be counseled. Patient leadership potential can be discovered and encouraged. Activities can be evaluated objectively as promoting
or hindering friendly interaction. Patients can be taught the technique and
can chart their group progress from social disorganization to social integration. The ramifications are infinite.

What must be constantly kept in mind is that the ward society is not
a static one, but a dynamic, changing one. Only as we keep well aware of
this factor can we intelligently introduce changes which will be constructive.

ESTABLISHING RELATIONSHIPS WITH INDIVIDUAL PATIENTS. With our emphasis on socialization and group living, we must not lose sight of the individual. Many patients are not ready to relate to others and need much assistance before they can feel a part of the ward group. For these patients, individual therapeutic contact over a fairly long period may be necessary. In the
majority of hospitals there are too few psychiatrists for any but the newly
admitted, acutely ill patients to receive individual psychotherapy. Hence, the
responsibility for seeing that they have therapeutic relationships falls chiefly
to nursing personnel.

These relationships are quite different from what is classically thought
of as psychotherapy. Emphasis is focused on *current* problems of the patient's
living with others in the ward setting. The nurse deals with conscious material
and does not make interpretations. She helps the patient to view realistically
his hospitalization, the personnel, his fellow patients, and himself in his *present*
role.

The place for such relating is in the ward area where the patient is
presently living with others, rather than in an office or elsewhere removed
from the ward. The aim differs also. The nurse does not seek to form a prolonged, dependent association with the patient, but rather works toward enlarging the scope of the patient's relationships, until he can interact independently with others (personnel, patients, visitors) in a satisfying and socially

acceptable manner and become a part of the ward society. The length of the relationship is entirely dependent upon the needs of the patient. In many instances, the nurse finds it necessary at first to just "be with" the patient, sitting quietly beside him, waiting until he is ready to reach out to her. She may begin to participate in activities with the patient long before any verbal exchanges between them are possible.

In short, the nurse strives to promote a one-to-one relationship with the patient as a first step toward his subsequent integration into the group; she does this by starting where the patient is and then slowly begins to offer more complex social experiences, first with her and then with others.

Problems arising out of such relationships must have a place where they can be brought up for discussion—perhaps in a weekly meeting devoted to this purpose, where leadership can be provided by the ward physician or by a nurse who has had advanced psychiatric nursing preparation.

In addition, a worthwhile policy would be to have all newly admitted patients experience an individual relationship with a member of the nursing personnel. Not only would the patient receive valuable assistance in adjusting to his hospitalization and in becoming aware of the interest of the personnel and of their helping qualities, but also much could be learned *early* about the patient and his problems in living with others that would aid in the planning of his nursing care. If every member of the nursing personnel devoted some time each day to relating individually to at least one patient, the numbers of patients so contacted would be sizable.

RELATING TO GROUPS OF PATIENTS. The nurse has many opportunities to relate to groups of patients. There are planned formal groups which meet regularly—patient government, remotivation groups, discussion groups, activity groups. In these, nursing personnel are often called upon to provide leadership, at least until leadership among patients can be developed. Many of these groups approach the level of group therapy, with discussion of such topics as family relationships, handling angry feelings, making friends, working and competing with others, attitudes toward authority, and the like. Other groups may confine themselves to talking about current events, hobbies, music, books, films, and so on.

Patients and personnel may, in groups, undertake projects which will improve the ward physically—painting the walls, repairing furniture, making ashtrays or wastebaskets, growing plants, building bookshelves. Nurses accompany patients on trips, picnics, walks. Many of these excursions take the patients into the community where much influence can be exercised in both directions. People in the community can begin to see patients as they really are, not so different than they are themselves; and patients can be introduced to interesting places ("Y's," museums, parks, public libraries, churches, theaters) and friendly people who can accept them and assist. Or outside groups can be brought into the hospital—to talk with patients, play games, provide education and recreation, or just to become acquainted with the hospital and the people within its environs.

Many group endeavors are spontaneous, arising out of a circumstance of the moment—a discussion of a news topic on television, for example, or the handling of a disagreement between patients. In all of these relationships —structured and unstructured—the patients are learning to cooperate with others, to get satisfaction out of group projects, to think of "we" instead of "I." Nursing personnel must be alert to opportunities for utilizing whatever lends itself at the moment to furthering patients' competence in group living.

As a result of their close and prolonged contact with patients, nursing personnel today are in a position to exert considerable therapeutic influence in the ward setting. They have a unique contribution to make, a role to play which does not conflict or compete with those played by members of other disciplines, but rather supplements these efforts and makes ward living a therapy with 24-hour-a-day possibilities.

REFERENCES

1. Engel, Leonard. *New Trends in the Care and Treatment of the Mentally Ill.* New York, National Association for Mental Health, 1959.
2. Briggs, D. L. Social psychiatry in Great Britain. *Amer. J. Nurs.* 59:215-220, Feb. 1959.
3. Catney, J. L. *A Study of Small Group Assignment in a Mental Hospital.* Ft. Lyon, Colo. Veterans Administration Hospital, 1960.

31

Creative Nursing in
Day and Night Care Centers

Marguerite J. Holmes, Doris Lefley, and Jean A. Werner*

In this psychiatric unit, patients are encouraged to assume responsibility for their own lives, behavior, and treatment . . . and nurses and other personnel are encouraged to share their own lives, feelings, and reactions with the patients.

The Day and Night Centers at the Illinois State Psychiatric Institute occupy a unit originally designed as an 18-bed closed ward for patients requiring full-time hospitalization. They are a part of the University of Chicago Service at the Institute, share the physical facility, and are under one administration. Otherwise, the centers are separate treatment units, each with its own patients, staff, program, problems, and attributes.

The day center operates from 8:30 A.M. to 5:00 P.M., the night center from 4:00 P.M. to 8:30 A.M. Both function Monday through Friday and are closed week ends and holidays. The day center is staffed by a psychiatric resident, three nurses, two male psychiatric aides, an activities therapist, a social worker, and a ward clerk. The night center is staffed by two psychiatric residents, a social group worker, three nurses, and two male psychiatric aides on the evening shift, and one nurse and an aide on the night shift. The chief

*From *American Journal of Nursing*, Vol. 62, No. 9 (September, 1962).

All three authors are associated with the University of Chicago Service at the Illinois State Psychiatric Institute and have worked together in developing the program at the day center. Miss Holmes (B.S., M.N., University of Washington) is nursing supervisor: Mrs. Lefley (Washington University School of Nursing, St. Louis, Mo.) is head nurse of the day center; and Miss Werner (Seattle University School of Nursing; B.S., Seattle University; M.N., University of Washington) is nursing educator. Both Miss Holmes and Miss Werner also share the responsibility for the night center program.

of service, nursing supervisor, and nursing educator have over-all responsibility for both centers.

These two centers were established to provide treatment facilities for patients who need hospitalization on less than a full-time basis. This includes patients unable to profit by individual psychotherapy or for whom outpatient treatment is insufficient. It also includes individuals who, after being hospitalized on a full-time unit for an acute psychiatric illness, have recovered sufficiently to return home each night and on week ends, or are able to resume employment or school, but who still need the benefits of an intensive treatment program.

An integral purpose of both programs is to assist patients to maintain themselves by helping them learn how to talk about and cope with feelings and problems concerning life in particular segments of their community.

PHILOSOPHY AND THERAPEUTIC APPROACH

One of the basic tenets in our philosophy is that patients should be trusted and encouraged to assume responsibility for their own lives, behavior, and treatment. A second is that the patient's continued participation in family and community life aids his progress in the therapeutic program in that it (1) limits regressive behavior by providing fewer opportunities for him to develop unhealthy dependency on the hospital; and (2) provides him with ongoing opportunities for experiential learning in daily contacts with family and community.

A third belief is that therapy is a continuing process involving the patients, the staff, and the patients' families, rather than being an exclusive function of the physician. Patients and all members of the staff share responsibility for the treatment program. Participating together in group therapy, activities projects, and the everyday vicissitudes of life on the ward constitute the core of the therapy, with considerable importance being placed on "the group."

An essential element in this approach is that personnel take part in the patients' daily activities. As much as is possible, nurses, aides, physicians, the activities therapist, and social workers are encouraged to help plan and actively engage in the program with the patients. The degree of interest the patients show in the group therapy sessions and in the recreational, social, and activities programs, as well as their willingness to utilize these forms of treatment, are directly related to the interest and involvement of personnel. Nursing is vitally important in this approach, since the nursing personnel are the most constant participants in all aspects of the patients' day.

Our goal is to provide an atmosphere and experiences in living that will help the patient learn to develop satisfactory relationships with other human beings. Supposedly, people trained in psychiatry should be best able to help others in this respect. Unfortunately, the tradition-bound training received by the majority of people in various fields of medicine and nursing, including psychiatry, often precludes this.

In many schools of nursing, students are taught that the appropriate, acceptable behavior is to talk about, at, or to the patient: that is, to make the patient the focus of attention at all times. The traditionally "good" nurse does not give personal information or express her feelings overtly. As a result, patients may feel that the nurse is not interested in them, and they may regard her as some sort of superhuman at work, without feelings, problems, goals, or personal achievements. Such an atmosphere makes it very difficult—indeed, threatening—for a patient to attempt to express his own feelings or problems. To do so would be to admit a weakness or loss of control if the supposedly "well" people around him act as if they have no feelings or problems (no "self") at all.

In many psychiatric hospitals the emphasis is on custodial care: protection of the patient from himself and from others, especially from others on "the outside" who made him ill. Too often patients are told, "we trust you, you must trust others (us)," while at the same time we watch him carefully to make sure he swallows his pill.

Of course, there are elements of truth in these traditional teachings, but too often these beliefs are considered to have universal application, rather than being adapted to the real situation.

The philosophy of the day and night centers attempts to refute some of these traditional psychiatric beliefs and practices. For example, we trust people with their own pills and their own lives. The other part—trusting them with ourselves—is more difficult to accomplish. So our next major task, one which we have only partly achieved, is to learn to trust ourselves and the patients enough that we can be free to share ourselves with them. There are few enough tools to work with in psychiatric nursing. One of them can be better, more therapeutic use of ourselves.

EXPERIENCES ARE SHARED. In all aspects of our program, the nursing staff has both the opportunity and the responsibility to interact with patients therapeutically. For instance, in the day center, the morning coffee hour can be used very effectively to help the whole group learn to communicate, not just the patients to communicate with each other. This is a time when people can share their feelings or problems and discover that it is possible to talk about anything—not just about symptoms but about themselves—and enjoy doing it. They can talk together as human beings with assets as well as human beings with problems.

The staff, however, must learn to share *their* feelings, thoughts, and opinions with the patients. This is important, because it indicates that symptoms and problems are not the only subjects for conversation, but that people can communicate with each other in a more healthy way. Patients can also learn from this that laughing, joking, and fantasy are not necessarily bad, hostile, or directed at them in a destructive way, but that these kinds of communication can be enjoyably shared with others.

Much of the staff's ability to utilize this kind of experience for patient growth, however, depends upon their own orientation to role and function. We are the ones who must provide the example of interaction. To do this, we must feel free to express ourselves, rather than feel that it is bad or nontherapeutic to talk about experiences we have had away from the hospital.

If we are to help the patient learn to talk about and deal with feelings and problems concerning his everyday life, then we must be able to integrate ourselves, our lives, and our community into the group situation. If we are unable or unwilling to do this, we are then showing the patients how to avoid dealing with everyday situations in living. We thus sabotage one of our most important goals—resolving problems in living through group discussion—a goal which differentiates the atmosphere of the day and night centers from the traditional, encapsulated social system found in most psychiatric hospitals. If this happens, both nurses and patients fall into the old pattern of adjusting to the institutional system.

Learning how to get along with others in a structured group program is important in itself but, in addition, the patient must relate what he learns about living "on the inside" to living "on the outside." To help patients relate these two things, nurses and other staff members must be able to share part of their personal experiences in daily living and be able to relate these to similar situations taking place within the group. There are many ways in which we can draw patients into discussions of this nature. One way might be to ask the patient if he has ever had an experience similar to the one we have just described. The discussion need not become "staff centered" nor lose sight of the patient and his needs.

If the personnel are made to feel that they should not participate with patients informally and socially (that is, introduce a part of their outside lives into the conversation), then cliques may develop. It is very easy for a small, cohesive staff to move away from the patient group to discuss what movie they saw, what they thought of it, and so forth, rather than involve patients in the discussion. The latter then feel left out and tend to form cliques of their own. These small groups of patients can gain some support and pseudo relief when they verbalize complaints, distortions, fears, and frustrations, but this does not help them work through their problems. Instead, it tends to perpetuate or reinforce the patterns of defense that they have previously used to avoid dealing with conflictual situations.

THE NURSE IN GROUP THERAPY

Nurses in the day and night centers have a somewhat unique role in group therapy in that they function both as co-leaders, working with the resident, and also as group members. More than any other staff member, the nurse is in a position to serve as a bridge between the leader of the group and its members. Because she is involved in almost every aspect of the program, she observes, interacts, and intervenes in individual or group problems throughout the ongoing situation.

For example, group therapy sessions are held three times a week, but the nurse is also present at other meetings and activities during the week. Since the resident is not necessarily present at these times, part of the nurse's function in group therapy is to clarify, elaborate on, and question the material discussed when it seems related to other events taking place on the unit. In this way, the group is better able to look at the whole issue or problem area and not at just the isolated segments. We believe that group therapy is more meaningful when it is part of an integrated experience.

Nursing personnel who have participated in patients' group therapy are also in a better position to evaluate the kinds of learning experiences that might be most helpful to these patients during the rest of the day. From the point of view of nursing, this unorthodox approach to group therapy seems to have some distinct advantages.

It could potentially have some problems, too, but we have not been particularly impressed with these so far. Difficulties might arise, for instance, if the resident physician were insecure enough to feel threatened by the presence of nursing personnel who are also capable of helping the group of patients by making thoughtful and perceptive comments. Or another sort of problem might develop if a member of the nursing staff were so in need of help herself that her participation became that of one seeking help rather than that of someone offering help to another.

The nurse's function in the group thus encompasses three aspects of interaction: observing, interpreting, and responding at the feeling level when it seems appropriate to do so. The concern that the nurse's role in group therapy may confuse the image that patients have of her seems unfounded. The three aspects of the nurse's role are not differentiated in the actual situation. The major consideration is to avoid the *all or nothing* mode of interaction: for example, the nurse must not fall into a pattern of using interpretive responses to the exclusion of her own feelings and observations. When the nurse learns to balance these three modes of interaction, patients are able to accept her in this role.

We feel that it is useful for patients to know that staff members have feelings. It is sometimes difficult for them to accept this at first, because of the distorted impression that "to be well" is the same as "to have no feelings." Often a concern of this nature is brought into the open only when patients hear the nurse express feelings, and indicate that they feel it is not her right to do so. When such distortions arise, the therapy session is an appropriate place to deal with them.

SPONTANEITY IS ENCOURAGED. Confronting patients with their problems is perhaps most legitimately done in a group therapy session, but the staff may express their reactions to patients, other staff, and the group outside of group sessions, too. In all the patient-staff interaction that goes on during the day or night, the nursing personnel must be genuinely themselves. They should express their feelings about the patients and each other quite spontaneously, and endeavor to help the patients do likewise.

This does not mean that the personnel are encouraged to throw tantrums or anything of the sort. It does mean, however, that if a patient's behavior is annoying or irritating, the group members, including the staff, should respond like normal human beings. The nurses must not only attempt to understand patient behavior, they should respond in ways that will help the patient learn what effect his behavior has on other people.

Sometimes nurses find it difficult to be spontaneous with patients. Undoubtedly, this comes partially from our training and previous experience in nursing. Another factor operating in this situation is the expectation that therapy should be a continuous process, going on all day long and not confined to the hours of group therapy. This expectation is likely to make us feel that we must perform at our best at all times and that our every comment must be "therapeutic." We tend to forget that more spontaneous human interaction can be therapeutic, also.

WORKING WITH THE GROUP. In the day and night centers the focus of psychiatric nursing is shifted from working primarily with individual patients to working primarily with patients in a group. Because the more conventional psychiatric treatment relationship is with individual patients, few of us are adequately prepared to deal effectively with a whole group or to respond to an individual in the group situation. It is much easier, safer, and considered more acceptable to take an individual off in a corner or to an office to talk over a problem privately.

If we deal with problems in the open, we fear others may get hurt, or even ourselves. As a means of protection, we find it easier not to have an audience either to defend or attack if we are in any situation where we are vulnerable, likely to be made fools of or be put "on the spot," or "lose the round" by having to admit error, mistaken judgment, faulty interpretation, or the like.

It takes considerably more skill and courage to discuss openly in the group problems between individual patients, conflicts among staff, or problems between patient and staff. We are likely to feel much more self-conscious and inadequate in the group situation, where everything we do or say will be seen or heard by everybody in the group. In bringing up and handling problems in the group, we have to be able to let the whole group see us as we really are. Most of us would like to give the impression to others, if not to ourselves, that we have no serious problems with other people. This may be related to the persisting but erroneous idea that if we have problems with another person, then our ability to help patients with their problems is somewhat questionable.

There are other difficulties involved in working primarily in groups rather than with patients individually. How fast do we move with a group, for instance, not just in group therapy, but also in the hour-to-hour group experiences? It is generally accepted that the patient sets the pace for his own treatment and progress. How can this idea be adapted to a group of patients, each of whom can move or change only at his own rate? In activities, should the most aggressive patients always be the ones responsible for having the ideas and organizing activities?

Is it useful to the more active patients to encourage or allow them always to be the leaders? What happens to the quiet patients in the shuffle? In any case, how should the nursing staff respond?

In group work, neither the activity level nor the group goal should be geared to the highest or lowest capabilities of individuals in the group. If the group goal is geared to the highest capabilities, the people who are already capable of taking responsibility and following through with a task will do all the work for the group, perhaps both liking and resenting this responsibility. Often this ability, while real, is used by the patient, with the tacit permission of the group, to avoid dealing with the problems that brought him to the hospital.

For example, one patient seemed unable to talk about his fear of girls and of his own sexuality until the group recognized and dealt with some of his fears of losing responsibility in the group and his tendency to view himself as the only one capable of assuming the role of spokesman or leader for the patients.

Another patient hid behind a facade of being a capable, responsible man and an authority on many subjects. Staff and patients alike not only allowed this, but in some instances perpetuated this kind of behavior. Although this was recognized as a problem and discussed by staff on many occasions, because of our own anxiety, the patient was permitted to seemingly fool himself and us. By permitting this, we allowed him, for some time, to avoid dealing with his debilitating dependency problems.

At the other end of the spectrum are those patients who persistently try to reinforce the idea—to themselves and to others—that they are completely incapable of understanding or doing anything. These feelings are reaffirmed by other patients who are better able to understand, talk about, and do things. The less capable ones then sort of give up, saying to themselves, "I knew it all the time. I can't do anything and I'll never get better." Whenever the staff allows this to happen, they imply that taking over or giving up are the only alternatives available to patients. A more useful solution would be to help both groups of patients learn other ways of dealing with themselves, their problems, and other people.

How can we help patients learn better ways of coping with problems and relating to others? Much of the teaching of healthy human relationships is done by example. A "do as I say, not as I do" attitude on the part of the staff implies that we don't believe in what we say, which must be discouraging and frustrating to patients. We must not only be able to talk with patients about their problems in relationships, we must also demonstrate effective working relationships, problem solving, and resolution of conflicts among ourselves.

If learning is to take place in the manner described, the milieu should be permissive enough to encourage the group members to operate freely. Only when patients feel free enough to react as they should ordinarily, will they develop the necessary involvement with other patients and staff. It then becomes possible to make use of their reactions and involvement with various people to help them understand how their behavior affects us, the rest of the group, and most probably the significant people in their lives outside the hospital.

INTERVENTION WHEN NECESSARY. Providing a permissive milieu, however, does not mean that the staff cannot intervene in a situation involving a member of the group. On the contrary, staff must be allowed to intervene in situations when they see the need, if they are to help patient members understand their actions in particular situations.

A permissive milieu, although often more effective therapeutically, is also more difficult for both staff and patients. Anxiety mounts as patients struggle through the tortuous process of gaining mastery of themselves and their impulses. Group controls are set up as required, and both staff and patients are given the responsibility to live within the limits accepted by the group.

How to deal with the "intellectualizations" of patients is another problem for the nursing staff. Nothing is gained if we help the patient learn what some of his responsibilities are, what kind of person he might really be, and what kind of people live in the world around him, but at the same time permit him to remain isolated and to view these bits of learning from a purely academic point of view.

We can, of course, set up rules and impose our own values of socially acceptable behavior on patients. If we do, though, some patients will respond by soon learning to act "as if" they were well. They respond at the intellectual level only, because they know all of the appropriate answers, but they have not learned to express real feelings. If the staff is unable to recognize and deal with these intellectual responses, these patients may be left at this level without ever having touched upon their real problem. They have learned one thing—to meet the needs of staff to see improvement. Obviously, this will produce no lasting therapeutic benefits.

WHAT ARE THE BENEFITS?

There are distinct therapeutic advantages for patients in a unit of this nature. As a former day center patient expressed it, "This kind of hospitalization gives me the chance to go out and practice what I have learned almost immediately, without having to wait several days or weeks for a week-end pass. Then, too, if problems arise when I am outside of the center, I can come back and talk about my feelings and problems with the group."

Part-time hospitalization in this kind of setting discourages dependency on the staff and on the hospital, serves to limit patients' regression by keeping them actively involved with their lives outside the hospital, and helps prevent them from getting so comfortably settled in the hospital that they give up trying to resolve their problems in relationships with others.

Another advantage—one which probably affects patients and staff about equally—involves motivation. Both patients and staff are able to invest more effort, interest, and enthusiasm in a therapeutic program that is limited to the length of a working day, or to an evening and night. Not being bound to the center and the nursing staff 24 hours a day allows patients a freedom to move away, try new approaches to old problems, and come back each day for a re-appraisal of difficulties and progress.

Involvement of all personnel is an essential aspect of the therapeutic program in the day and night centers. We do not necessarily lose our abilities to be helpful to patients when we step out of our conventional and stereotyped roles. In many psychiatric settings there is a tendency to limit the therapeutic potential by limiting the area of functioning. By working together in therapy and activities at the day and night care centers, we are trying to refute the idea, which may be either implicit or explicit, that doctors, nurses, and others do quite distinctly different things in order to be helpful to patients, and that each must continue in his traditional, isolated ways without regard for the patient who experiences his day in its entirety, not just in its segments.

32

Group Work Method in Psychiatric Nursing Practice

Elaine Kirshenbaum and Douglas Glasgow*

Introduction of milieu therapy in a psychiatric hospital offered an opportunity for the nursing staff to experiment. Nursing staff members became group leaders and learned how to function comfortably in a role which formerly had been foreign to them.

Changes in the structure and function of the psychiatric hospital, and emphasis on the systemized use of groups—arising from the development of the therapeutic community concept—have affected the work and attitudes of all those concerned with the care of psychiatric patients. The nursing staff particularly have had to alter their concepts about their traditional ways of practicing and have had to find new ways to make an effective contribution to the treatment of psychiatric patients.

At Hillside Hospital during the past two years, there has been an increasing use of milieu therapy as an adjunct to psychotherapy. Although milieu therapy is often associated in the minds of many professional and lay people with shortages of qualified staff, the milieu therapy program was initiated at Hillside Hospital as a matter of choice; Hillside has not been plagued by problems of staffing which other psychiatric hospitals have had

---

*From *American Journal of Nursing*, Vol. 64, No. 10 (October, 1964).

Mrs. Kirshenbaum who is a graduate of the Brooklyn Jewish Hospital School of Nursing, N.Y., and has earned both a bachelor's and a master's degree from Adelphi University, Garden City, N.Y., is associate director of nursing in charge of inservice education at Hillside Hospital, Glen Oaks, N.Y.

Mr. Glasgow who has a master's degree in social work from Columbia University, New York, N.Y., was a supervising psychiatric social worker at Hillside and taught at both Adelphi and Columbia Universities. He now is with the Southern California Kaiser Permanente Medical Group in the Department of Psychiatry.

to face. However, the initiation of a milieu therapy program does require changes in traditional staff roles, attitudes, and practice methods, and therefore the staff as well as patients at Hillside have been affected. The patient's day no longer is organized around finding ways to occupy his time between psychotherapy sessions; his routines—how he uses his free time and meets his various responsibilities—have become significant.

Descriptions of role changes within the various disciplines following the use of milieu therapy have been published. Occupational therapy, traditionally a one-to-one therapeutic process, was transformed into a work group experience. Group social work no longer is concerned with creating social activities only to fill time, but now assumes responsibility for using the patient government structure as an instrument of environmental control and as a treatment modality for ego development. Psychiatry has begun to accept responsibility for giving direction to the management of situations outside the individual psychotherapeutic sessions and has begun to use milieu therapy programs as an adjunct to psychotherapy.

Nursing has been dramatically affected by the milieu therapy program. Nursing traditionally has emphasized three aspects of care: intimate bodily care, assistance with medical care, and psychological and emotional care. In the psychiatric hospital, where milieu therapy is a major treatment modality, intimate bodily care is usually minimal in the traditional sense. Most patients are ambulatory and do not need intimate bodily services such as bed baths and back rubs. However, many psychiatric patients do require guidance, encouragement, and education to help them meet their own bodily needs, as well as the care and organization of their personal possessions.

Medical care, while not her primary function, plays an important part in determining the nurse's role in a psychiatric hospital. The nurse assists with such physical treatments as insulin shock therapy and electroconvulsive therapy. She is alert to symptoms of medical or surgical conditions which should be brought to the doctor's attention; she administers such first aid as is needed in any active group of people; and she is ready to assist in all emergency situations. Since the advent of tranquilizing drugs, the administration of medications, including observation of the patient for effects and side effects, has become increasingly important.

The psychological and emotional care aspects of nursing are of primary importance in the psychiatric setting. Here, there is a potential for enlarging and deepening the nurse's therapeutic role. Although this aspect of care in a therapeutic milieu program is not an exclusive nursing responsibility, the psychiatric nurse is in a unique position to use her interpersonal skills therapeutically. But, to do so effectively, she must be willing to accept changes in her traditional location, work roles, and interdisciplinary contacts.

In a milieu therapy program, where the philosophy of treatment focuses on social organization, relationships, emotional climate, and communications, less value is attached to task orientation: nurses doing things for or to the patient. Members of the nursing staff spend less time in the nursing stations; ward day rooms and recreation rooms become the centers of interaction—not only between patients, but also between patients and members of the nursing staff.

AN EXPERIMENTAL PROJECT

In order to be effective agents of behavioral change, nurses must acquire new skills and function in new ways. Since the controlled use of groups is a basic ingredient of milieu therapy, nursing staff members at Hillside, with the support and supervision of a group social worker, explored the possibilities of working with organized groups of patients and proceeded with an experimental project.

The project was confined to one unit and involved 19 of the unit's 54 patients. This unit is divided into two living areas, one for men and one for women. The patients, most of whom were diagnosed as schizophrenic, ranged from 15 to 62 years of age. The prognosis for most was guarded. They came primarily from middle class backgrounds with a white collar vocational outlook. All had a prescribed activity schedule as an integral part of their treatment program. Many of these prescribed activities required membership in organized groups so that the 19 patients who participated in this project also were members of other organized groups.

The nursing personnel involved in the project ranged from unit supervisor to unit psychiatric aides. In order to be selected for the project, personnel had to have had a working relationship with the patients to be included in the groups, a knowledge of the patient's social roles on the unit, a knowledge of the various treatment goals, a knowledge of and ease in the use of a specific type of group activity, and a willingness to risk the experience of an ongoing group. Personnel with competence in four subjects were chosen and four groups then were formed: cooking, sketching, Spanish conversation, and reading.

Each group met for a minimum of one hour a week from September 1962 to June 1963. These groups were not modeled on the traditional group psychotherapeutic model. Although verbal communication was important, the emphasis in each group was on "doing," performance, and achievement. The project was designed to fulfill four basic purposes: to increase social interactions and break isolation, provide a group experience in experiential learning, increase esteem, and encourage the emergence of individuality.

In the course of fulfilling their group tasks, patients' feelings often were expressed, verbally or otherwise. If these feelings were related to the "doing" role necessary for group functioning, the feelings were handled on the spot; if they stemmed from deep-seated pathology, the nursing leader discussed them with the doctor for exploration during the patients' psychotherapeutic sessions.

The nurse, as the group leader, relied upon the group social worker as a consultant in the use of the group method. The group social worker and nursing staff members had often worked together in the wards. The social worker had also led seminars for nursing supervisory personnel on the role of groups in a milieu therapeutic program. A cooperative relationship, therefore, had existed between this worker and the nursing staff before this project began.

In the seminars, which served as a basis for working with the experimental groups, the nurses discussed the formal and informal group patterns of patients on the various units. They learned to recognize and understand that informal groups serve many purposes for patients. They also learned how to work with such groups in the treatment of patients. For example, a nurse may be faced with a group of patients who will not go to bed at a reasonable hour. If she has learned to examine the situation, and can pinpoint the leader and the followers, she then has a basis for deciding whether she will work with the leader to persuade the patients to go back to bed or, perhaps, separate the followers, one by one, from the leader of this informal group to accomplish her purpose.

SKETCHING GROUP. The first group to meet was a sketching group of five patients, three women and two men. Several of these patients had asked to sketch, draw, paint, or become involved in some art form as a means of expression; each had exhibited severe difficulty in verbal communication and in interpersonal relationships in general, but were somewhat motivated to become members of the sketching group.

The goals for this group, in addition to answering the expressed desires of the patients to sketch, were to provide an experience that was essentially pleasurable; to allow the patient, through the use of very simple props, to express what he saw in his own form; and to allow the group and its leader, through discussion, to set limits and define reality.

The group sessions lasted for one hour and 45 minutes. Initially the members were permitted freedom of expression until they became comfortable in handling paints, charcoal, and paper, and in dealing with each other. After the second session, the patients were given simple objects which the leader, who was a senior nursing aide, encouraged them to draw while he moved from one to another offering help and suggestions. Soon all were able to put on paper some picture of the objects they saw. Distortions in perception were evident. The leader then helped the patients correct their distortions. For example, when the group was drawing a desk containing a lamp, telephone, and book, the size of each object in relation to the others, the spacing between them, and the size of the total area was pointed out. In this way, attempts were made to help the individual patient see the objects as they really were.

Such a group provided an opportunity for socialization as well as providing a nonverbal means of expression. It offered one adolescent young man a new way to relate to the people around him. This patient, whose behavior was extremely infantile, had not been able to find an area of living in which he could be successful, yet he was quite talented artistically. He derived satisfaction from the admiration of his work and, using his art as a vehicle of communication, slowly began to relate to people in a more positive way.

The leader's role in this group was to define reality, help patients talk to each other by using their drawings as a basis of discussion, and provide a pleasurable experience for the group as a whole. In so doing, his own relationships with the patients deepened. He often shared with a patient moments of heightened clarity or a difficult moment, such as that in which a patient experienced the confusion of a lamp not being a lamp and simply could not distinguish between her own distortions and reality.

CONVERSATIONAL SPANISH GROUP. The conversational Spanish group, led by another senior psychiatric nursing aide, was composed initially of four

227

patients who had expressed an interest in learning to speak Spanish. This desire reflected their need to perform more adequately in an intellectual sphere. It was the staff's view that more adequate performance in this area would increase their self-esteem.

A practical aim of this group, obviously, was to learn enough Spanish to be able to carry on a simple conversation. In addition, interaction and conversation between the participants in this learning situation would provide a form of socialization.

To facilitate learning, a nonthreatening atmosphere with minimal pressures was established; competitive procedures, such as grades and tests, were not used. Despite this approach, the patients found it necessary to test the competence of the group leader by consulting Spanish textbooks and selecting sentences to present for translation. The leader, recognizing their fear of involvement, did not respond to the testing with anger. Instead, he accepted the challenges. His answers to the many inquiries actually helped the patients gain a degree of comfort in their relationship with him and established confidence in his ability. After the first few sessions, the group settled down to more serious work.

The group's goals were partially achieved as the patients learned enough to carry on simple conversations in Spanish. Their self-esteem was enhanced and the staff person began to gain a new view of the patients' behavior. The staff member saw himself in a role other than that of the parent surrogate or "controller" and "limiter" often required in the ward setting. He was, instead, the teacher and helper.

COOKING GROUP. The size of the cooking group, led by a staff nurse, was largely limited by the space and facilities of the cottage kitchen; five women patients comprised the group. The cooking was done during the hours between supper and evening activities.

It was hoped that this group would help the patients do more comfortably those things they would be expected to do at home, such as planning menus, shopping, and preparing food. Specific goals were set for each individual patient.

The patients in this group differed somewhat from those in the other groups: they were more reluctant to become involved in the project. However, membership in the group had been prescribed for them and participation was listed as part of their regularly scheduled weekly activities.

The first few sessions were devoted primarily to getting patients to attend. Establishing motivation and insisting upon attendance absorbed the time and energy of the leader. One woman voiced fear of exposing her lack of skills in the kitchen; a middle-aged mother hesitated because she believed the group would only heighten her feelings of inadequacy. In the beginning sessions, the group leader explained why membership in this group had been prescribed. Because she recognized their fears, she suggested that their first endeavors be simple.

In the sessions following, the group's efforts became more involved. They used the end of one session to prepare for the next, discussing ingredients needed, and organizing a shopping trip to town. The patients soon participated more comfortably. They began to be pleased about having baked a fine cake, pie, or casserole. As their comfort increased, they began to share some of their cooked food with the other women in the cottage. They were complimented by the other patients. Soon the food they prepared was much sought after. Sharing the fruits of their labor soon became a regular practice; it was served, usually with coffee and quiet socializing, after check-in time at night.

The goals of this group were achieved in varying degrees. Eventually, all the patients were able to sustain themselves in the group for the length of the project. For one patient, this was her first experience with baking; for another, her first meaningful social group experience. One married woman, sought out by others in the group because of her knowledge about cooking, became able to work more easily in the kitchen and, as her self-esteem was raised, began to express feelings of greater adequacy. The nurse leading the group gained new insight and closer contact with these patients, and was able to make a greater contribution to the treatment team.

Seeking ways of motivating patients to attend the group required an understanding of the psychodynamics of each patient as well as ingenuity and perseverance on the part of the nurse leader. Closely related to this were her efforts to help the patients overcome their fears of role performance. Cooking is so closely associated with the female role in the home that it inevitably evoked many of the conflicts experienced before hospitalization. An awareness of the undercurrents of conflict, combined with a constant refocusing of the patients' attention to the job at hand, helped to overcome some of the immobilizing fears relating to their specific role performance as members of a cooking group. Helping the patients achieve acceptance in their social environment was another aspect of the nurse's role as the group leader. She did this by helping each patient find a role within the group that would be both comfortable for the patient and acceptable to the other members. The nurse also helped the group as a whole find acceptance in the cottage through the sharing of the prepared food.

READING GROUP. The reading group, led by the unit nursing supervisor, was composed of five severely depressed, withdrawn patients. Membership in this group also was prescribed. Three of the group were so poorly motivated they had to be escorted to the sessions.

The group leader set out to encourage interaction with others, strengthen the patients' self-respect, and foster self-confidence and a sense of personal worth. Since this was a group of highly literate patients, reading was believed to be a nonthreatening activity. It required little or no personal investment on the part of the patients to read a small selection out loud. Reading in rotation to complete a story was the method used to provide them with experience in cooperating to achieve a goal.

The leader provided opportunities for social interaction throughout each meeting. At the start of the session, the leader often initiated talk about hospital and ward activities or events experienced by all the group members. The social interaction during the course of the meeting was related to the reading itself: one person read and the others listened. When one person finished reading, he would hand the book to the person sitting alongside and show him where to continue. Occasionally, someone would ask the meaning of a word. The group leader directed such questions to the patients and one of them often would volunteer the definition. At the end of each meeting, the reading material would be discussed.

This group began with the nurse leader clearly outlining the procedures to be followed: time, place, length of the meeting, and the expectation that the members would attend regularly. Participation in reading one paragraph aloud would be encouraged, but not be required of those who felt unable to do so. At the first few sessions the nurse leader selected the material to be read. As the group progressed, the members assumed this responsibility. The selections often reflected the preoccupations of the patient. One young man repeatedly brought in stories of violence. An obese female patient selected stories about eating.

Success in this group was marked. The participation of one member is described because it so closely parallels the course of the others.

Miss Abbott refused to attend the reading group at first and came only when escorted by her doctor. She selected a chair nearest the door and outside of the group. She smoked continually. She was introduced to the members of the group and the group's purpose and procedures were explained to her. For the first few weeks she selected the same chair which made it necessary for the person handing her the book to get up and walk over to her. After being shown the place, she would read just a few sentences, excuse herself, pass the book to someone else, and go out for a drink of water. At times she would pass the book in the middle of a paragraph or the middle of a sentence and not show the other person the place. At one of the meetings another patient who was also very much of an isolate asked Miss Abbott if she would like to sit beside her. Miss Abbott said she would stay where she was but when the meeting ended she walked back to the cottage with this patient. Gradually, with gentle encouragement and no demands, she became part of the group, read louder, and was able to show the next person where the place was. She eventually joined in the discussion of future material to be read.

The primary role of the nurse leader in this group was to help the patients give up their defense of withdrawal without directly attacking this defense. She did this by creating a climate of acceptance and respect for each individual and utilizing a medium (reading aloud) that in itself caused interaction. Information about the patients' interactions and the reading material each selected was brought to the attention of the treating doctors by the nurse leader.

EVALUATION

These formal groups contributed to the treatment of the patients and provided a basis for new kinds of relationships with staff members and other patients. It provided an area for the nursing staff members to help the patient examine his responses to a new situation or to problem situations that might arise within the context of the group, and to help him to find new ways of responding when this was desirable. Through staff intervention, alertness, ingenuity, and knowledge, the group experience was made meaningful to the patient and changes in his behavior were made on the basis of experiential learning.

Recognition of the nursing staff's contributions to the treatment program was evidenced by the value which was attached to their communications at team meetings about patient behavior and progress in the groups they led. Making a significant contribution to the treatment of patients increased the staff's self-esteem and sense of belonging to the interdisciplinary treatment team. However, a nursing staff needs to be properly prepared for this role. Some of the lag in nursing practice results from a lag in education. Since theory, education, and practice never seem to keep pace with each other, the hospital or treating institution must provide ways for bridging the gap between educational preparation and functional expectation. Inservice education is an attempt to meet this need. However, since the expectation is for interdisciplinary functioning, perhaps some type of interdisciplinary education would be a more efficient way to create a more versatile paramedical staff.

The nature of the relationships between the disciplines concerned with treating patients are bound with tradition and long-standing attitudes; changes in these relationships bring problems. We clearly saw the need for the nursing staff to draw upon the skills of persons in other disciplines who had training and experience in group work. In this particular project, the nursing staff drew upon the practice skills of the group social worker—a relatively cooperative endeavor stemming from previous working relationships. But, what happens during the cooperative endeavor when it is necessary for a member of one practice profession to supervise another? Implied in a supervisor-supervisee relationship are subordinate and superior positions. Such a provincial concern interfered with providing the best and most thorough supervision of all nursing personnel in our project, creating a situation in which the group leaders often felt that they had to flounder for want of specific guidance.

Adjustment to the role of group leader was less difficult because as members of the nursing staff these leaders already had information, knowledge, and patient contact. They knew the patients' socioeconomic and educational backgrounds which was helpful when they attempted to help patients face reality. Knowledge about patients' problems in social adjustment alerted the group leader to possible problem areas and to areas where he might need to intervene. Personal contact with each of the patients had established a relationship prior to the group experience, but adjustment in the staff's relationships with those in other disciplines was required for adequate group participation.

A number of organization bottlenecks arose as we proceeded with the project. The nursing department's lack of access to supplies (art materials, paints, cooking utensils, and so forth) often caused inconvenience. Time for the nursing staff member to meet with their groups required planning, scheduling, and continual follow-up to be certain that nursing staff members leading groups would not be called upon to perform routine nursing duties during the time of their group meetings. In spite of such planning, when a staff member's interest in leading a group slumped, more traditional nursing duties often were allowed to impinge upon the group leader's meeting time. Only one group, however, was discontinued as a result of the lessened interest of the group leader.

We believe that our nursing staff members look forward to this new way of functioning. It appears to answer some of their needs to be thought of as contributing members of the treatment team. Further, the groups were helpful in changing the behavior of patients. Although we are not able to say with all certainty that group experiences were the decisive factor in behavioral change, significant changes did occur while psychiatric patients were participants in these groups.

BIBLIOGRAPHY

Glasgow, Douglas, *Ego Psychology and its Application to Working with Patient Government and Task Oriented Groups*. (Paper presented at a conference on ego psychology and its application to social work with groups at Hillside Hospital, Glen Oaks, New York, June 1963.)

Greenberg, Irving and others. *The Development of a Resocialization Milieu Program*. (Paper to be presented at the First International Congress of Social Psychiatry, London, England, August 1964.)

Hurteau, Phyllis. Street clothes or uniform, for psychiatric nursing personnel. *Nurs. Outlook* 11:359-360, May 1963.

Pinsky, Sidney, and others. *Use of Therapeutic Groups for the Resocialization of Ex-Mental Patients*. (Paper presented at the 8th Annual Institute and 21st Annual Conference of the American Group Psychotherapy Association, London, June 23-25, 1964.)

Rappaport, Robert. *Community as Doctor: New Perspectives on a Therapeutic Community*. Springfield, Ill., Charles C. Thomas, 1961.

Wachspress, Morton, and others. *Impact of a Patient Work Program on a Psychiatric Ward*. (To be published.)

33

A New Admission Procedure

Philip R. A. May and Mary A. Wilkinson*

Mechanization and thoughful planning have made the admission of psychiatric patients a prompt, friendly, and therapeutic service.

In the often complex and prolonged sequence of events from the onset of the first symptoms of psychiatric illness to the beginning of definitive treatment, the admission process of a psychiatric hospital is a critical experience that may well influence the subsequent course of a patient's illness.[1] Here the patient's fantasies, fears, hopes, and expectations of hospital treatment are brought to the first test of reality; here are presented the first official and unofficial attitudes and reactions of the hospital to his illness and its treat-

*From *Nursing Outlook*, Vol. 11, No. 5 (May, 1963).

Dr. May is director of clinical services at the Neuropsychiatric Institute, and associate clinical professor of psychiatry, University of California at Los Angeles, and was research director at Camarillo State Hospital, Calif. He received his basic medical education in England, and holds a doctorate of medicine from Stanford University, Calif., as well. His past experience includes psychiatric work in the Royal Army Medical Corps, British Army; and in Colorado Psychopathic Hospital; U.S. Public Health Service; and Camarillo State Hospital.

Miss Wilkinson (Johns Hopkins Hospital School of Nursing; B.A., Rochester University, N.Y.) retired last May from her position as superintendent of nursing at Camarillo State. She had been superintendent of nursing at Boston State Hospital, and supervisor and associate professor of psychiatric nursing, Stanford University. Following her retirement, she traveled abroad, and has now returned.

[1]In this article a distinction is made between the admission *suite*—the physical location where a patient is first received; an admission *ward*—also a physical location; and the admission *service* which is that functional division of the hospital that has to do with admitting patients.

This is the first of two articles discussing the nursing role in the admission procedure.

ment; here is the opportunity to start with a positive therapeutic experience and to set the tone for subsequent treatment.

Esther Lucile Brown, in her book, *Newer Dimensions of Patient Care* (Russell Sage Foundation, 1961), comments: "Can anyone doubt that the manner in which a patient is received when he enters the hospital may have a profound effect upon his perception of whether he is welcome as a human being or is only the bearer of a disease to be treated? Before he even gets to the designated floor of the institution, a level of expectation may already have been set in his mind of the care and attention he will receive."

Much has been written about intensive treatment and custodialism as they apply to the patient's ward experience, and about the subtle interaction of role and expectation that insidiously and remorselessly determine the development of chronicity, but little consideration has been given to the role of the admission service in this regard.

Dr. Brown, in the same book, points out that this is not a simple matter. "To provide an admission service that attempts to maximize its therapeutic potential on a day-by-day basis, however, is a difficult task. Even to attempt to achieve such an end requires that more attention be given to it than at present, not only by hospital administrators but by medical social workers, nurses, physicians, and any clinical psychologists or other social scientists on the staff, who are interested in how every part of the hospital can . . . furnish positive psychological aid. To achieve this goal also requires that those members of the staff charged with responsibility for the daily reception of patients and their families receive help and recognition if they are to be able to maintain a climate of genuine interest and sympathetic understanding."

The obviously vicious is easily corrected, but there are more subtle, less obvious influences that, masquerading as good treatment, engender in patient and staff attitudes of passivity and resentment and which induce anxiety and expectations of chronic, prolonged care. A critical study of admission procedures is necessary to determine to what extent they are truly therapeutic, and to what extent they obstruct the patient's recovery potential.

NURSING ROLES IN PREVIOUS ADMISSION PROCEDURES

At Camarillo State Hospital (Camarillo, California), as in many of the larger psychiatric hospitals, nursing service personnel, with minimal participation by other services, welcomed and processed male and female patients separately. The male and female admission suites were attractive, comfortably furnished, and provided with liberal supplies of coffee and cookies. The staff were efficient, kind, devoted to and proud of their work; and apart from the fact that there was not enough space to accommodate satisfactorily the bus load of admissions that arrived daily from Los Angeles—the source of over 80 percent of the admissions, on the whole there was generally the appearance of a good job well done, in adequate surroundings.

In the evolution of therapeutic patient care, this was certainly a great advance over the old-time system of cheerless degradation into anonymity. But it is necessary to examine critically the deeper implications of this well-intentioned hustle and bustle. Beneath the therapeutic façade, in many ways subtle and not so subtle, a sick, helpless, dependent role was implanted in patients, and nursing service was cast in an authoritarian, custodial role.

Helplessness and expectations of passivity were exemplified in the actions of the sheriff handing the patient over to nursing, while crisp nursing uniforms prepared him for a traditional physical nursing role.

The admission process was carried out by nursing alone. There was no team functioning. By default, nursing was forced to assume the roles that should have been played by medical, social service, clerical, medical records, and business services. The impression was created for the patient that the nurses and the legal authorities were responsible for his admission and the medical role was merely a subsidiary one of verification.

Actions such as undressing the patient, bathing, shampooing, changing clothes, and inspecting for vermin reinforced the roles of the mothering nurse and a helpless, physically sick child to be cared for, and there was minimal opportunity for independent or cooperative action by the patient.

Restriction of freedom of speech and action, only partly due to limited time and space, initiated an authoritarian approach. Physical removal of patients from the admission suite at the first sign of disturbed behavior was peremptorily carried out in full view of other patients, inevitably creating patient and staff attitudes that disturbed behavior is an expected and intolerable accompaniment of psychiatric disorder.

It was customary for the nurses to take away the patient's personal property and clothing to be marked or stored without even giving him a personal receipt. This further established the nurse's authoritarian role.

Critical examination of these accepted roles toward newly admitted patients was difficult because there was great pride in the tremendous amount of hard work that the admission suites accomplished—busyness has ever been a sought-for nursing role. In addition, the appearance of kindly consideration and friendliness concealed the harm to the patient, yet met staff needs.

RATIONALE OF THE ADMISSION PROCESS

One aspect of the therapeutic task of the psychiatric admission service is the facilitation of continuous care by one treatment team in one location as rapidly as possible. In this context, the functions of the admission service are to decide whether a patient should be admitted; to select a suitable treatment ward and treatment team; to order whatever treatment is necessary until that team can assume responsibility; and to prepare the way for treatment.

To carry out the last function adequately, the medical information that comes with the patient must be sent immediately to the ward where it can be of some practical therapeutic value, rather than stored away in some central file, accessible only to those who have least responsibility for treatment. The admitting doctor and nurse should transmit to the treatment team their additional observations about the patient that might be of importance in treatment. It is also important that they do only that which is necessary for the proper treatment of the patient until the treatment team can take over. Examination or treatment over and above this minimum is not only unnecessary duplication of effort, but may actually interfere with subsequent treatment by creating a closer relationship than necessary and then breaking it. Physical examination by doctor and nurse should be limited to the minimum necessary to determine whether the patient has a physical illness which would require immediate treatment in a general hospital if the patient were not mentally ill. Detailed physical and psychiatric examination should be the responsibility of the treatment staff who must have direct knowledge of the patient's total condition for adequate planning and medical management.

In the admission suite and during the first few weeks of hospital care, an extraordinary number of forms, cards, and folders need to be filled out for each patient—laboratory and x-ray requests and reports, medical records, property records, nursing notes, physical examination and dental examination forms, notification of different departments, and so on. Each of these requires at least the patient's name and hospital number, usually age, sex, and other simple data, so that the total time spent by nursing staff in just writing the headings is astronomical.

By proper use of machine operation and teamwork with clerical personnel, all these routine forms can be headed by machine and distributed from the admission suite, thereby releasing a large block of nursing time for therapeutic interaction with the patient, both in the admission suite and on the ward. But even if over-all time savings were small, this use of machines is justifiable per se—the attitude is created for patient and for staff that interaction with the patient is the important function of nursing staff, not filling in forms.

It is important at the time of initial contact with the patient to do something for him that he would not normally do for himself and not to leave him alone. Creating a sense of personal attention and active work on the patient's problems is of great practical, supportive, and symbolic significance and will enable him to maintain his sense of identity and personal worth. Another function of the admission suite, therefore, should be to carry out immediately those tasks which can be done more efficiently in a central location to expedite or to facilitate treatment on the ward. For example, few persons realize how much time is consumed in arranging routine laboratory tests, x-rays, photographs, and so on, and in taking the patient to and from the areas where these are done. Even in the most efficient hospital, all these tests are rarely done within 24 hours; in the less efficient hospital, they usually take several days or weeks, which offers a ready excuse for delaying therapeutic action.

Arranging for the tests to be done immediately in the admission suite eliminates delay and time wastage. It also gives ward personnel more time for therapeutic contact with patients and is of immediate therapeutic benefit to the patient in the admission suite. The procedures can be efficient without being impersonal, and they offer an excellent opportunity for therapeutic interaction between patient and admission staff in a recognizably medical, supportive, structured situation. Their swift and efficient carrying out symbolizes the antithesis of custodialism—the hospital's determination to get down to business right away, that time is of the essence, and that something is going to be done carefully, thoroughly, and immediately. This is extremely important, especially to the paranoid patient whose position is aggravated by the delays and inefficiencies of the usual admission process. Whether or not he agrees with the act of admission, swift, sure service establishes a rational basis for his relationship to the staff.

The handling of clothes and personal possessions on admission is usually considered to be purely a business procedure, but it is actually of great therapeutic significance. Too often in the past patients have been initiated into an anonymous, incompetent, custodial role by being stripped of their clothes and belongings, which were then stored away—at best, with the promise that they would be returned "as soon as they are marked." This could take hours, days, or even weeks. It is of special importance to the paranoid and the confused, as well as to relatives and staff, to make it clear immediately that clothing and property are important because they are *personal,* that the patient is important as an individual, that his identity must be preserved, and that he should wear his own clothes and keep his own property. The clothes he is wearing, and those which he will take with him to the ward, should be marked at once with his own name, while that which he does not need or that which is valuable should be carefully looked after. A personal receipt for stored property should be given to the patient to keep on his person as well as to the person who accompanied him to the hospital.

Personal hygiene is important, but it is unlikely that the patient came to the hospital because he needed a bath. It is therapeutically preferable to offer the patient a bath or shower on his treatment ward at a time when it might be more appropriate than to insist on an "admission bath." Inspection of the skin may be included as a part of routine physical examination on the treatment ward. A dehumanized routine of inspection, bathing, shampooing, cleansing, and delousing in the admission suite will merely convey to patient and staff the attitude that he is an unclean subhuman and that his appearance is more important than his worries and concerns. Filth and vermin are fortunately rare in our culture and, in any case, physical cleanliness and hygiene are more properly the considerations of the treatment team who will care for the patient than the admission team.

A very important admission suite function is the management of the family and of family affairs. Those patients and families who are urgently in need of social casework must be identified, and all patients need preparation for meeting the social worker on the treatment team. Thus, it is far more important for staff on the admission service to arrange for the *treatment team* social worker to see the patient or family immediately on arriving on the ward, than to take a detailed history that must later be duplicated. There is danger of creating the impression that only the admission service knows enough to understand the patient's problems, that once away from there he is only another custodial case.

REORGANIZED ADMISSION SUITE
AND NEW NURSING ROLES

In planning for a radical reorganization of the admission service, we established two goals:

One, from the moment of a patient's arrival, all nursing action should be realistically adapted to the situation, so that he will experience in the admission suite a prototype of the nursing roles he will meet throughout his hospital stay. These roles should emphasize: *a*) self-activation of the patient to the maximum degree permitted by his intellectual, physical, and emotional capacities; *b*) support and substitution of nursing action for the patient's self-action only when it is clear that he is unable to act for himself; and *c*) non-authoritarian (but clear) interpretation of reality, with limit-setting and guiding actions which will, in all aspects of his hospital experience, help him to help himself.

Two, a true psychiatric team should be developed in which the nurse can develop her differentiated functions of hostess, receptionist, and interpreter of reality; observer and recorder, performer of special examinations; and dispatcher of records. In so doing, she can activate and support each patient through each admission activity, and clarify reality as needed; she then can escort the patient to his treatment ward.

In this setting, the nurse becomes a team member who assumes certain limited and defined functions, which thus permits the other professions full opportunity for their own specialized activities. This team's balanced action can represent to the patient most effectively the strength and quality of the hospital treatment team who will try to help him get well.

NEW NURSING PROCEDURES

The new service which opened at Camarillo State Hospital on August 1, 1960, combines the former male and female admission suites into one admission service. It extends the team concept to the admission service, with the inclusion of business services and medical records on the treatment team. All members of the team have offices in the admission suite—medical records, nursing, trust (that section of business services which has to do with patient's clothing, personal property, money, insurance, veterans affairs, hospital charges and related matters), social service, and physicians. Ambulatory patients enter the admission suite through an attractive patio with a comfortably furnished reception room where cookies and coffee are available; the doors are open and patients are free to be indoors or outdoors in the patio. The senior nurse assigns a nursing employee to help each patient individually throughout the entire admission procedure. This starts with an informal interview to complete the admission questionnaire, giving the hospital basic data about the patient's social history and his financial affairs. The admission procedure and the function of social service are explained to the patient, and he is asked whether he wishes to see the social worker both at this time and later as things come up during the admission process.

After this, the various other services do not follow any particular sequence. They include an interview with a psychiatrist; chest x-ray; temperature, blood pressure, pulse, and respiration; blood taken for serology and blood count, and urine for urinalysis.

The patient does not disrobe or change clothes. His personal property and clothes are checked and listed. Any excess clothing beyond the complement required on the ward is stored in the hospital storage area. A receipt is given to him, as well as to the person who came to the hospital with him. Labels are prepared for the clothes that he is wearing and for the others that he will take with him to the ward. These are sewn on at a convenient time after he arrives on the ward.

It should be noted particularly that our patients are routinely permitted to keep in their personal possession: wallet, identification cards, plain band rings, cosmetics, combs, brushes, bobby pins, hair ornaments, purse, religious medals (with or without chain), $5.00 in money, stamps and stationery, electric razor, transistor radio, hearing aid, glasses, teeth, eye medication, magazines, and phonograph records.

The patient is photographed, in a natural pose, with a Polaroid camera which provides two pictures from a single shot. We do not require him to hold a number before him, much in the fashion of a convict, when the picture is taken. One photograph is attached to the ward card and the other to the abstract card in the central case folder. These help ward staff and others identify the patient as a person and to recall him as an individual when they read the records.

The social worker interviews family members and, if indicated, the patient. She also has the important function of maintaining liaison with those hospital and other agencies that are the source of many of the admissions.

It has been our experience that in this type of admission procedure, nursing staff have preferred to dress in ordinary clothes, neat and business-like but less formal and less likely to provoke a nurse stereotype than a uniform. All nursing persons can function in any nursing activity interchangeably so that, except for staff needs, no authority patterns exist. Nursing has a team role that exemplifies its place on the treatment team.

No team members attempt to assume the clearly defined responsibilities of other members of the team, yet all give mutual support to each other. Medical records staff prepare and type medical records, and handle functions related to statistical reports. The physician deals with the patient's reasons for admission, ward selection, and immediate treatment prescription. Social service functions in developing a casework relationship with patient and family. The trust section of business services is responsible for property, clothing, valuables, insurance, veterans affairs, hospital charges, and related matters. Thus, nursing staff are freed for their particular responsibilities.

Because the sheriffs and other accompanying agents conduct their necessary official transactions with the medical records, clerical, and business office staff, and not with the nurse and doctor, the patient is helped to distinguish between the often painful and anachronistic legal-administrative process and the process of psychiatric treatment.

MECHANIZATION OF PAPER WORK. Paper work has been reduced and the repetitive transcribing of patients' name case numbers, and other information has been mechanized by installing a high capacity Addressograph plate making machine and a high speed imprinting machine in the admission service area. Much identification information can be put in five lines within a 1-inch by 3½-inch plate, which can be made in two minutes. When patients are committed by court action or are transferred from other hospitals, this information is telephoned to the admissions service who then can prepare plates and imprint the forms before the patient arrives.

A substantial advantage to this one small bit of mechanization is that the information (if the plate is properly made) is correct no matter how many times the plate is used. This eliminates thousands of hours previously spent in proofreading and checking hand- or typewritten data.

By revising our forms, we were able to reduce the total number from 55 to 35 for each patient. (The skeptic should count the number of forms and sheets used in his own hospital for each patient during the first few weeks of hospital stay before he labels this as a fantastic figure.) All 35 documents, pre-assembled in folders, are imprinted in two minutes. The only clerical work now done by nursing personnel is supervising document flow through and out of the admission suite.

The psychiatrist's and social worker's admission notes are dictated, transcribed, and signed in the admission suite, so that the patient arrives on the treatment ward with the initial part of the ward record completed and with all the forms that will be used routinely during the initial period of hospital care properly headed and prepared.

Any patient who comes to the hospital during normal weekday working hours can complete the entire admission procedure and be taken to his ultimate treatment ward within one hour after arrival. Those patients who arrive at night or on weekends, are housed temporarily on a ward until the next working day. They are then returned to the admission suite to complete the admission procedure.

EFFECT OF THE NEW PROCEDURE. The patient has a more positive experience in the admission suite, and so does the staff—previously harassed and frustrated by paper work and blurring of roles. The patient gets immediate attention, and experiences efficiency combined with understanding and humanity, with the general impression that he will receive prompt, good, and thorough treatment by a well-coordinated treatment team. At a deeper emotional level, he derives support and release of tension from this structured, active program. Fears that patients might be bewildered or antagonized by efficiency have proved unjustified. Patients who have been through admission procedure elsewhere (or who had been admitted before under the old system) commented favorably on the change. In the first year of operation, with approximately 5,800 admissions and returns, there were only two instances in which the patient was so disturbed that it was not possible to complete the procedure.

Nurses who had worked under the old system commented that neither patients nor staff seem to get as disturbed as they used to. The atmosphere of the admission suite, even at peak hours, is so deceptively casual and unhurried as to convey the misleading superficial impression that nothing is going on.

The new admission process operates with exactly the same staff as the old system, but it carries out or eliminates many duties previously done by ward staff. These were: escorting patients to x-ray, laboratory, and photography; filling in the headings and identification data on the routine forms; and escorting patients from the admission wards (which no longer exist) to their treatment wards. Some idea of the magnitude of the savings may be gained by considering that it was estimated that 8 nursing staff members were spending a total of 33.5 hours a week at a cost of $4,800 a year (1959 salaries), escorting patients to x-ray. This aspect is particularly important since Camarillo State Hospital had been understaffed in nursing service for many years and had the lowest budget per capita of any hospital in California for nursing service.

To sum up, procedures in the admission suite of a psychiatric hospital commonly operate in a subtly untherapeutic fashion to initiate a pattern of chronicity and to place nursing service in authoritarian, unproductive, inappropriate, and untherapeutic roles. Our new, more efficient, treatment oriented, admission procedure emphasizes team operation, and eliminates paper work by a combination of procedural change and the use of mechanized equipment. This has resulted in changed, more satisfying nursing roles and a more positive therapeutic experience for the patient.

34

Admitting a Patient Is Therapy

Philip R. A. May and Mary A. Wilkinson*

The nursing role changes when the admission procedure in a psychiatric hospital recognizes the individual worth of each patient and makes of his admission a therapeutic process.

In the previous article about procedures in the admission suite of a psychiatric hospital, we pointed out that admission procedures commonly operate in a subtly untherapeutic fashion.[1] The material further notes that such procedures initiate a pattern of chronicity and place nursing service in authoritarian, unproductive, inappropriate, and untherapeutic roles. The change in the procedure altered this negative philosophy and made the nursing role therapeutic.

It is appropriate to examine the operations and nursing roles on the admission ward—the physical setting where admission service is offered to all patients newly admitted or readmitted for psychiatric treatment and care. To what extent are they truly therapeutic and to what extent might they engender anti-therapeutic attitudes in patient and staff or otherwise damage patient-staff relationships? Every patient has a recovery potential—the least one can do is not to interfere with it.

It has been customary in larger psychiatric hospitals—and, indeed, in some smaller ones—to send patients to special admission wards where they are the subject of a diagnostic evaluation that may last one to four weeks, and which includes physical examination, psychiatric history and examination, various laboratory tests, perhaps psychological testing, dental examination, and x-rays. Finally, there is a staff conference, a treatment plan is proposed, and the patient is transferred to a treatment ward for the execution of this plan. In the evolution from custodial to therapeutic patient care, such a sys-

---

*From *Nursing Outlook*, Vol. 11, No. 6 (June, 1963).

tem represents a great advance. It symbolizes recognition of the importance of proper diagnosis and treatment. The façade of procedural efficiency, however, conceals serious anti-therapeutic efforts.

A prolonged period of diagnostic evaluation implies from the very outset, to patient and to staff, that time is unimportant and the patient's illness is necessarily chronic and ominous. Moreover, by a medical version of Parkinson's Law ("work expands to fill the time available"), diagnostic evaluation is prolonged to fill the time available and the maximum period for work-up is soon established as a minimum.[2] The nurses insidiously come to believe that it takes a week to get an x-ray, or two weeks for a laboratory report; that the doctor is so busy he cannot see the patient until tomorrow; and that the typists will be doing a good job if they have the history ready the day before the final conference. We have observed, however, that where it is customary to commit a patient for 48 hours, observation and diagnosis is completed in 48 hours; where the period is 7 days, it takes 7 days; where it is 90 days, it takes 90 days.

Whether the patient's reaction to prolonged diagnosis is irritability, resentment, apathy, resignation, complaining, or escape, precious time is wasted and a pattern of chronicity is initiated. To compound the injury to the patient's recovery potential, hardly has he become used to the staff of one ward when he is transferred to another. The continuity of the therapeutic process is interrupted and most, if not all, of the work of the first few weeks is undone. Even if he remains in the care of the same doctor (and this is by no means always the arrangement), there is little justification for adding to his anxiety by an abrupt change of locale and nursing staff. If the ward transfer does involve a change from one physician to another, the second will probably prefer to carry out his own evaluation and develop a treatment plan that is more closely related to the assets and liabilities of the new treatment team.

In particular, the treatment plan must be realistically adapted to the number of nursing personnel available on the treatment ward, to their level of training and to their individual special skills. In this context the nursing recommendations of the admission ward must often appear to be meaningless stereotypes, routinely entered into the record and routinely ignored.

PREVIOUS NURSING ROLES

A brief, historical review of the nursing roles in admission wards and treatment wards seems important at this point. At Camarillo State Hospital, the patient turnover and work loads on the admission wards were incompatible with good psychiatric nursing; there were 5,811 admissions per year with an average of two weeks' residence on the admission wards. A typical 100-bed admission ward had a nursing staffing pattern of 8-6-3 (for the 3 shifts respectively) to handle more than 200 admissions a month, and the roles of nursing were reduced to the best accomplishment possible of overwhelming admission routines and rituals. Nursing participation in observing and recording symptomatic behavior and the patient's reactions to various interpersonal approaches (one of the most important nursing roles) was necessarily minimal. The patient had little freedom for expression of feelings, and disturbed behavior was always manageable by transfer to one of the two "acute disturbed" admission wards. This opportunity to slough off nursing responsibility for acute patients' needs was, perhaps, the most damaging factor to the nurse's role. The patient culture rapidly implanted notions of institutional behavior—how to behave in order to be sent to a "good ward" and how to adjust with minimal staff intervention. Alternatively, the patient's anxiety in this turnover situation became manifest in disturbed behavior, suicidal drives, confusion, or feelings of abandonment. His dependency overwhelmed and estranged the overworked nursing staff.

All admission ward staff operated on the concept that they were fulfilling a valuable function in "diagnosing and beginning treatment." At formal staff conferences, the patients were properly labeled diagnostically and a formalized routine of treatment was prescribed. Both were commonly disregarded by the staff on the treatment ward, who preferred to prescribe treatment as a result of their own evaluation and who might well be in disagreement with the admission ward recommendations. The careful selection of the ward to which the patient was to be transferred, on the basis of behavior, inevitably sponsored the good and bad *patient* and good and bad *ward* myths which the patient culture accepted and perpetuated—and nursing had a part in these unfortunate designations. Although those with Army experience might have questioned the real state of morale in such a transit camp, there was great apparent pride in the tremendous amount of hard work that the admission wards accomplished, and the appearance of kindly consideration and friendliness concealed the harm to the patient. The inability of nurses to have a satisfying relationship with patients was evident on the days when an exhausted staff transferred patients to their treatment wards with a great sigh of relief, and the patient experienced feelings of being got rid of.

These unhappy connotations were further perpetuated after the transfer. The ward staff who finally received the patients from the admission wards were in no position to make that first all important relationship with patient and family. They were presented with a stereotype of the patient in terms of a formal diagnosis in psychiatric nomenclature; an informal diagnosis of "good" or "bad"; no knowledge whatsoever of the patient as an individual; and a formalized treatment prescription.

The presumption that the patient had been oriented on the admission ward led, again, to the further abandonment of the patient in large measure to the patient culture or to mass responses. The continual movement of patients by interward transfer was most frustrating to those nurses who sought to meet individual patient's needs; attachment to a patient from admission until discharge was a rarity and there could be none of the satisfaction which results to all from continuity of care.

THE OLD ORDER CHANGETH

Organization of the admission ward along "therapeutic community" lines, as conducted by Wilmer, may be successful in reducing anxiety and behavioral disturbances and in mitigating some of the therapeutic atrocities that are perpetuated in the admission ward, but this is still a palliative approach[3]. It does not strike at the heart of the problem—the inherent viciousness of the concept of the admission ward. With the exception of those few patients who need special neurological or physical examination procedures (and these can be accomplished rapidly), there is serious question as to whether there is anything to be gained therapeutically from a separate period of diagnostic study on a separate ward.

There is a strong argument for the abolition of the admission ward and the development of a plan whereby the patient can be admitted directly to the care of one treatment team under whose care he will remain until he is discharged. Conservative treatment and careful observation—the essence of watchful waiting—are certainly a necessary part of the therapeutic armamentarium, but they are better presented to patient and staff as a positive therapeutic maneuver rather than as a custodial delay made necessary by elaborate work-up.

Attention has recently been focused on decentralization and the regional distribution of admissions to produce stable and continuing patient-staff and team relationships, for example, the Clarinda plan, and the Kansas plan.[4,5] We believe that decentralization alone is not sufficient to produce a truly therapeutic admission process. In addition to decentralization there must be three other actions: therapeutic organization of the reception process in the admission suite[6]; abolition of the admission ward concept; and abolition of the distinction between "intensive treatment" and "continued treatment" wards. Any distinction between services should be on the basis of the varying needs of different types of patients (children, adults, geriatric patients) and not on the basis of acute or chronic, good or bad behavior. Nursing roles, also, must alter accordingly.

THE NEW PROCEDURE

Since August 1, 1960, all patients admitted to Camarillo State Hospital have passed through a single admission suite described in our preceding article. This new procedure has a philosophy which is therapeutic. It aims to admit the patient as rapidly and as efficiently as possible, and to take him immediately to the treatment team which will care for him during his entire hospital stay.

The treatment oriented admission procedure emphasizes team operation and the elimination of paper work by a combination of procedural change and the use of mechanized equipment. In this way it is possible to receive the patient on an individual basis, and to take him to his treatment ward within one hour of his reception at the hospital—in his own clothes and with his own personal property, with adequate medical and nursing information and with the following eight procedures having been completed:

1. Preparation and heading of all forms that will be used in the first few weeks of hospital care.
2. Listing and reception of clothes and personal items, with preparation of making labels.
3. Completion of social background and financial questionnaire.
4. Chest x-ray.
5. Photograph.
6. Collection of specimens for blood count, serology, and urinalysis.

7. Interview by psychiatrist (and social worker, if indicated).
8. T.P.R., B.P. and nursing observation notes.

The distinction between "treatment" wards and "chronic" or "continued care" wards has been abolished. All wards are treatment wards, and patients are assigned to wards by a rotation roster that spreads new admissions evenly throughout the hospital, and not on the basis of the duration of his illness or his behavioral characteristics. The patient will remain under the care of the same doctor and treatment team for his entire hospital stay, providing stability of contact for himself and his family. Thus there is no realistic basis for a patient or a ward to feel that they are being discriminated against. The attitude is set that everybody is a treatment case and that every ward is expected to do active treatment and to send patients back home.

SHORTENED HOSPITAL STAY. Under the revised procedure, treatment by the ward team is recognized as starting on the day of admission instead of after a lag of one to four weeks. In addition to eliminating the lag period, prompt treatment might reduce hospital stay in another way, or at least improve the efficiency of the treatment period; the patient comes to his treatment ward at an earlier stage of his illness and his treatment can be planned continuously by one team. In the old method there was always the possibility of a change of plans at the time of transfer from the admission ward to the treatment ward.

Without statistical research studies, we can only speculate as to financial savings, but if only one hospital day, or only one week, were saved for each patient, the over-all financial saving would be considerable to the hospital, not to say what it could mean to the patient or his family.

USING SPACE MORE EFFECTIVELY. Formerly, 384 beds were used to accommodate new admissions during the initial period of diagnostic evaluation. Under the new procedure only 10 to 12 beds need to be kept on the admission suite, and these for admissions at night and on week ends. Therefore, approximately 370 beds were made available for other purposes. These beds are now used for research, for neurological patients, and for a much needed expansion of the medical-surgical service. In other words, 370 additional beds were made available for use without adding a single bed to the hospital. Quite clearly, the number of patients in the hospital and the total number of beds have not changed (except, perhaps, indirectly through shortening of hospital stay); therefore, there has been no cash saving in the hospital budget, but there has been more efficient utilization of space. It might be reasoned that the only other way to add these treatment beds to the hospital would have been to build them at a cost of over $3,000,000 (at the conservative estimate of $8,500 for the cost of a bed).

TRANSITION TO NEW NURSING ROLES. The reader should not imagine that such a radical procedural revision can be easily and smoothly put into effect. The reaction to a sudden appearance on the ward of newly admitted patients in their own clothes and carrying their own suitcases covered the range from near panic to the remark "about time, too." Any change is always a potential stress and some difficulty is to be expected. Ward staff are required to assume new roles, to change established patterns, and to carry out old routines at new times; the change of designation from "continued care" to "treatment" ward may cause anxiety; relief from paper work may precipitate uncertainty about what to do instead. These are all natural human reactions and must be appreciated as such.

The staff on the wards and in the admission suite at Camarillo showed great forbearance in handling and correcting the errors of omission and commission that were necessarily made in the early stages. None of the fears as to the possible effect on patients' suicide and assault rates came to pass and none of the difficulties proved to be insurmountable. During the first year, there was no suicide attempt by a newly admitted patient and fewer new patients became disturbed; figures show that the incidence of serious assault is less common in the newly admitted patient than in patients who have been in the hospital longer.

Since they were left to their own ingenuity in devising methods of handling the situation, the staff have gradually assumed responsibility for orienting patients. Soon patient groups in the wards were organized to work with nursing staff in meeting the first needs of new patients; outside the wards, nursing service and the patient government association joined in a weekly welcome night for new patients. We begin to see the patient more closely related to staff—aware of and under treatment in a new way.

His living facility, though limited, at least has a chance now of being his home ward throughout his hospital stay, a particular spot to call his own, a particular place to be and to go back to. This gives both patient and treatment team a feeling of security and continuity. Perhaps, most of all, the new role of the ward doctor, who is now responsible for the entire hospital care of the patient, may make possible fuller utilization of modern psychiatric nursing and all of its techniques.

REFERENCES

1. May, P. R. A., and Wilkinson, Mary. New nursing roles in the admission service of a psychiatric hospital. *Nurs. Outlook* 11:355-358, May 1963.
2. Parkinson, C. N. *Parkinson's Law and Other Studies in Administration.* Boston, Houghton Mifflin Co., 1957.
3. Wilmer, H. A. *Social Psychiatry in Action.* Springfield, Ill., Charles C. Thomas, Publisher, 1958.
4. Jackson, G. W., and Smith, F. V. The Kansas plan—a proposal for mental hospital reorganization. *Ment. Hosp.* 12:5-8, Jan. 1961.
5. Garcia, L. B. The Clarinda plan—an ecological approach to hospital organization. *Ment. Hosp.* 11:30-31, Nov. 1960.
6. May and Wilkinson, *op. cit.*

35

The Group Culture
and Nursing Practice

Anne G. Hargreaves*

> *Yesterday's nurse could be primarily concerned with the individual; today's nurse must concern herself with the individual-within-the-group.*
>
> *Group work has become much more than a form of therapy for psychiatric patients. Instead, it is proving an increasingly useful technique for enabling many different groups of individuals to work through their problems. Conflicts can be externalized—the individual finds out what is going on inside by looking outside himself. He has the opportunity to test the reality of his perceptions—his thoughts and actions—and to experiment with alternative ways of behaving. Group work is a social experience, with standards emerging from the group.*
>
> *All of this indicates an altered role for nurses. A nurse with over 20 years' experience in group work explains why this is so, identifies the principles and procedures of group work, and describes the varied groups with whom she has worked.*

*Reprinted from *American Journal of Nursing*, Vol. 67, No. 9, September 1967, pp. 1840-1846, by permission of the author and The American Journal of Nursing Company. Copyright September 1967, The American Journal of Nursing Company.

Mrs. Hargreaves (Boston City Hospital School of Nursing; B.S., M.S., Boston University) is associate professor at Boston University where she is also enrolled for doctoral study. Married and the mother of two young sons, she manages also to be active in several professional associations. She is currently chairman of the Nurse Practice Committee of the Massachusetts Nurses Association, a member of the MNA Committee on Education, and secretary of the Boston University Chapter, American Association of University Professors.

Part I: Concepts

The group movement has been described as uniquely American since it came about as the result of the pragmatism of psychiatry in this country. Interestingly enough, however, the first reported instance of group therapy was not with psychiatric patients: it was with a group of seriously ill and discouraged tuberculosis patients, described in the early 1900's by Dr. Joseph Pratt, an internist. Since then, the principles and processes of group work have been explored by many distinguished workers in the field of mental health and illness—among them, Herbert Mead, Harry Stack Sullivan, Carl Rogers, Jacob Moreno, and Kurt Lewin. More recent names, especially in perceptual work, are those of Muzafer Sherif and Solomon Asch.

Anyone contemplating an active role in group work may be initially dismayed by the multiplicity of concepts and approaches within this field, each with its own theoretical background. Yet, while there are contradictions, there is also considerable overlapping; the differences are sometimes no more than a matter of relative emphasis. Eventually, as you become familiar with the various theories and as you, yourself, gain experience in working with groups, you will find yourself developing your own frame of reference. Whatever theoretical framework you choose, however, keep in mind the nature of the group you are working with, your own personality, and how the two interact. This is each nurse's unique, creative opportunity.

There are many definitions of group therapy. I like the simple one: "Group therapy is a process led by someone significantly less involved in pathology to ameliorate the problems of group members in relationship to themselves and society." Slavson defines group therapy as a corrective emotional experience operating through libido distribution and redistribution, ego strengthening, adjustment of the superego, and correction of the self-image, and involving transference, catharsis, insight, reality testing, and sublimation.[1]

Regardless of definition and theoretical orientation, three common denominators or factors generally characterize the group process: (1) an intellectual factor—listening, explaining, watching, imitating others; (2) an emotional factor—transference between patient and therapist; and (3) an actional factor—interaction, catharsis, and reality testing.

APPROACHES

The therapist's conceptual framework determines the relative emphasis on these three factors. Carl Rogers and his nondirective counseling approach reflects a high degree of the emotional factor; Jacob Moreno and his utilization of psychodrama emphasizes the action factor; other therapists tend to concentrate on the intellectual or didactic factors.

The approach adopted in group work will depend largely on the leader's frame of reference and on the expectations and goals of the group. The following rough categorization of approaches may help to clarify your thinking on the subject.

First, there is the *repressive inspirational* approach, which has the emotional appeal of a revival meeting and somewhat of a salesmanship quality. An example of this is the Alcoholics Anonymous meeting.

---

[1]Slavson, S. R. *Textbook in Analytic Group Psychotherapy*. New York, International Universities Press, 1964.

In the *psychoanalytic* approach, there is uncovering of unconscious conflicts, leading to insight on the part of the patient. Patients learn the roles of formerly repressed ideas and feelings as these manifest themselves in pathologic behavior. Forgotten memories are recalled by the technique of free association. Discussion is free, and sensitivity and skill are needed to guide interpretations.

The *spontaneity* approach is best characterized by Jacob Moreno's psychodrama technique. Here you have a stage, an audience of patients, a core of trained personnel as auxiliary egos, and a patient who is encouraged to act out his problems or to recapitulate significant childhood experiences. This technique offers a means of regaining freedom, spontaneity, originality, creativeness.

The *client-centered* approach implies giving of one's self, a willingness to listen and to understand. It holds to the idea that individuals have a potential for growth under proper circumstances and that unsuccessful behavior stems from faulty perception of reality. The group is therefore encouraged to find its own solutions. Exploration brings group members to an understanding of reality. The method is nondirective: no interpretations, advice, or probing suggestions or questions. Direction is left to the group; the therapist follows.

In the *direct* approach, there is free discussion by members, with the leader striving to understand goals. When this understanding is achieved, the leader points out to the individuals in the group how they are operating and why. They then change their aims as indicated or meet them in a more effective way. This approach calls for a more assertive role on the part of the leader.

THE PROCESS

Today individuals in all age groups from preschool through the aged—in almost every conceivable kind of situation and in a variety of settings—are benefiting from the group process. The nature of the relationships within the group constitutes the interaction that holds the group together; this, in turn, influences the relationship. The topical content is determined by each group's experiences and problems.

Conversation ebbs and flows from past to present to future, but is most frequently in terms of the now. Often the leader does not know exactly what is going on in the group. You need flexibility and an ability to tolerate not knowing. Discussion takes place at many levels, conscious and unconscious.

Not all persons do equally well or derive the same benefits from group work. The capacity to adapt to the group process seems to involve a number of ego traits not directly related to traditional concepts such as ego dysfunction. A person can be very seriously disturbed with primitive defenses and do very well in group work. Another person, much better integrated and with more adaptive defenses, will find the group process intolerable. A more crucial issue seems to be whether the patient can become comfortably interdependent with another human being, and be able to learn to share. Some persons seem able to do this and some do not.

Generally speaking, individuals and the groups of which they are a part move through four more or less distinct phases in the course of group work.

1. During the initial phase individuals test limits with group members and leader. They may do so by being overtalkative, by interfering with initiative on the part of any other member, or by being hostile toward the hospital, the group experience itself, or the leader. Occasionally some timid soul may try to communicate support to the leader and register disapproval of the anger, but most members will join together in verbal and nonverbal expression of resistance and aggression. They fail to attend, come late, engage in chit chat. Expressed resentments such as "no one really cares" or "the meetings don't help" provide for considerable agreement and group unity.

Leaders have to learn to be comfortable with such negative reactions and to understand that members may need to deny feelings that are there. The leader's task is to encourage freedom of expression—to clarify and find common ground for differences. Members will say, "No, that isn't the way it is," or distort the situation: "It's different than it looks." They may project: "That's just the way *you* see it." All these statements work against cohesiveness, and many of them come from an individual not knowing where he stands in relation to the others.

The leader becomes the focus of much of the thinking and feeling. Members question how free they can be with what they think and say. Will the leader or members retaliate? Will the leader live up to the agreement? A period of being loved and hated sets in. Competitiveness is stirred; cliques may form or the group may unite against the leader.

Gradually, as feelings are worked through, more positive attitudes emerge and an atmosphere for constructive work develops. With time and effort the members of the group and the leader start to feel more comfortable with each other.

2. A freer expression of pathology characterizes the second stage of the group process. Members become more tolerant of each other's thinking, however different from their own. Communication develops as they learn to initiate and listen, to send and receive nonverbal signals, and to be inwardly moved by the communication of others. As personal experiences are related and opposing views are shared, the air often becomes charged.

The leader's work is cut out for her as communication becomes an organized network. She does best to focus on a story for the day, grasping and organizing an enormous amount of detail, but keeping the focus on a problem common to the group. She offers the members opportunities to identify with each other and helps them move toward a common goal. Members gradually give up cherished points of view in light of other persons' experiences.

3. In the third stage of the group process, members become reflective and seek answers in terms of themselves. The group then serves a real purpose in providing opportunity for the individual to critically appraise himself as reflected by others. This stage becomes a period of considerable growth.

4. The final phase is separation. At this time there is a marked decrease in hostility, a looking to the future, and an application of lessons learned from past experiences that previously had been too painful to look at.

To summarize, the views and the experiences of the individual members constitute the content of the group process. The members' task is to share opinions and feelings. The leader's task is to create an atmosphere where there can be freedom of expression, an exchange of ideas, clarification of meanings, and identification of a common ground for differences. Group life and growth do not move forward in an orderly fashion; progress takes place in spurts.

THE NURSE LEADER

It may throw some light on how I perceive the nature of group work if I describe my own background and development in this field. I'm the oldest in a family of nine and I learned early, through interaction, about intimate cooperation in groups. Although I later joined such groups as the Girl Scouts, the church choir, and the gang on the corner, I still prefer to work in groups of about nine members.

Upon entering nursing school I was out to prove I could stand alone but found little inner freedom in the next three years. We students did find some comfort in banding together against authority, forming a group of sorts, and complaining. Nevertheless, we welcomed the strict rules and regulations since we were stirred by thoughts and feelings we could not comprehend and which I now know were related to the process of change in ourselves. We learned to rely on prescriptions to solve problems and lived in terror of making a mistake. Relationships were seen as a source of pleasure or displeasure and not as opportunities for growth. We received little help in conflict resolution.

The operating room pleased me most: things were clear there. This field therefore became my career choice when I joined the Army Nurse Corps. As the nurse on a surgical team I learned a great deal about the task-oriented group. Through collaboration, I gradually became aware of a "something" in relationships which influences behavior and I requested a transfer to a psychiatric setting. There, for the first time, I saw patients sitting with a doctor in group discussions.

Upon discharge from the service I pursued my interest at the Boston State Hospital where Dr. Elvin Semrad was pioneering in group psychotherapy with psychotic patients. He encouraged the nurses to participate. Scared to death, I took on a group of 12 disturbed women in a back ward. We met three times a week, an hour at a time, sitting on hard benches in a smelly cold room behind locked doors. The patients proceeded to teach me what I didn't know about mental illness and group therapy.

Weekly, we nurses met with Dr. Semrad and other group leaders, admitting our frustrations, indecisions, and ignorance. Our aggravations and uneasiness gradually gave way to small successes. For the first time I found myself asking many of the same questions that were asked by those from other disciplines. As we pooled our experiences we became a group; we learned the painful tasks of collaboration.

My graduate work was at the Massachusetts Mental Health Center during the period when social psychiatry was emphasized. It was here that I found that patients develop a world of their own, meaningful once you get close to it. The best way to learn about it, I found, was to join a group concerned with the daily living problems in that world. And I have since discovered that this also holds true in relation to other groups.

Today, as a faculty member at Boston University School of Nursing, I am still active in group work. Nurses in the clinical setting there—among them, myself—serve as leaders for all kinds of groups: hospitalized and partially hospitalized patients, autistic and retarded children and their mothers, prisoners, undergraduate nursing students, adolescents, and the like. As a result of these experiences, I would like to share my impressions of the qualities needed by a nurse leader.

PERSONAL QUALITIES

First of all, you need that "third ear" we hear so much about today, as well as a "clinical eye"—the sensing of latent significance in a situation. Equally important are the personality characteristics that enable you to feel comfortable in a group: a measure of security, ego strength, and freedom from excessive worry. The person you are is more important than what you actually do. Group members will be alert to your qualities as a person, to what you say and don't say, as well as to what you do. The more you have met and effectively dealt with problems in living, the more effective you will be.

You must maintain an empathetic, yet objective, attitude—feel and express warmth and concern but not reinforce or identify with individual dilemmas. You should be able to tolerate frustration, to perceive and react appropriately in a given situation, to withstand the always present hostility, and to deal directly when it's called for. Spontaneity at times is necessary as well as an ability to tolerate confrontation.

A group approach calls for ability to grasp and organize an enormous amount of detail. You must be prepared and willing to explore references to yourself and recognize opportunities to initiate communication among others, yet leave the development of the group experience to the members themselves.

In summary, then, the following qualities in nurse leaders seem important: efficient perception of reality, an openness to experience, spontaneity, expressiveness, a clear identity, objectivity rather than self-centeredness, creativity, an ability to fuse the concrete and abstract, a democratic attitude, comfort with a variety of human beings, ability to listen, to initiate communication and to arrive at a consensus, and—last but not least—capacity for love, imagination, and humor.

Unfortunately, our present focus on pathology in both general and psychiatric nursing education leaves much to be desired in the education of the nurse group therapist. Rather than the traditional prescriptive approach, we need to understand how persons grow and develop and to use this understanding to help them achieve their potential. We must learn how to recognize and help with anxiety, with needs to know and not know, problems of control and limits, and environmental interplay.

Refocusing our educational programs in the direction of health and of inner fulfillment for all individuals would give us a nurse who would understand love and independence; would have mastered aggressive drives; resolved her own psychosexual identity; and assumed adult patterns of thought and behavior. In the process, she also should have learned considerably about the operations of the ego.

A personal experience as a group member is fine preparation for leadership; so is observing groups in action led by competent therapists. You can, of course, read about groups, but taking on a group for actual practice is perhaps the most meaningful learning experience you can have. You could then meet with other group leaders to compare experiences. You might keep written reports and tape recordings which could be shared and discussed, utilizing an experienced group therapist as consultant.

Part II: Groups in Action

Each group develops its own personality. Each one, too, will have its own special area of concern. It is erroneous to think of group work as limited only to those in need of psychiatric therapy. Individuals in many different situations can benefit from group work as the following examples of various groups, all led by nurses, illustrate.

COLLEGE STUDENTS

Undergraduate students at Boston University School of Nursing meet in groups of twelve for one hour a week throughout their four academic years. They receive a total of eight credits for this experience, which is considered the "integrated" part of the psychiatric nursing program. The group leaders are primarily psychiatric nursing faculty.

This group experience provides an *esprit de corps* without which students in a large university would feel isolated, lonely, and removed from the teacher and each other. In a group, they find it easier to communicate their individual intimate problems when others are communicating theirs and receiving friendly, understanding support from the leader, other members, and the group as a whole. Radical changes occur in the student as she moves from the dependence of early adolescence to the independence of the adult. The group work is therefore focused on the student's relationship with herself and others as maturing persons who can deal with the pressures of living; the goal is to teach students to use the capabilities they have.

Students' responses to the college situation are in part a function of their psychological perception of the situation and, in part, patterns of defense against the anxiety it may arouse. Situations they meet can challenge further intellectual and emotional growth or cause them to retreat from such growth. The purpose of the groups is to provide opportunities for the former.

PSYCHIATRIC PATIENTS

When group therapy was first initiated at the Massachusetts Mental Health Center, there was considerable resistance from patients and staff. The former said: "Why should I tell my personal problems to so many people?" "I have my doctor." "Is this just another gripe session?" The nonverbal resistance took the form of refusing to attend, arranging appointments with doctors and social workers at meeting times, or showing a sudden interest in the work program. The doctors at first questioned the nurses' ability to lead groups and ignored or deprecated their reports.

Today, however, every patient in the hospital meets once a week in a group led by a nurse. These sessions provide opportunity for them to become acquainted with each other, to develop a sense of belonging, and to establish a relationship with at least one staff member. In the meetings, patients practice verbal and social skills, test out positive and negative feelings about staff and treatment, check the reality of their thoughts and reactions, and consider how they will work their way back into their homes and job situations.

Today group meetings are well accepted by patients, families, and staff. They enhance the ward's spirit, provide for socialization activities, and represent a setting wherein patients can test their thoughts and feelings. Group work has become an integral part of the therapeutic milieu.

PRISONERS

For two years now I have been leading an experimental group at a county prison, which meets once a week for two hours. The membership is limited to twelve (there is a waiting list), and admission is by unanimous vote of the members of the group. So far 60 members have participated in the experience, leaving as their sentences are finished. We meet in the library, sitting around a table with an oil painting of the previous sheriff looking down on us. The group members through their own devious connections always arrange coffee.

Within the group are all patterns of emotional disturbance, but some consistencies seem to emerge. Almost all the members have been deeply rejected in their childhood and gain attention by aggressiveness. Their emotional relationships are meager and disturbed.

Their history is generally one of considerable disagreement between parents, with usually overprotective mothers and fathers who don't seem to care very much; a fellow ends up feeling pretty insignificant. Insecurity and fear are always present and all members underrate their own personal value, although sometimes they cover this over by haughty resentful behavior. They need no lectures on right and wrong but considerable help in ego strengthening; they have most punitive superegos.

We work to get in touch with the deeper emotional accompaniments of experience. Our talk is direct. It includes the crimes they have committed, the stresses that may have precipitated or accompanied the acts, the guilt they may feel. We explore the contempt they feel for themselves and the guards; their interrupted relationships with families and friends; and survival techniques during the prison experience.

We direct a good deal of our effort toward the future, pulling out the positive aspects of living and how these can be built on. We work on what it is they want for themselves out of living, on learning to trust persons in authority and each other. The group members, in studying the situation of each person, help themselves, each other, and me to identify and work on the personal and social factors that create difficulties for them.

HEAD NURSES AND SUPERVISORS

At a typical state hospital in Massachusetts—typical, that is, in having many patients and few nurses—an experiment in inservice education was started some two years ago: group work. As leader I met every other week with two groups: one of nurse supervisors and another of head nurses.

The project was voluntary to the extent that the nurses could choose this experience or one of three more formal courses in sociology, psychology, or psychiatric nursing. We kept no records, made no reports to the administration· the purpose of the groups was the nurses' own development, and our discussions focused on problems nurses meet in their daily practice.

At the first meeting, the 11 head nurses sat far apart from each other, paper and pencil in hand, grumbling about taking time from their busy work schedules. It quickly became evident that they did not know each other, had much resentment about past educational experiences, and a sense of helplessness in their current work situation.

The supervising nurses were an older group of eight women, long associated with the hospital and with a cohesion of sorts. Their initial attitude can best be described as cynical; they were extremely skeptical of the group approach. They had brought their knitting and clarified immediately there would be no homework.

How could we get these nurses to learn to face together and solve the problems of their apartness, their noncommunication with each other and lack of helpfulness, their status problems and other differences? I was sure we had to focus on relationship problems if we were to get to the problems involved in their jobs, but I was not prepared for the exacerbation of my own painful nursing experiences in the months that followed.

The exploration of disillusionment and cynicism opened up a need to lean on the hospital structure and to deal with inner lives. Doctors and administrators were seen as not living up to expectations and making excessive demands on the nurses. There was little trust and the nurses saw themselves as helpless children at the mercy of "good" or "bad" authorities.

Hospital rules—rules that had long outgrown their usefulness—were seen as law: routine twice-a-day temperatures; equally routine weights, recorded in a time-consuming manner. The nurses were abiding by policies to which many did not subscribe. Small wonder that they felt ambivalent toward patients who over the years had lost their social identity as they had lost their professional identity. Long overdue was the opportunity for these nurses to perceive their own feelings and reactions to the hospital situation, to feel in control of themselves, and to move purposefully where they wanted to go.

We pushed through the first phase of group work with more than the usual negative response to the leader. In the second stage, actual exploration of problems led to these nurses' looking at their own roles. The supervisory group became especially active in noting breakdowns in communication: they reinstated communication with an evening supervisor that had been cut off for several months, organized themselves into a group to meet with administration to work out policies, and became actively concerned with pressure groups influencing nursing practice. They worked out, and submitted to the director of nurses, a plan for reallocation of work loads; to their surprise, it was accepted and used.

At one point the head nurses and supervisors joined forces in insisting that nurses have a part in treatment planning for patients rather than operating according to a plan laid down by others. All the nurses now seem to enjoy standing on their own feet; they have gained in stature and feel more free to express the talent that was always there.

Two comments made by group members seem to me significant:

"You sure moved us the day you called us a bunch of contented cows sitting around chewing our cud. We were mad, but we moved. . . ."

"I don't know what happened—I began to talk and haven't stopped since. It feels so good. Four times in the past when I was fed up I would clear my desk, pack up and go. Not now—we work it out with all the varieties of feeling involved and I like it."

ADOLESCENT GIRLS

For over a year now, I have been meeting with a group of girls, aged 14 to 18, on an outpatient basis. (Their mothers and fathers attend group sessions led by a social worker.) The problems which brought them to the clinic varied: failure in school, arguments, drinking, drugs, lying, stealing, running way, overweight, depression, and phobias. We meet once a week for an hour and a half after school hours, in a bare, nondistracting room with chairs arranged close together around a table, and talk about problems introduced by individual members and the group itself as a living experience.

Problems are consistently dealt with as a group matter. In times of stress, voices are raised, chairs pushed back, windows opened, and trips to the bathroom—always in groups of two—increase. We move rapidly from very grown up to very immature situations. One time we discussed earrings, boy friends, and more adult hair arrangements, while lollipops were passed around and enjoyed. Another time, while heatedly discussing the demands of mothers, some of the girls chewed and snapped their bubble gum with vigor and delight, with everyone carefully watching the leader's reactions. The most mature discussions will disintegrate while the group breaks into giggling, poking each other, or sharing secrets from which the leader is excluded.

Things are seldom as they appear to be and the members are quite disgusted if you accept them as such. Much more is communicated through behavior than through words. A sad mood can turn quickly into joy at the poke of a peer, or a supportive smile and a reach of the hand from the leader. Things are *all* good or *all* bad.

They check out reality with each other and the leader. Frequently, however, they ask point blank: "What do you think about smoking, petting, drinking?" and, sadly, "Will I ever grow up?" At one meeting, with hesitation, they shared a dirty joke; this was followed by a poem one girl wrote about her warm feelings for her mother, and then one girl encouraged another to sing a love song to close the meeting. It was indeed a meeting of shared feeling.

Toward the leader are expressed hostility, demanding dependency, identification, respect, and affection. Tolerance is tested over and over. "Don't get scared when we are," they make clear, and check time and again to make sure you are not.

I talk directly and honestly with the girls—adult to emerging adult. I show no disappointment when an individual or the group slips back, which happens quite frequently. I'm expressive about a new hair style or dress. While encouraging something they are working toward, I try not to overexpect. It's their goals, not mine, we work on.

They want things better. They question me about being a nurse, my husband, my children. We share pictures, their dreams of what it will be like when they get married, the "hunk" they are going to meet some day, while they show off their new chino pants or collapse into gales of laughter as they are caught up in the contagion of the moment.

The theme is always the same: "growing up is a scary business." We take two steps forward and one back. For technique, simple friendliness goes a long way. I listen, talk to them, and do things with them. They watch for lack of interest, but resent prying. Tone and facial expressions are important. They resent criticism, talking down, and preaching.

One girl sat in sullen silence for three months while I talked *at* her. She warmed up first to the members. I persisted and today we are the best of friends. In such unresponsiveness it is uncomfortable to ramble on, but I do with this group by telling stories and sharing experiences. It works better than the silence so often intolerable to the adolescent. It's amazing how often, after such monologues, they will say, "you really understand our problem." We have connected in persistence.

MENTAL HEALTH CLINIC STAFF

Group meetings for staff in a community mental health clinic, we have discovered, provides optimum conditions for learning, change, and creativity, and seem to indicate that a group's effective functioning depends on the members' relationship to one another. The staff consists of a doctor, social workers, nurses, psychologists, a nursery school teacher, and an administrative assistant, representing a wide range in age, educational and ethnic background, and traditions.

With a consultant in group work serving as leader, we started to explore the barriers to free communication in a group which focused on the problems members were having in groups they were leading. Each person brought to the discussion his own professional language, conceptions, and expectations; this led to antagonism and confusion.

After several months the medical director joined the group and was immediately subjected to pressures to make unilateral decisions that would clear up the confusion. These were resisted, however, and members gradually began to look at their work as a group, at the assumptions different professions make about each other, and at their relationships to patients.

There were the typical questions at first with respect to rank and privilege: office space, decisions about treatment plans, and who was going to make the coffee. Now we look more to the consequences of our actions and the variety of our attitudes, sentiments, beliefs, and values. We have become better able to explore and question the traditional role of medicine as more meaningful kinds of approaches have been worked out. As we progress, professional roles are becoming less rigidly defined and protected.

As we, ourselves, change, we change in our ways of coping with situations and seek new ways to work effectively together to care for people. Such a process is not without pain as we try to resolve issues, but the experience has convinced me that people can become rational about the problems of their work only as they become rational about relationships in trying to think and work together.

36

What Is REALISTIC
Emotional Support?

Gertrud B. Ujhely*

With compassion, wisdom, and simplicity, an expert psychiatric nurse unfolds here her own view of what the nonspecialist reasonably can expect of herself in offering emotional support. She explains what it means to look for themes in a conversation, how to put one's own feelings to good use, and when to ask for help.

Certain questions concerning nurse-patient relationships are voiced over and over again by nurses who are not psychiatric nursing specialists and who feel caught between Scylla and Charybdis when they attempt to offer patients emotional support. They fear being dashed on the rocks of silence and resistance if they offer too little support, or being pulled under by a complicated whirlpool of feelings if they offer too much.

*Reprinted from *American Journal of Nursing*, Vol. 68, No. 4, April 1968, pp. 758-762, by permission of the author and The American Journal of Nursing Company. Copyright April 1968, The American Journal of Nursing Company.

Miss Ujhely, associate professor and director of the graduate program in psychiatric nursing at Adelphi University, Garden City, New York, is especially interested in helping practicing nurses to be reasonable about their expectations of themselves and of patients, as this article indicates. A graduate of American University, Beirut, Lebanon, Miss Ujhely has her B.S. from Hunter College and her M.A. from Teachers College, Columbia University, both in New York City. She is currently a doctoral candidate in psychiatric-mental health nursing at New York University.

This article is adapted from a speech presented at Wagner College School of Nursing, Staten Island, N.Y., in November 1967. It presents, in part, content from the author's forthcoming book, *Determinants of the Nurse Patient Relationship*, to be released in May by Springer Publishing Company, Inc., New York.

General questions of this type are:

What kind of emotional support can the nurse who is not a specialist in psychiatric nursing give patients?
At what point should a specialist be called in?

More specific questions are:

How do I know what message the patient is trying to get across to me?
How can I prevent him from asking more of me than I can handle?
What am I to do if my own feelings get in the way?
How do I know that I have the whole message?

Such questions often are based on the belief that there is or should be a clear-cut line between what the specialist and the nonspecialist can do. I believe this is not true, either in nursing or in any other professional discipline. For what today is the domain of the specialist should tomorrow become the property of the entire profession, for how else can the level of practice of a profession be raised? In nursing, for instance, techniques of patient counseling were first utilized and developed by public health nurses; now, in many schools of nursing, freshmen in the first semester are exposed to this area of knowledge.

I would say, then, that the general practitioners within any one specialty should be able to extend to patients the amount and kind of emotional support that is known to the profession at large at a given time.

I also believe that the emotional aspects of care are a responsibility of the specialists in the various clinical areas, and should not be separated out and left to psychiatric nurses. I believe that, by assuming this responsibility, each nursing specialty can produce knowledge that will be useful in other areas. Consider our loss if we had reserved counseling techniques for use only in public health nursing!

Obviously, I believe that any nurse, for example one who practices as a staff nurse on a medical-surgical service, can provide patients with some emotional support. How much this individual nurse will be able to help her patient with his emotional needs will depend mainly on her theoretical background, on the amount of experience she has had in this clinical area, and on her ability to make adjustments to a given patient.

USING THEORY

In spite of the American Nurses' Association position that all nursing education should be placed in institutions of higher learning, the controversy still rages as to whether a nurse needs or does not need theory to do her job. The real issue, however, is not whether one needs theory or not, but rather what kind of theory and how many theories. For everyone uses theory, not only in patient care but in daily living, whether he is aware of it or not. For, in order to understand a given situation and deal with it we compare it, knowingly or not, with generalizations about similar situations stored away in our memories. Even though we may have little formal theoretical knowledge, we still have generalizations to back us up. These are drawn from common sense, from what we pick up in our contacts with others, from hearsay, and even from old wives' tales, proverbs, and the like.

The nurse who has completed a basic program in nursing is usually familiar with a number of theoretical concepts. Nurses who undergo the rigors of graduate study are exposed to a greater variety of theories. The broader a nurse's theoretical background the more able she will be to choose from many possible explanations the one which will best fit her particular patient's case. The nurse who has only one answer must either hope that her answer is correct or bend the data to fit her theory.

Take, for instance, a patient who, after careful deliberation, has decided to go through with his operation and signs the required permission slip. The moment after he has signed the slip, he becomes extremely anxious. He wonders whether he has made the right decision after all. The nurse who relies mainly on common sense and personal experience might think, when seeing the patient in his quandary, that he is afraid of the operation. She will probably try to reassure him that he has nothing to worry about, his doctor is a great surgeon, and so on. But this patient, instead of relaxing, becomes furious with her, because he has thought through all this himself and does not need her to repeat it.

The nurse who has learned selected concepts may deduce that this patient indicates, by his restlessness and his vacillating behavior, that he is in conflict. She knows that conflict presupposes the existence of at least two incompatible goals. Hence, she proceeds to help him become aware of the goals he finds so difficult to reconcile. The patient might appreciate her efforts, for he had to go through this process before he made up his mind, but he still is no closer to knowing why he should be so uncomfortable and beset with doubts.

Suppose a nurse takes care of him who has had the opportunity to sit through a course in social psychology. She too will think that the patient might be afraid or that he might be in conflict; but she also will be struck by the fact that his uneasiness did not occur until after his decision. This phenomenon —"cognitive dissonance"—though similar to conflict, is different from it. It characteristically occurs after a person has committed himself to one of two or more goals, none of which is entirely satisfactory. By recognizing that this concept applies to this patient the nurse has found a way of helping him. First, she can indicate to him that his discomfort has less to do with the kind of decision he has made than with the fact that he has made a decision. She can also let him know that this is not unusual, and she can show him how he may rid himself of this state—by encouraging him to dwell further on the good aspects of his decision and on the negative aspects of the alternative.

Thus, the more knowledge the nurse can bring to bear on a given situation, the greater is the likelihood that she will hit the nail on the head. There is, of course, no limit to what anyone can know. New knowledge is created faster than any one of us can assimilate and put to use. Each one of us can, however, keep adding to our learning and applying what we have learned.

USING EXPERIENCE

How does the amount of experience a nurse has in a given specialty affect the way she can deal with a given patient? If she has seen a thousand patients give birth, if she has seen hundreds of patients go through the tribulation of learning crutch walking, or if she has seen many patients through the discomforts which follow surgery, she may permit herself to reassure her patients as to when their discomfort is likely to end. She may also permit herself to pressure a patient to exert more energy or self-control or endurance than he is exerting on his own. For, she knows from experience when the peak of discomfort is reached and when it subsides. She also knows from experience how much most patients can do in their own behalf, and she is able to recognize when the patient has really reached his limit.

If the novice nurse tries to reassure the patient in this way, however, he is likely to doubt her word and feel more forlorn than ever. If she tries to pressure him further than he is willing to go, she has no basis for judgment and she may tax him beyond his resources. The novice nurse, then, must take the patient's word at face value. She must desist from putting further pressure on him and should concentrate primarily on providing comfort for him, or at least on being with him while he suffers.

In other words, the beginning nurse will need to be more conservative and must expect to progress more slowly with her patient than will the nurse who has accumulated considerable experience in her field.

However, all nurses must be careful that they do not permit theory and experience to blind them to an existing situation. For, it is possible that a given patient will not fit the accumulated understanding of the nurse; he or his condition might behave differently from everything the nurse, even with years of practice, has ever seen. It is most important that this difference be recognized, acknowledged, and reported so that more expert help can be obtained.

CALLING FOR HELP

A specialist in psychiatric nursing or any other field pertinent to the problem should be called in when neither the nurse's background nor her experience are sufficient to explain the phenomena at hand. Ideally, of course, the nurse practitioner should call in her own clinical supervisor first and, if she too finds the situation beyond understanding, she will then see that a specialist from another area is called. Whether this specialist be first a physician or a nurse will depend on the problem, on the setting, and on the kinds of specialists available.

There are other occasions when the nurse should not hesitate to press for consultation: namely, when she "feels" that more is going on than meets the eye—something that may or may not indicate that the patient is in serious emotional difficulty. How does the nurse know this? Nine times out of 10 she does not know it, but she intuits it, as it were. She may feel a tingling at the back of her neck or have a premonition without being able to put her finger on anything specific. But for her a red light is flashing danger.

I believe firmly that the nurse should give in to her hunches, even if they turn out to be false alarms. Better two false alarms than one true one gone unheeded.

USING PREDICTION

The nonpsychiatric nurse who works in a specialty has additional information about patterns of illness which can help her provide meaningful support to the patients she sees every day.

That is, she is cognizant of the themes prevalent in certain conditions; for example (and I am generalizing), grief where there is loss of organs or limbs, or aggression where there is immobilization. She probably knows something about the kind of person who usually suffers from a particular condition, even though much of this type of information is still very tentative. For instance, in my experience patients with Parkinson's disease often have a history of seeking perfection, while patients with multiple sclerosis have often had—again in my experience—an almost inhuman determination to achieve what they have set out to achieve.

The nurse who works in a specialty is also aware that two patients with the same disease may have two opposite reactions to it. For example, many patients who have suffered coronary occlusions tend to deny the severity of their condition, while others become utter hypochondriacs. A patient who finds that he has cancer may either be glad it has been discovered in its early stages or he may want to jump off the nearest bridge because the term "cancer" means to him the inevitability of a life of lingering, unbearable agony.

Of course, what a patient's condition means to him will depend on the way he is able to perceive, interpret, and respond to it in light of his age, his socioeconomic background, his ethnic heritage, and his religion.

I realize that this is a tall order and that there is no ultimate in the knowledge that can ever be attained. Slowly and at her own pace, however, each nurse can build herself an arsenal of knowledge, revising it as new information emerges and according to the way it tests out when she works with patients.

LISTENING FOR THEMES

The more knowledge and experience the nurse has and the more familiar she is with the themes that are likely to come up, the sooner she will have some idea of what patients are trying to convey to her. If she is relatively inexperienced, she needs to handle the patients' fragments of communication as she would a jigsaw puzzle; slowly at first, not knowing where she is going, but sooner or later discovering a pattern. Then she can more actively look for the remaining pieces needed to fill in the design.

And, just as with a jigsaw puzzle, she must not allow herself to get frantic, for then she will be unable to distinguish the pieces; nor can she use only her head, but must, instead, allow her whole being to help her in solving the riddle.

Let me try to be more specific. Usually it is in his first encounter with the nurse that the patient lets her know the problem area in which he wants her help. He does not say it in so many words, of course, but, if the nurse lets him take the lead in the conversation and merely interjects phrases that let him know she is listening, or that she needs clarification on a particular point, he will tell her, by relating a variety of topics, what the *theme* of his problem is. By "theme" I merely mean the main idea which one can extract from a series of statements. Usually as the nurse listens, the patient will develop in front of her eyes, as it were, three kinds of themes: the *content* theme (the "what" of his story), the *mood* theme (how he tells his story), and the *interaction* theme (the way he relates to the nurse and, by reciprocity, sets up how he would like her to relate to him).

As a matter of principle the nurse should deal first with the content theme—with the story the patient is telling her. The reason for this is that the mood theme is usually related to the content and cannot be solved unless more information about the content has been obtained. For example, if a patient is very sad or angry because he is not allowed to go home when he was promised he would be going, dealing with the sadness or the anger will not get the nurse anywhere, nor will it solve the patient's problem.

On the other hand, finding out what the patient was told about not going home may give the nurse an opportunity to clear up misunderstandings, or to examine with the patient what his expectations had been in the first place. As these matters are clarified, there is a good chance his mood may change and become more positive.

But then again, if the nurse notices the patient's mood change suddenly, she should not hang on to the content discussed with him the last time she saw him, but should rather inquire what happened that might have led him to feel the way he does.

Another principle (at least for me) is that the nurse should not challenge the patient's way of interacting with her as long as he is able to present content to her which they can both examine. This will prevent the occurrence of a relationship that becomes so involved that the patient really offers the nurse more than she can handle, with the likely result that she must, in order to save her hide, remove herself from him. The only times a nurse should deal with the interaction per se are (1) when it blocks the problem-solving process—for instance, when the patient confronts the nurse with a stubborn silence—and (2) when the patient acts toward the nurse in exactly the same way that he does in the situations he describes to her as problematic.

The nurse needs to be careful that she does not automatically assume all the roles into which she is cast by the patient. If he says she behaves like a dragon or like his mother, she does not have to act these roles. Instead, she might ask him in what way she resembles a dragon or his mother and then, in what ways she might be different from them.

Along with our not having to take the roles a patient may wish to assign us, I would like to remind the nurse that, just because the patient asks us a question, it does not necessarily follow that we must come up with an answer. That is, when a patient asks a loaded question or reveals a heavy emotional burden, it may help the nurse with her own feelings if she keeps in mind that we cannot possibly lift a burden from a patient; we can only help him carry it himself. Besides—and this is even more important—he usually does not want an answer to his spoken question, but to something else which he may or may not ask aloud, depending on the way we handle his first question.

USING OUR FEELINGS

Patients, knowingly or unknowingly, arouse feelings in us in response to overt or covert messages. And frequently these feelings are not acceptable to us, at least not in relation to a patient. Hence, we may want to get rid of them and may find that, in order to do this, we have to disengage ourselves from the patient.

Our feelings might also be aroused by a given patient if he has, by word or behavior, violated a value we hold sacred. We may not even be aware that this particular value which happens to be our own is not shared by everyone.

A nurse is entitled to have feelings, regardless of what nature, toward a patient. We are not necessarily entitled, however, to express these feelings openly to him. There is a difference between having an emotion and expressing it. I think that some of our fears about experiencing emotions of love, hate, sympathy, or whatever toward patients have to do with the fear that we might let them know what we are experiencing.

But once we are clear on this difference, we can be grateful for experiencing emotions in relation to interaction with patients. For, how else would we know what is going on? The volumes written about the "therapeutic use of self" really do not say very much more than to use your emotions to assess what is going on, and steer the inquiry accordingly.

For instance, imagine working with a patient who has had a stroke and who keeps complaining about how unhappy he is. The chances are that for a while you will feel very sympathetic toward him; you will even go out of your way and do little favors for him. But after a while, you find yourself rather reluctant to go and see the patient; in fact, you usually find something more pressing to do. Then someone else picks up the slack, but sooner or later follows in your footsteps. And the patient remains the same, except that he now also begins to complain that staff show him interest for a while and then drop him as if they had discovered he had leprosy. You may find that you feel so guilty about this that you ask to be transferred to another ward.

Is this necessary? I do not think so. If, early in the relationship, you can acknowledge to yourself that you are irritated with him, you can then, before doing anything about it, examine the reason for your irritation. Is it that you were brought up with the belief that one should not feel sorry for oneself? If so, fine, as far as you are concerned. You need not feel sorry for yourself ever, but you must concede that other people were brought up differently. The moment you have gone through these mental gymnastics you will find that your annoyance with the patient has largely dissipated itself; instead, you might experience a certain amount of curiosity as to what makes this patient tick in the way he does. There may be cultural reasons which prescribe his behavior for him as your kind of behavior has been prescribed for you.

On the other hand, your anger may have been triggered by a disguised anger in the patient. He may not really be so sad about what he is going through, but he may be saying—and you will pick this up if you listen closely —"Look how I suffer! It is not fair that I should have been chosen to bear this fate; why not my neighbor, why me?" He is not really sorry for himself; he is really angry that this fate should have befallen him of all people. When you are reasonably sure that this is what he means you might ask him if, in effect, this is what he is saying to you. The chances are that sooner or later he will admit to it. If, then, you can agree with him that he might well feel this way, he will allow himself to express his anger more openly, and will thus have moved from one stage of grief about his condition to the next.

None of this might have been accomplished had you not been aware of your feeling of annoyance toward your patient: by acknowledging this feeling and using it, you have actually used yourself therapeutically.

When do you stop listening and start moving toward a solution? Usually, we move too fast toward a solution, long before we have heard all there is to hear about a patient's message. A rule of thumb might be—except in emergencies when you *must* act, and except with patients who are utterly helpless or who have serious handicaps in their ability to perceive, interpret, or respond to the world around them—that we take our time. The chances are that we have not heard all the facets of a patient's themes. And, if we come to his rescue too soon, the chances are that he has used us to take his chestnuts out of the fire. The chances are further that we will resent him for it, and that he will not have learned anything, nor will he be any better for it.

RESOLVING PROBLEMS

Suppose the patient has a problem communicating with the aides or with his physician. Don't do it for him. Let him describe what the problem is, what the other person does, and his own role in the impasse. It may not be the aide or the physician but the way the patient makes his requests known to them that is the problem. And—again, provided the patient does not fall under the exceptions listed above—helping him learn to communicate with others so they are willing to receive his messages will be of greater service to him in the long run than doing it for him. In fact, by conveying his request for him we really are enlarging the distance between the other persons and the patient instead of helping to reduce it.

Providing emotional support to patients, then, involves a nurse's accumulated theory and experience, her ear for themes, and the way she uses her feelings toward patients. She need not be a psychiatric nurse to provide meaningful support or, in turn, to experience the satisfaction that comes from having used herself therapeutically.

37

Changing of the Guard

Alice M. Robinson, R.N.*

Psychiatric nursing has entered a new era, and the nurse now has a real opportunity to do satisfying and constructive work.

Those of us who have watched long lines of men and women walk by each day in worn, disheveled clothing, with heads bowed and hands listless, find it difficult to believe that psychiatry is at least emerging from its dark corner. We are watching it become a real and lifegiving hope for hundreds and thousands of mentally ill Americans and we are watching it with no little wonder and gratification.

Not so long ago the psychiatric nurse was almost unheard of. Those few nurses who, for some reason or other, stayed in their offices in huge, rickety buildings, listening to the cries of unwanted human beings, are gradually becoming a part of the past. That past is filled with voluminous paper work, tales of brutal beatings by attendant "guards," and lonely, narrow lives.

Do not believe for one minute that these things do not still exist, for they do. But the pall has lifted, and there are now clean, tidy wards, well cared for patients, nurses and doctors whose lives are full, and mentally ill persons who go out of the hospitals improved or cured.

What has helped the psychiatric nurse to become this person of the full life, new courage, and a real desire to give care to patients? First of all, our changing philosophy of education in nursing has recognized the necessity for complete physical and mental care of patients. An integral part of this new philosophy has been the recognition that the patient not only has skin and

*From *American Journal of Nursing,* Vol. 50, No. 3 (March, 1950).

Miss Robinson (Duke University School of Nursing; B.S., Catholic University) is on educational leave from the Veterans Administration and is now taking advanced work in psychiatric nursing at Boston University.

bones and organs but that he also has emotions and thoughts and that he is a spiritual being with definite rights.

Thus nurses are beginning to understand *why* a patient is irritable or cranky or aloof. They are learning the meaning of one of the most important single factors in mental illness—fear! Fear makes the new mother feel strange toward her child; it makes a youngster who is posted for a tonsillectomy cry all night; it makes a man with a mild cardiac condition constantly ring his call bell.

WHAT MAKES A PSYCHIATRIC NURSE?

What in the nurse draws her toward the specialty of psychiatry? It is undeniable that some of us possess certain personality characteristics which others of us do not. To become interested in psychiatry, one must be *aware*. This awareness must be not only of the patient's total needs, but of one's own needs. For unless we can understand our own behavior, we cannot understand or appreciate the behavior of others. Awareness goes even further; it goes on to an appreciation of everyday things—beauty, and kindness, and humor.

There are those who believe that, in order to work with psychiatric patients, a nurse must have an "iron constitution." In a way, this is true, for the nurse must be strong within herself to represent to her patients the security and confidence they need so much. But it does not mean that she must shut herself up in a hard, narrow shell without expansion and without the "fresh air" that goes with a well rounded personality.

I remember well the first time this point was driven home to me. I was a senior nursing student and I was on night duty on the psychiatric ward of our general hospital. I worked with another senior student, a quiet young woman who from the beginning had shown an aptitude for nursing the mentally ill. A drunken, frightened prostitute was brought to the ward by two emergency room interns. Her profanity was awesome, and she fought, kicked, and scratched. When placed in a quiet room she stood, glowering in a corner, screaming abuse and threats. The other student and I looked at each other; we knew we must undress her and get her to bed. My friend and co-worker, who had known fear and bitterness in her own broken home, opened the door and walked in. As the prostitute advanced toward her my friend paid no attention whatsoever but sat down and began to talk quietly and in a matter-of-fact manner. In a very short time the prostitute had promised to undress if left alone; in less than an hour she lay asleep.

This entire incident could have been different and terrible. Certainly it is not advisable to enter, alone, a room in which there is a disturbed patient. But this nurse knew what the patient needed; and she knew it, not because someone had taught her and not because she had studied her text, but simply because she recognized in another person a reaction she herself had had and she knew how to deal with it. The nurse's own confidence was such that the whole room became pervaded with security—there were fours walls, it was quiet, and here was a friend. And, yes, this is a prostitute, but she still deserves the right to modesty, so let her undress alone; we are dutybound to watch through a crack in the door, but she needs to feel adult and independent, and then, too, sometimes a prostitute feels unclean in front of two starched, immaculate uniforms! These are the things one recognizes through a broadened viewpoint and that go unrecognized by the nurse of the "iron constitution" who says, "Okay, Babe, get your clothes off! And if you don't understand English I'll get some help and we'll show you what we mean!"

WHAT DOES THE PSYCHIATRIC NURSE DO?

Today the psychiatric nurse is an integral part of a group, and, as a member of that group, her value is being recognized and used to the fullest extent. She has established rapport with the doctor, the attendant, the social worker, and the patient's family. It is being realized at last that it is usually the nurse who spends the most time with the patient and who has many opportunities, not only to observe his behavior, but also to gain his confidence. In this latter respect she is the doctor's greatest ally, and doctors are opening their eyes to this fact. Now the nurse is given the opportunity to contribute her specialized knowledge to conferences, ward rounds, the training of personnel, and actual psychotherapy.

Psychotherapy is defined as "that form of therapy which employs psychologic methods in the treatment of functional nervous disorders: these methods include suggestion, persuasion, hypnotic suggestion, psychoanalysis, re-education, etc."[1] The nurse, of course, does not employ hypnotic suggestion and psychoanalysis, but she most certainly employs suggestion and persuasion and she is an important contributor to the patient's re-education. Many a patient has left the hospital feeling eternally grateful to a nurse who took the time to be especially understanding, especially kind when he was at his lowest ebb.

Once, for four months, I spent the greater part of my working hours with a catatonic patient. Mildred was a young woman who had been very ill for a number of months; she would not speak, was extremely negativistic, frequently required tube-feeding, and in general was a real nursing problem. Mildred first began to interest me because she spent an average of eighteen days out of each month standing in a quiet room. She was kept there because she was impulsively assaultive and frequently attacked both personnel and other patients.

It became my daily task to bathe Mildred and to see that she ate. She did not like me at first because, when she refused to go to the bathroom and get into the tub, I would pick her up and, amid a flurry of fisticuffs, would put her into the tub and bathe her from head to foot. She did not like me because, after at least an hour or two of work, I would finally succeed in getting her dressed each day. My success was consistently short-lived, for she would patiently remove every stitch of clothing as soon as she was left alone.

Getting her to eat was a full-time job, until I discovered that if her tray was put in a certain room at each meal time she would go in by herself and

---

[1]Dorland, W. A. Newman: *The American Illustrated Medical Dictionary*, ed. 21, Philadelphia, Saunders, 1947, p. 1200.

eat. Occasionally at noon I brought her pie and candy bars and these she would refuse; but if I left them beside her and went away, they would magically disappear. Mildred began to gain a little weight; she was in a quiet room only at night. I spent long periods of time sitting on the floor by the mattress in her room talking to her; there was never any answer to my conversation.

One day Mildred looked up and said, "That was good cake you brought me yesterday. Did you make it?" And later, as I thumbed through a magazine sitting beside her in the day room, she slowly reached over and took hold of one side of the page and began to comment on the pictures. This was the beginning of improvement for Mildred. I had to leave that ward after four months but just a short time ago I heard that Mildred was home on a probational visit with her family. I like to think that the patience and time I spent with Mildred has been of benefit to her. It has to me.

The well prepared psychiatric nurse has wide choice as to the particular division of nursing she wishes to enter. She is, for instance, invaluable in a public health program. Nowhere else does she come in closer contact with family life, social and economic conditions. Nowhere else can she practice preventive nursing as well. This is true also if she enters industrial nursing and private practice. Few of our mentally ill, however, can afford the latter. It is unfortunate because it is in an intimate relationship of this sort that the psychiatric nurse is at her best.

In the general hospital there is a real need for nurses who recognize emotional and mental stress as an inevitable accompaniment to physical illness. Such nurses are frequently given the opportunity to pass this valuable knowledge on to students. If there is a psychiatric ward in the general hospital, the advantage is increased a hundredfold, for here the nurse can help undo some of the tragic results of an incompletely cared for physical illness—hypochondriasis, a mental breakdown following childbirth, or an anxiety reaction or depression in patients with carcinoma or tuberculosis.

A grateful doctor told me recently of a nurse from the psychiatric ward in a general hospital who had visited one of his patients every day until the patient's death. His patient was a woman nearly seventy who was in the terminal stage of carcinoma. She had led an active and vigorous life during which she had experienced little or no illness, and her present pain and helplessness caused her to react in an extremely psychotic manner, so that she was becoming unmanageable on the gynecology ward. The doctor did not want to send her to the psychiatric ward but had made up his mind he would have to, when the psychiatric nurse began to take an interest in the old lady. Her experience in nursing the mentally ill had taught her that fear of the unknown flourishes when time lies heavy on the hands.

She visited the patient each day and frequently spent an hour or two of her own time with the patient when she stopped by on her way off duty. The nurse interested the woman in crocheting place mats for her daughter-in-law and also asked her to write out a different recipe each evening. In the morning these recipes were critically reviewed, and then the old lady would paste them in a notebook, which she later gave to the nurse.

It is not always easy to interest patients in such elementary occupational therapy. It requires a deep understanding of the reasons behind abnormal behavior and the ability to establish good enough rapport so that the patient will want to co-operate in small tasks. Such physical-mental breakdowns as this occur every day in the general hospital and, with a good in-service program which emphasizes psychological and emotional aspects of nursing care, the need to move a patient to the psychiatric ward may not even become a possibility.

Last but not least, the psychiatric nurse has a varied choice in her own field. In the small psychiatric unit of a general hospital or in the private mental hospital, she is more likely to see patients in the acute stages of mental illness, the bizarre behavior, and the most acute nursing care problems. She has a better opportunity for teaching, as she works with smaller groups of personnel, and she has a chance to become well acquainted with all of her patients.

Our state mental hospitals—in fact, all of our public mental hospitals—are desperate for well trained nurses. They are needed to help eliminate the "guard" system, which has prevailed too long; to help enliven the many dull hours for patients; to help in eventual improvement and recovery for more and more sick persons. They are needed in the special therapies, such as psychodrama and group psychotherapy, where, with specific training, their value can become inestimable.

The needs of all these hospitals are not only for general staff nurses, but for persons qualified for administrative and teaching positions. Psychiatric nursing demands a knowledge of smooth interpersonal relationships as well as varied and lengthy experience and post-graduate work in nursing education. A number of our universities and schools of nursing now offer advanced courses in psychiatric nursing. There are many job and leadership opportunities for the nurse who is adequately prepared and who is not afraid of new horizons.

The picture in psychiatric nursing is not all good. Here and there on the canvas are blurred spots, splotches of unwanted color. Too often the public hospitals are situated in remote districts. The work itself is hard and often unappreciated. For the most part remuneration is poor. And even the best psychiatric nurses will tell you it can become depressing. But every day, every week, every month, interested people are trying to overcome these drawbacks.

The public still remains much too ignorant of the needs of our mental hospitals. But through better public relations—use of radio, magazines, newspapers, even movies—people are learning. They must first become conscious of these needs, then they must have the desire to help. We nurses owe it to ourselves and to our patients to help create this desire. Our participation in community life can do much to foster good public relations and that participation can be effective in producing the awareness so vitally necessary to the recognition and prevention of mental illness.

It is gratifying to walk into a psychiatric hospital today and see nurses working with patients where, not too many years ago, there was only the echo of the nurse's footsteps as she hurried from building to building. Today it is not strange to see attendants playing ball or having a smoke and quiet talk with patients, where once they stood grim and challenging at each exit.

Psychiatric nursing is achieving a new freedom. And with this freedom many trained, experienced psychiatric nurses are extending a welcome to those new graduates who are willing to accept a challenge, who want to find that particular satisfaction in work which comes from being part of a group who have mutual respect for each other and who can strive together toward a goal of human kindness.

38

The Psychiatric Nurse
and Psychotherapy

Jane A. Schmahl*

By no haphazard selection or accidental afterthought are we called "nurses" and our profession, "nursing." Without patients to care for, there would be no nurses. This statement is so obvious as to seem ridiculous, yet the nursing profession faces a grave crisis and challenge. Are nurses going to take care of patients, or do something else? All nurses are responsible for taking a definitive stand on this issue and for initiating action to implement it.

Fairchild identifies the nurse as a person who meets certain basic needs of patients until they can care for themselves and others. He warns that: "Indeed, some of the needs I have noted could be met at least partially in other ways. If they are, I will risk a prediction. Should you elect to direct your major function and action into areas and methods divorced from meeting the basic needs . . . , like cultures that abandon their genetic roots—you, too, will run the risk of becoming only historic. Should this happen, I would predict that a new group would emerge. . . . I would further predict that these people would be known as nurses and their profession as nursing."[1]

Unless we plan for our future, then, we shall find ourselves in the precarious position of having lost it. Fairchild's warning has particular relevance for psychiatric nurses because of a current trend that appears to take the form of involving nurses more and more in the practice of individual psychotherapy. In view of Fairchild's comments, and this trend, the immediate question that

*From *Nursing Outlook*, Vol. 10, No. 7 (July, 1962).

Miss Schmahl (Frances Payne Bolton School of Nursing, Western Reserve University, Cleveland; B.S., M.A, Teachers College, Columbia University, New York) holds the certificate for teachers from William Alason White Institute, New York, and is a lecturer there in psychiatric nursing. She is, also, associate professor of nursing at Skidmore College Department of Nursing, where she works with the faculty in integrating psychiatric principles throughout the basic nursing curriculum. She wishes to express her gratitude to Montague Ullman, M.D., and Miltiades L. Zophiropoulos, M.D. for their help in the preparation of this article.

arises is: Can the psychiatric nurse utilize psychotherapeutic theory and technique without jeopardizing her role as a nurse, and if so, how?*

The historical development of psychiatric nursing is in part a reflection of the growth of nursing as a profession. Furthermore, the development of psychiatric theory and practice also has left its mark on psychiatric nursing. In the last three decades, psychiatry has shifted from a primary emphasis on the organic and hereditary sources of mental illness to an increased focus on the interpersonal and intrapsychic processes. Instead of viewing the mental hospital as a house of detention with the chief purpose of restraining, protecting, controlling, subduing, and maintaining the patient, it now perceives the hospital as a specialized social system dedicated to providing the patient with therapeutic experiences designed to modify a mentally ill way of life. The mental hospital ward with its collective living arrangements is a reality world in miniature, thereby becoming the nexus with the less protected life outside.

In the United States, increased understanding of the psychotic process has been intimately related to the specific insights and techniques of psychoanalysis, particularly the recognition of the importance of the transference phenomenon. Notman, commenting on the application of these factors in the treatment of patients in mental hospitals, says:

The doctor-patient relationship and the therapeutic hour was thus the model for utilization of this new knowledge. The prestige of both the doctor in the hospital hierarchy, and the value assigned to "cure with insight" over "symptomatic improvement" have both contributed to "borrowing" of these techniques in modified form by other therapeutic disciplines.[2]

Both patient and personnel are apt to feel that the real treatment of patients takes place in those cloistered sessions.

When psychotherapy is exalted to such lofty heights, it is inevitable that a split occurs between ward personnel and the psychotherapist, which results in accentuating the differences between the custodial and therapeutic roles. In the competition for autonomy and prestige, and in fear of being plunged into therapeutic nihilism everyone—psychiatrists, psychologists social workers, and now psychiatric nurses—is scrambling to practice psychotherapy.

As one way of giving more effective nursing care to patients, the profession has put increased emphasis on nurses working with selected patients in a one-to-one relationship over a protracted period of time. And, because psychiatric nursing is apt to involve little or no physical care, it becomes more difficult to define the qualitative differences between a one-to-one nurse-patient relationship and the patient-therapist relationship in individual psychotherapy.

---

*The descriptive role category of "psychiatric nurse" includes the graduate of a basic professional program in nursing, who practices nursing in a psychiatric setting. One purpose of this paper is to provide an operational model for all nurse-patient relationships in a psychiatric setting. However, it must be recognized that the levels of operation will vary from nurse to nurse according to her professional education and training, experience, and skill. But, also, it should be expected that all professional psychiatric nurse practitioners will be able to demonstrate most of the identified skills at a beginning level.

In discussing the supervisory process in psychiatric nursing, Switzer says that "it is only to be expected that misunderstandings, misconceptions, disagreements, and misapplications will exist until the borrowed theories and concepts are restudied and reformulated to fit the particular needs of nursing education, which are in many ways vastly different from those of individual supervision in psychiatry."[3] This comment may apply as well to the differences between the practice of psychiatric nursing and psychotherapy.

In a sense, nurses used psychotherapy with their patients long before it was given a name. They recognized the role of emotional factors in illness and suffering, and referred to this aspect of nursing as comforting, protecting, reassuring, supporting, mothering, encouraging, and helping. They learned that when they permitted the patient to talk out his problems, and when they listened with understanding and compassion, the patient often felt relieved and perceived his problem in a new light. This was good therapy.

In another report, I have raised the problem of role differentiation in psychiatric nursing and psychotherapy.[4] The important question is: How does the practice of psychiatric nursing differ from the practice of psychotherapy? Another is: How does the nurse utilize psychotherapeutic theory and technique to establish her role of nurse vis-à-vis the psychiatric patient? The answers, in a sense, lie in the definition of terms.

There are as many definitions of psychotherapy as there are schools of thought on the subject. Inevitably, most definitions include the goals, methods, and techniques of psychotherapy, which are apt to leave the reader more confused than enlightened. In a broad and general sense, we can say that psychotherapy takes place in all verbal and nonverbal transactions that help to release the constructive potential of the individuals mutually involved.

In this general context, psychotherapeutic interaction with a patient may occur in relationships not only with the doctor but also with the nurse, attendant, family, or housekeeping, kitchen, and maintenance staff. It may occur under many different guises, and will utilize reassurance, physical care and presence, closeness, listening, and socializing.

If we are to clarify the relationship of psychotherapy to the practice of psychiatric nursing, it is important to differentiate this broad interpretation of being psychotherapeutic from the practice of technical and scientific psychotherapy. Wolberg defines psychotherapy in its scientific and technical sense:

A form of treatment for problems of an emotional nature in which a trained person *deliberately* establishes a professional relationship with a patient with the object of removing, modifying or retarding existing symptoms, of medicating disturbed patterns of behavior and of promoting positive personality growth and development.[5]

Fromm-Reichmann identifies the goals more operationally when she says intensive psychotherapy is:

Alleviation of patients' emotional difficulties in living and elimination of the symptomatology, this goal to be reached by gaining insight into and understanding of the unconscious roots of the patient's problems, the genetics and dynamics, on the part of both patient and psychiatrist, whereby such understanding and insight may frequently promote changes in the dynamic structure of the patient's personality.[6]

275

In a technical sense, then, psychotherapy is a form of treatment distinguished by psychological rather than physical or chemical means. It is a highly specialized type of relationship that involves the deliberate application of particular theoretical and technical considerations designed to enable an individual to treat psychiatric illness. In view of this, the practice of technical psychotherapy requires a special and unique kind of training. The psychiatrist so trained is concerned with carrying out specific functions in order to eliminate symptoms and to bring about constructive personality change.

The psychiatric nurse has not been trained to practice scientific psychotherapy. She is trained to practice psychiatric nursing—the practice of nursing in the psychiatric sphere, in which she makes use of certain psychotherapeutic theory and practices to further her goals as a nurse. These goals include establishing contact with the patient, seeing that his basic needs are met, and dealing with obstacles that limit his effective adjustment to the ward and hospital. Within the practice of nursing, all her functions and ministrations contain the potential for constructive change or psychotherapeutic effect. The nurse has an ancillary role in psychotherapy through which she creates infinite possibilities for the cure of the patient to take place.

An analogy to this problem of who practices psychotherapy can be found in the practice of medicine. Some of the functions carried out by the physician may be delegated to members of other professions, as for example, the administration of medicine by the nurse. Strictly speaking, this is a medical function; however, in no way is it inferred that when the nurse gives medicines, she practices medicine. Because a nursing function has medical or psychotherapeutic relevance, it cannot be equated with the practice of medicine or the practice of psychotherapy.

The roles of the psychiatrist and nurse cannot be clarified exclusively on the basis of who is concerned with psychotherapy and who is not. The goals of a particular psychotherapeutic relationship must be considered and only in relation to these goals can the level of skill, training, and experience differentiate between the psychiatrist's role and the nurse's role.

THE NURSE'S ROLE IDENTIFIED

The goals of a psychotherapeutic nurse-patient relationship can be identified, and the roles of the nurse and psychiatrist can be differentiated in the following condensed report of nurse-patient transactions.*

Daniel was in the hospital for the fourth time. His deeply entrenched rituals made it impossible for him to care for himself, nor would he permit others to care for him. His food intake was hardly enough to keep him alive, and he took two or three hours to eat even that little bit. He made repeated demands for independence even as he regressed to complete infantile dependence.
My first contact with Daniel was accidental. I found him hiding in the dormitory, sitting in a chair by his bedside, preoccupied and untidy. He was unshaven; greasy hair straggled around his ears; his skin was yellowish, eyes glassy, and his lips parched. His lips moved as if he were hallucinating. Although his eyes met mine

---

*These transactions took place at Veterans Administration Hospital, New York City, where the author received individual psychiatric nursing supervision from Gertrude Cherescavich, assistant chief, nursing education.

several times, he appeared out of contact with reality. I said, "I've noticed you and would like to know you better." Tapping his foot impatiently, he responded with, "OK, OK, leave me alone." After introducing myself, and some hesitating conversation, I told him I would return next Friday.

My automatic response was to get away as fast as I could, but my interest was roused and I decided to work with Daniel.

The patient presented a broad problem of complete isolation, withdrawal, and regression; he had removed himself from the human race. In response to him, the staff felt helpless, and this in turn led to their withdrawal from the patient. Such an unloved and uncared for patient can die, and it was crucial to break through Daniel's isolation and get him to eat.

The psychiatric nurse's responsibility is to deal resourcefully with the patient's tendency toward regression. Daniel's regression, his systematized rituals—organized as his defense against intolerable anxiety, and a lifesaving device—had become slow suicide through starvation. The mere presence of another person became the source of interference with the system. Yet, the nurse had to intervene.

One aspect of the psychiatric nurse's role is to work with the patient's unrealistic demands and expectations. At times, the nurse must deny these or grant them only in part, as when Daniel's nurse accepted his wanting to be alone but let him know that she definitely would keep in touch with him.

Another function of the nurse is to provide closeness, but Daniel's rejection of the nurse made this difficult. A meeting with the nursing personnel highlighted the need for closer collaboration and communication with the total psychiatric team. Obviously, this patient could be helped only to the degree that the ward became a therapeutic community in which each member worked toward compatible goals.

During my later contacts with Daniel, he continued to dismiss me and insisted that I not talk. Although I remained silent, I communicated my desire to be with him. When he insisted, I left, but I always reminded him I would be available if he wanted me.

After four weeks of this type of exchange, Daniel showed a change in his behavior. Following one visit, about two hours after dismissing me, he came out of the dormitory with head downcast as he lifted each foot slowly and carefully. He came to the nurses' station where I sat directly facing him. He looked at the clock and "through me," without a sign of recognition, and walked slowly toward the dining room out of sight. Then, he returned, lingered a few moments with his profile toward me, peeked at me, and quickly looked away. He seemed to have taken a step in finding out who the nurse was. This was Daniel's first voluntary attempt to move toward anyone in the environment.

Several weeks later, following my return from a 2-weeks' absence, another significant incident occurred.

For 20 minutes, I observed Daniel standing as if frozen at the dormitory entrance. As he lifted one foot and then the other, it became obvious that he was engaged in an agonizing struggle of whether or not to move. As I walked up to him and stood where he could see me, he shouted angrily, "Leave me alone; I'm terribly disturbed now." I said, "Yes, I know you are suffering. That's why I came over." I said I would go, and added, "But I want you to know we would like to help." Daniel remained fastened to the dormitory entrance for five more minutes and then made his way to his bedside chair.

This experience became a turning point for the nurse in her relationship with Daniel. She had managed to convey to him that the staff was aware of his suffering and that he was important. Perhaps this communication of concern helped to unfreeze him to mobilize him into action. Her record of this experience notes:

My heart went out to him today. As I could feel the pain of his struggle, I wanted to take him in my arms and comfort him. I have wanted to help him but felt powerless to do so. Previously, I have dreaded seeing him because I was afraid of his rejection. Today my tears are not for myself. Now that I have a clearer idea of what he is going through, perhaps I can let go of my search for a miracle."

Before the nurse-patient relationship could take on any therapeutic meaning and value, the nurse had to empathize with Daniel, had to feel with him his emotional turmoil, and experience him as a person. Moreover, the nurse had been unconsciously involved with her own partially confused interpretation of the descriptive categories of "patient," "mentally ill," and "schizophrenic," rather than with Daniel as a person, not too unlike herself. Just as Daniel viewed himself as not quite human, so did the nurse. Feelings do get conveyed to patients, and as Daniel sensed her reactions, his own sense of desperate and unrelieved loneliness was fortified. As the nurse's appraisal became less stereotyped, Daniel's dismissal of her took on new meaning. Because of this, subtle changes in his behavior started to occur. He answered her greeting with "hello," and when she asked how he felt, he responded, "pretty well." He continued to dismiss her, but only after she was with him for a longer period of time. His foot-tapping had stopped completely in his sessions with the doctor.

Concomitantly, personnel evidenced their more positive feelings toward Daniel. They wrote fuller notes about him; more frequently popped their heads into the ward and made small talk with him about the weather, and so on.

The slight change in Daniel had moved personnel to respond by expecting him to handle problems still beyond his ability—eating, loss of weight, the weighing procedure, and showering. The nurse's relationship with him came to a standstill. Not knowing how to use the nurse further, Daniel attempted to get rid of her once again. She, in turn, became more unsure of which direction to move.

The altered relationship required further exercise of nursing skills. Somewhere within this total situation, a change was necessary—a potentially explosive one—to let Daniel know the staff cared about what was happening to him. The time had come for the nurse to personalize her relationship, to help him verbalize his anger and annoyance. With these goals in mind, an important milestone was reached.

Daniel appeared physically ill, depressed, and agitated now. Sitting at the foot of his bed, I told him, "I've been very worried about you. You have had such a rough time these past weeks."
He responded by yelling and looking at me directly, "I'm upset, so leave me alone. I'm so tensed up." I replied, "I know, and today I want to talk about this with you."

This was the first time I had not accepted his dismissal. I remained, and tried to put into words some of what he might be feeling about me and his experience. "You sure are angry. I guess all of this must be pretty painful for you and you are feeling miserable." At this, Daniel told me he didn't want any of my help, and told me to get out. I responded by telling him, "I've been coming to see you for two months, and have always left when you asked me to. But today, I can't leave until I tell you how I feel about what's been happening." He screamed at the top of his voice for the head nurse, attendant, and doctor, "Take her away. I have to do this myself." I remained silent, concerned with how the staff would handle this. When he quieted, I said, "I guess it must hurt to have people try to get close to you." Angry and bewildered, Daniel continued to scream and yell that he didn't want any of my "goddam therapy or sweet talk—you stupid, banal bitch. Can't you understand English?"

With bright eyes and clenched fists, Daniel then leaned forward in his chair, and screamed threats at me. "Get out of here or I'll hit you with this water pitcher." He turned to get it, touched it, but did not lift it from the tray. His rituals were forgotten; he was a very different picture from his usual withdrawn self. Simultaneously, as I realized that all along I had been frightened of being assaulted, I recognized that it was crucial for me to stay with him during his barrage.

Suddenly, Daniel slumped in his chair as though exhausted. He appeared relaxed. Together we sat in pregnant silence for five minutes. Then, suddenly, he seemed to "fall apart." He started to cry, stopped, started again, and stopped. He looked like a helpless and lost child. Was he crying because he had experienced the delicious surprise of being treated gently and tenderly? This can be even worse than being treated with contempt because this arouses hope and trust, and—also—panic that these might miscarry.

After more verbal threats followed by periods of silence, I said, "I have to go now, but I'll be back to see you on Wednesday." Daniel threatened, "If you do, I'll smash you right in the face." After a thoughtful pause, I told him, "I'll take that chance." He mumbled an almost inaudible, "Thank you."

At this point it was difficult to know if Daniel was thanking the nurse for having stayed with him, for accepting his anger, or if he was thanking her for the promise of coming back. The important thing was that Daniel had at last poked his head out of his cage of loneliness.

The patient, who had been closed in and suffocated, for the first time openly expressed the rebellion he felt. It was the beginning of experiencing himself as a real person among other persons.

By staying with him, the nurse had created a possibility for Daniel to learn that he could not destroy other people with his anger. Perhaps most important of all, as he demonstrated in later behavior, he learned that he would have to begin to take care of himself if he were to get personnel "off his back."

Movement from physical and emotional suicide was possible for Daniel only when he could begin to crawl out of the vacuum he had created with his protective rituals. The explosion was a definitive step in this direction. Its timing was crucial and took place only after a long period of accepting the patient on his terms and granting his request to be alone. After this experience, the relationship was characterized by episodes in which Daniel showed increased acceptance of the nurse alternated with dismissals that ranged from mild and automatic to cursing and screaming.

The nurse's role here is seen to provide the patient with acceptance, understanding, and clarification of his feelings. Simultaneously, this patient began to reach out to other personnel and to develop a meaningful relationship with an aide who liked him. The patient never completely accepted the nurse, but partly through her, he was able to choose for himself other significant persons in the environment with whom he could be more comfortable. The nurse, therefore, through her one-to-one relationship with Daniel, became a bridge to other people in the environment who could help him in more direct ways.

ROLE IDENTIFICATION CONFUSED. The similarity and differences between the practices of psychiatric nursing and psychotherapy are determined for the most part by the specific objectives of each discipline. In Daniel's situation, the psychiatric nurse's role is very much in keeping with the generalized concept of the nurse's role in other areas, particularly as it relates to meeting those needs associated with physical well being and survival. This similarity in role is based on the assumption that the nurse has and uses the knowledge of psychodynamics particularly as it relates to her own reactions. It is especially difficult, however, to define the role of the psychiatric nurse with a patient who is able to function on a more integrated level of social participation and whose interactions with individuals are much more complex. In such situations, the objectives of psychiatric nursing tend to become obscure, and role confusion is inevitable. The following material will illustrate just such a complicated situation.

This was Bob's first hospitalization for which he admitted himself voluntarily. He was tall, attractive, and neatly dressed, in his early thirties, and had a wife and two children. He went home weekends, and the chief nursing problems were associated with his periods of extreme anxiety during which he would go off by himself to study, sleep, or just sit. At these times, he became annoyed at any attempts by nursing personnel to be with him. He alternated these periods of withdrawal with being constantly "underfoot," asking numerous questions, and being extremely seductive and flirtatious with the nurses. The nurses responded by dismissing and avoiding him during the withdrawn periods, or by also being seductive and provocative.

Bob was sitting by his bedside, cleanly shaved and scrubbed, apparently deep in study when I introduced myself to him. Drawing up a chair to face him, I commented on his involvement. He responded almost inaudibly, in a flat tone, "I'm studying math. It was during this hospitalization that I found out what I have been really missing—engineering." Sensing some feeling of loss, I asked, "You're not in engineering anymore? What happened?" Looking at me directly, he vehemently blurted out, "My mother! She is one of my chief problems. She spoiled me rotten so I've been afraid to do anything on my own."

Playing nervously with his fingers, his face lined with anguish, he expressed concern that "I'll do the same thing with my children." After some gentle urging, he talked about his children. His eyes lit up as, in a tone of unmistakable fondness, he said of his 3-year-old girl, "She's going to be a real heartbreaker. Have you ever read *Lolita?*" He continued to discuss the story, and the author's description of little girls between nine and fourteen who "have a special kind of spark. The author calls them nymphets." In a teasing tone, he added, "I tell my wife that our little girl is a little nymphet."

I was acutely aware of being uneasy, and disturbing questions intruded on my consciousness. Was Bob merely joking, or expressing vital concern? Concern for his

daughter, for himself, or both? Was he crying out to me for help? Abruptly, I shifted the discussion from his daughter to his son, and as the time came for me to leave, I brought the conversation back to less emotionally charged subjects. "Perhaps we can talk some more next week. I'll want to know how the math is progressing."
He rose from his chair and responded, "I'd like that. It was so good talking to you," and shook my hand. As he did, the pressure was a bit too long and hard, and I had the disquieting feeling that somehow I had been "courted" throughout this contact.

Unlike Daniel, Bob exhibited genuine awareness of his problems and some peripheral insight into the sources of them. They seemed to center on his crippling dependency on his mother, concern about his relationship with his children, and preparation for a future job in engineering. A different, but related problem, was of immediate concern to the nurse, and was within her sphere of influence. This was the necessity to deal with the patient's seductiveness with nursing personnel and their difficulty in handling it effectively. The nurse, in her first extended contact with the patient, had experienced the forceful impact of his seductive manipulation and had been aware of the anxiety it had roused in her. This enabled her to understand the problem, and do something constructive about it.

Several weeks after the nurse's first contact with the patient—during which he was off the ward doing work in the hospital—another interesting episode took place, at the second contact.

I sat next to Bob during a patient government meeting, and he asked, "Are you a dietitian? You aren't here all the time." Wondering if or why he had forgotten our previous meeting, I clarified my role in the hospital. Scrutinizing me, he commented, "Oh? So, you're a nurse." After a preoccupied pause, he added, "You have beautiful eyes and your eyelashes have a strange blue tinge to them. They're very attractive."
During the protracted silence which I allowed to follow, I ruminated about the possible meanings of this exchange. He sat in silence, but appeared quizzical, as though pondering an issue. Was he deciding in which direction to move? To court me? Or to use me as a professional helper?
When I finally replied, I refocused the attention and concern back to him. "How have things been going for you since last I saw you?"
Thoughtfully, Bob replied, "A little better. Anything is better than before I came into the hospital. I was so depressed and couldn't concentrate on anything. I know I have the ability to achieve much more than I have. Ever since I was a little boy, my whole interest has been engineering. I even used to build airplanes when I should have been studying. Now I have nothing to fall back on." He sounded sad and remorseful.

The patient had difficulty in establishing who the nurse was, her role with him, and what he might expect of her. This uncertainty and discomfort led to his reverting to his pattern of flattery and seductiveness as the only way of gaining control in a situation in which the patient felt stripped of any power. He had developed this pattern as a defense against his mother's smothering overprotection and covert, but persistent, rejection of him.
In handling the problem, the nurse had worked through her initial anxiety while, at the same time, she gained some understanding into the dynamics

of the patient's behavior. Consequently, she did not find it necessary to reject Bob, a response he appeared to fear and expect. Neither did she exploit his provocativeness to bolster her own needs for approval and admiration. Her waiting in silence did not cut him off, but allowed time for both the patient and the nurse to think about what they wanted from the relationship and how to go about achieving it. The nurse supported the patient in his apprehension about the direction in which to move, by refocusing the attention back to him. Thus, she identified herself as a professional person intimately concerned with the patient's welfare. Having been neither rejected nor exploited, Bob began to accept his status as a patient, and an avenue was opened up whereby he could share his problems with the nurse. This was a definitive step toward working through his relationship with all women.

Objectives of psychiatric nursing and psychotherapy. The behavior of both patients presented obstacles to their receiving the help they needed. In both situations, the nurse's concern was in limiting herself to help them deal with the daily reality of life in the hospital.

The crucial issue in Daniel's care was physical survival. Consequently, both nurse and psychiatrist directed and limited their efforts to helping him organize and perpetuate life-saving activities into his pattern of compulsive rituals. Each had to intervene in Daniel's destructive isolation—each in activities of his own discipline. When Daniel was so "frozen" he could not get on the scales, the nurse lifted him on. She focused on three specific nursing areas: meeting the patient's needs appropriately, helping him communicate, and helping him participate socially in the hospital situation.

The psychiatrist helped Daniel by tube-feeding him when he was unable to eat enough, and further helping him supportively when he was regressed beyond much social participation. He was not yet able to accept any psychiatric dealing with such aspects of his life as the unconscious motivation behind his inability to eat.

During the treatment period, the practice of the psychiatrist and the nurse converged on the issue of handling the immediate basic needs. For the psychiatrist, they were only a transitional means to an end of curing the patient. For the nurse, however, the handling of these needs is an end in itself. Both the nurse and the psychiatrist used the same principles, tools, and technique derived from the science of psychotherapy, but they combined them with their unique and respective skills as a nurse and a physician.

Because Bob participated socially on a higher level than Daniel, his care presented a different problem. He was able to communicate well and to withstand a moderate degree of anxiety, and so, the psychiatrist could focus on the patient's gaining insight into the unconscious motivations of his behavior with the significant people in his life. The psychiatrist could utilize the historical data for understanding Bob's irrational motivations in the present, and his task was to clarify for Bob his infantile wishes to appease, control, and manipulate—to be dependent and move away from relationships when he was frightened. He focused on and utilized Bob's transference to him as a way of helping him modify his poor self-concept.

Bob presented a more difficult situation for the nurse, particularly as it related to defining and differentiating his role. Her primary objective was to help him relate with her and the other nurses more realistically. She could do this by focusing on a specific area of his life—his behavior as it related to the nursing staff, other patients, and so on. At the same time, she had to avoid exploration and interpretation of his behavior with other persons, as for example, his incestuous feelings for his daughter. Stubblefield comments, "It is precisely in these areas that I think a great deal of competition develops between the nurse and therapist. This creates many of our communication problems and results in lack of clarity about therapeutic goals."[7]

Psychiatric nursing is primarily concerned with the vicissitudes of the patient's life in the hospital. Thus, the nurse's role with Bob was as mother surrogate and protector, administrator, and teacher; it was her task to channel rather than interpret, to dilute rather than stimulate, Bob's transference to her. She did this when she refocused his attention from herself without any attempt to press for further elucidation of his feelings about her. It was also her task to support him when his anxiety was related to what was going on in psychotherapy. She did this by listening to him and accepting his feelings, even the negative ones directed toward the psychiatrist.

In this situation, psychotherapy and psychiatric nursing had different objectives. The psychiatrist's efforts extended to the ultimate goal of the patient's living more productively in the community. The psychiatric nurse was concerned with the management of Bob's manifestations of irrational motivation in the daily experiences of ward living. She had to do this while avoiding participation in the irrational aspects of the transaction and reflecting acceptance and support of the patient.

As a first step in clarifying the relationship between psychiatric nursing and psychotherapy, I have been concerned primarily with exploring and clarifying several psychotherapeutic, nurse-patient, one-to-one interactions.

Another aspect as crucial as the clarification of the nurse-patient, one-to-one interaction needs to be explored. How does the practice of psychiatric nursing communicate with all of the other positive treatment forces? How does this communication enrich and enhance the therapeutic force of the nurse? These questions need to be explored further.

FURTHER CONSIDERATIONS

I said earlier that the nursing profession as a whole is unclear about the role identity of the nurse. One effect of the confusion is that the professional nurse gives away many of her unique functions to non-professional workers. But this seldom results in her taking on medical functions to replace lost nursing responsibilities. This does not seem to be true in psychiatric nursing where nurses are said to be taking on medical functions, namely the practice of psychotherapy. Why does there seem to be even greater role confusion in psychiatric nursing?

The nurse-patient data presented and analyzed here demonstrate that many aspects of psychotherapy become involved in psychiatric nursing, just as aspects of medicine become involved in other areas of nursing. These include recognizing and dealing with the transference that operates between a patient and a nurse, understanding the unconscious motivations underlying a patient's inability to eat, interpreting and clarifying of the patient's behavior limited to the context in which it occurs, and so on. Unlike nurses in other areas, however, the psychiatric nurse is totally and exclusively oriented to the mentally ill patient. Because of the inherent nature of the psychiatric problem, the nurse must necessarily be directly involved in psychotherapeutic technique and theory to a much greater degree than nurses in other areas of practice must be involved in medical technique and theory. At the same time, the psychiatric nurse has to use the techniques differently. It is the special application of psychotherapeutic theory and technique that differentiates psychiatric nursing from psychotherapy, thereby establishing role identity.

The limitations of the psychiatric nurse's role exert powerful influences on her acceptance or rejection of the role. Because of the complexities involved in behavior disorder, at best, the results of any psychotherapeutic effort are slow, if not imperceptible.

As the nurse becomes engaged in the process, she has a mounting awareness of the difficulties present, as when the nurse accepted Daniel and simultaneously became aware of the depth of his problem. The nature of the psychiatric nursing process, the nurse's personal and professional involvement in it, and her increased awareness of difficulties, all affect her own effectiveness which can lead her to fall for the speciousness of some issues or to become awed by the vastness of some others. There is ensuing anxiety because of the absence of an easy remedy or resolution.

The psychiatric nurse's role as described implies some definite limits and therefore may not be conspicuously self-aggrandizing. Thus, the temptation of the psychiatric nurse to reject her role and assume a different one. I believe it is this intrapsychic aspect of the conflict—as compared with and differentiated from the essentially externally imposed elements of social prestige, value, and others—that is the source of role rejection by the psychiatric nurse.

From all of this, several implications for psychiatric nursing practice can be identified. Rather than being the source of role rejection, the limitations here can become a primary source of the nurse's deep and lasting satisfaction. The nursing role is characterized by its intimacy and physical proximity. The nurse's native skills are chiefly concerned with the process of "caring for" and include all the aspects of physical care plus giving reassurance, comfort, support, and so on. Her acquired skills aid her in using this role as an instrument to collect data concerning the patient's problem, to search for the meaning of behavior, to intervene as necessary, and to put hunches about behavior to the test of validation.

I suspect that the desire to utilize the "capacity to care for" within a professional and scientific framework probably is the single, most important factor in the choice of nursing as a profession. Analysis of the patient situations demonstrated how the objective of psychotherapy, the *cure* of the patient, is inevitably related to the objective of psychiatric nursing, the *care* of the patient. This concept has far-reaching implications for nursing education, which, however, go beyond the scope of this article.

It has been demonstrated that the psychiatric nurse's primary instrument is her ability to establish successful interpersonal relations. In her discussion of the preparation of psychiatrists, Thompson focuses on the need for them to understand themselves.[8] This fact raises an issue of the importance for the nurse to thoroughly understand the instrument she must use the most—her own personality. To understand this instrument better, I believe that psychiatric nurses must begin to reckon seriously with the value of personal psychotherapy as a bona fide part of their professional experience, although a personal psychoanalysis can never replace training for psychotherapy.

Because psychotherapy is an autonomous specialty, as is nursing, I believe it is impossible for the psychiatric nurse to become a practicing psychotherapist and at the same time retain her identity as a nurse. In attempting to do so, she becomes a kind of two-headed creature who is neither nurse nor therapist, and thereby relegates herself to the position of a second-class citizen. On the other hand, I am certain that there are some psychiatric nurses who have the necessary personality attributes to make a valuable contribution as trained psychotherapists. There is nothing, however, in the professional heritage or the clinical education of the nurse to justify her practicing psychotherapy without intensive, specialized, and formalized training. It is important to recognize that if the nurse becomes a trained psychotherapist, she has shifted her professional base and her primary professional identification.

The skills of the psychiatric nurse and psychotherapist are based upon the same principles of behavior and theory of psychopathology. But in deriving her own techniques from her understanding of the principles of psychotherapy, the psychiatric nurse must observe the distinctions in function and structure between her role and that of the psychotherapist. To the extent that the psychiatric nurse merely imitates the psychotherapist, she throws away the wealth of opportunities that her role as a nurse provides for her to help patients utilize to the fullest the therapeutic facilities in the hospital and community.

REFERENCES

1. Fairchild, L. McCarty. Discussion of the identification of the components in a therapeutic nurse-patient relationship, by Theresa M. Fernandez and Libby Zagorin. In *Psychiatric Nursing Concepts and Basic Nursing Education.* Proceedings of the Conference at Boulder, Colorado, June 15-18, 1959. New York, National League for Nursing, 1960, pp. 116-117.

2. Galioni, E. F., and others. The nature and purposes of mental hospital wards. In *The Patient and the Mental Hospital,* ed. by Milton Greenblatt and others. Glencoe, Ill, The Free Press, 1957, p. 335.

3. Switzer, Robert E. Discussion of Individual supervision: a method of teaching psychiatric concepts in nursing education, by Dorothy E. Gregg and others. In *Psychiatric Nursing Concepts and Basic Nursing Education.* Proceedings of the Conference at Boulder, Colorado, June 15-18, 1959. New York, National League for Nursing, 1960, p. 74.

4. Schmahl, Jane A. Discussion of Nursing therapy in the acute and post-acute phases: an atypical case, by June Mellow. In *Three Reports of Nurse-Patient Interaction in Psychiatric Nursing.* Presented at the 1959 convention of the National League for Nursing. New York, National League for Nursing, 1959, pp. 21-23.

5. Wolberg, Lewis R. *The Technique of Psychotherapy.* New York, Grune and Stratton, 1954, p. 3.

6. Fromm-Reichmann, Frieda. *Principles of Intensive Psychotherapy.* Chicago, University of Chicago Press, 1950, Introduction, p. (x).

7. Stubblefield, Robert L. Discussion of individual supervision: a method of teaching psychiatric concepts in nursing education, by Dorothy E. Gregg and others. In *Psychiatric Nursing Concepts and Basic Nursing Education.* Proceedings of the Conference at Boulder, Colorado, June 15-18, 1959. New York, National League for Nursing, 1960, p. 73.

8. Thompson, Clara. A study of the emotional climate of psychoanalytic institutes. *Psychiatry* 21:45-51, Feb. 1958.

Providing a Therapeutic Community

39

A Therapeutic Milieu
for Borderline Patients

Estelle I. Carleton and Joan Canatsy Johnson*

Nurses in a new type of psychiatric hospital assess their experience in an intensive treatment program.

The Mental Health Center of America, believed to be the first free, private, psychiatric hospital in the United States, was opened in Denver, Colorado, on July 1, 1958. The Center is on the grounds of the Ex-Patient's Sanatorium, a hospital which served for 50 years as a rehabilitation center for patients with tuberculosis and chronic disease. When medical advancements and improved care reduced the number of beds needed for these patients, the board of trustees decided to convert the extra buildings for use in the badly needed area of treatment of the mentally ill.

Although sponsored by a Jewish organization, the hospital accepts, from anywhere in the country, patients who fit the criteria for admission. Every part of the patient's hospitalization is free, including room, meals, and treatment. The hospital is supported by donations from groups and individuals all over the United States.

This hospital is unique also in that only a particular kind of patient is treated here—the "borderline" patient. Borderline is a designation for that group of illnesses which fall between the psychoneurotic and the psychotic. These are often referred to as pre-psychotic, ambulatory or latent schizophrenias, severe neurotic, and pseudoneurotic schizophrenias.

---

*From *American Journal of Nursing*, Vol. 61, No. 1 (January, 1961).

Miss Carleton (Kansas City, Mo., General Hospital School of Nursing; B.S., M.S., University of Colorado) is director of nursing services at the Mental Health Center of America.

Mrs. Johnson (St. Luke's School of Nursing, Denver; B.S., University of Denver) was formerly head nurse at the Center. She is now at the University of Washington in Seattle, working for her master's degree.

Borderline patients may appear psychoneurotic, presenting obsessive-compulsive, hysterical, or psychosomatic defenses. But they can also manifest paranoid states and depressive reactions. Both neurotic and psychotic symptoms are present and can be demonstrated by careful clinical evaluation. Sometimes the psychotic symptoms can be observed in a diagnostic interview, but often they are not apparent except on psychological testing.

The outstanding characteristic of the borderline patient is a weak ego, and treatment goals are centered on strengthening the ego. Knight has described three attitudes which a healthy person must maintain: "(1) self-esteem, (2) a sense of responsibility for his behavior, and (3) a feeling of maintaining inner controls over himself."[1] The loss of any of these is a realistic danger for the borderline patient. Knight believes that a therapeutic, open-hospital setting is important in helping the borderline patient regain or strengthen these attitudes.

It was to meet such a need that the Mental Health Center of America was established as a small, open-door hospital offering a type of milieu therapy. Its milieu offers the patient a therapeutic environment and therapeutic relationships 24 hours a day. The treatment program includes individual psychoanalytically oriented psychotherapy, group psychotherapy, occupational therapy, recreational therapy, and intensive contact with all staff personnel. The amount of time each patient devotes to each part of the program is individually determined, according to the patient's tolerance and needs. Tranquilizers are used as adjunctive therapy, but we have no electric shock, no insulin therapy, no hydrotherapy, and no locked wards.

PHYSICAL FACILITIES

Patients' rooms and staff offices are on the first floor of a remodeled building. Occupational therapy and recreational facilities are in the basement. An auditorium and other recreational facilities are in an adjacent building, and spacious grounds allow for other kinds of recreation including vegetable and flower gardens initiated and cared for by some of the patients. Administrative offices, kitchen, and dining room facilities are in yet another building and are shared with patients in the Ex-Patient's Sanatorium building.

About half the patients' rooms are single and half are double. They are furnished with modern, hotel-type furniture rather than conventional hospital furniture, and patients are encouraged to add pictures, draperies, bookcases, and the like, of their own choosing. The hospital atmosphere has some of the flavor of a college dormitory.

The staff includes two psychiatrists, one part-time clinical psychologist, one part-time psychiatric social worker, one occupational therapist, four nurses, and two nursing assistants. This size staff is considered the very minimum necessary to provide adequate treatment for the 14 patients in the hospital. The team concept is in effect here and there is frequent sharing of roles.

---

[1]Knight, R. P. Management and psychotherapy of the borderline schizophrenic patient. In *Psychoanalytic Psychiatry and Psychology*, ed. by Robert P. Knight and Cyrus R. Friedman. (Austen Riggs Center, Publications, Vol. 1) New York, International Universities Press, 1954, p. 115.

For example, one of the group therapy groups is led by a psychiatrist and a staff nurse; the other is led by the head nurse and the psychiatric social worker who also does casework with the patients' families. The clinical psychologist does the testing, but also has some patients in therapy.

For patients to be admitted to this hospital, they must meet certain definite criteria. They must be (1) referred by a physician, (2) between 21 and 50 years of age, (3) ambulatory, (4) in the borderline category, (5) able to function in an open-hospital setting, and (6) able to profit from treatment on an inpatient basis in six to eighteen months.

Although the five men and nine women who are patients here now are from nine different states and vary in age from 21 to 38 years, they make up a fairly homogeneous group. Nearly all of them fall into the "above average to superior" range of intellectual functioning and most of them have had education beyond high school. All have shown signs of illness for several years and many of them have had previous psychiatric treatment including hospitalization and shock therapy. A few of these patients have had an acute schizophrenic episode, but have reconstituted so that they again fall into the borderline category.

NURSING ROLE IN THE MILIEU

Some of the nursing functions are quite conventional and include observation and recording, passing medications, and carrying out treatments. But these functions take up a relatively small amount of the nurses' time on each shift. During the patients' waking hours, each nurse has from four to six hours which she spends with the patients.

An important function of the nurse in this milieu—one which is generally accepted as a nursing function but is not yet carried out in many psychiatric hospitals—is using herself in a therapeutic relationship with the patients.

Since the borderline patient has a weak ego, many of the ego functions—such as reality testing, mediating between the superego and the id, and utilizing healthy defense mechanisms—are impaired, sometimes grossly. The relationships these patients have with other people are rigid and inadequate, and their own self-concepts are narcissistic and depreciatory. Through her relationships with patients, the nurse tries to create for them new learning experiences which will help them learn to trust other people, acquire self-confidence and self-esteem, and progress from dependence to interdependence. The nurse also helps patients identify and work through the practical aspects of what they learn in psychotherapy, for example, learning to work or play with a group of peers.

Another function of the nurse is connected quite directly to relating therapeutically with the patients—enforcing the hospital structure. Since the hospital is unlocked, there are few rules and few restrictions on the patients' activities. The staff has attempted to keep the structure at a minimum. However, there are some rules which patients need to abide by, such as getting up on time and being present for required activities. As with all contacts with patients, enforcing rules can be done therapeutically or punitively, and the way in which it is done can have an important effect on the patients' treatment.

PROBLEMS IN NURSING CARE

Having a very small hospital with a selected borderline population has presented a variety of problems which affect the nursing care of the patients. The ward structure is such that there is rather close contact between patients and staff over a long period of time. This close contact in such a small group appears to intensify the transference situation. The nurses are quite obviously seen as mother figures, and patients view each other as siblings competing against one another. Numerous situations arise in which the nurse uses herself and her relationship with a patient in order to help him learn to share her with others, or to be less dependent. The nurse must constantly guard against favoritism which would cause more problems.

Connected with the transference situation is the ambivalence which most of the borderline patients feel toward relationships with others. Although they need and long for close, giving relationships, they resist attempts by other people to form relationships with them and they express a great deal of suspicion and hostility toward those who make such attempts. Obviously, this strong admixture of negative and positive feelings makes it very difficult for a therapist to establish lasting, positive transference. The ambivalence that the patient may express toward the nurse therapist as a mother figure is trying and often quite discouraging.

These patients have difficulty believing that someone is really interested in them and cares about them. They do not accept this as a matter of course and the people who are involved in their treatment must do more than go out of their way to prove their interest. To lessen the distance between staff and patients, the nursing staff encourages informality. Nurses do not wear caps, and both nurses and patients are called by their first names. We have found that this does not endanger therapeutic effectiveness and seems much more natural in these long-term relationships.

One of the characteristics of a borderline patient is a tendency to regress. Many of them would like to go to bed and be cared for. Just being in a hospital often encourages regression and active steps must be taken to counteract it. Anti-regressive measures focus on encouraging patients to assume responsibility for their own treatment; however, these patients do show a definite reluctance to assume much of the responsibility. This reluctance is a by-product of their regression, passivity, and withdrawal. We have some specific methods which we use to discourage regression—having the patients keep their own rooms and persons neat, making them get up by a specified hour in the morning, get to their own milieu activities on time, and pick up their own medications from the office at specified times. Some of the patients are encouraged to hold part-time jobs in the community.

One of the major roles of the nurse is to encourage group activities. Although these patients have many things in common—their illness, their common backgrounds, interpersonal problems, and feelings—they resist identification with each other, are very intolerant of one another's problems and characteristics, and do not readily support or try to help each other with their problems. To the staff, they often appear as little islands. A nurse may go from one to another, hearing identical fears and problems. Yet she will be unable to get them to share these with each other or even believe that anyone else could be having any of the same problems. Among the few times the patients function as a group is when they are united against the staff or hospital structure, or at a time of crisis such as the early discharge of another patient who cannot benefit from further treatment at the hospital.

Almost all the group activities, such as picnics or skiing trips, which are initiated by the staff are met with resistance, but the patients are unable to organize or agree on anything themselves. They are much better able to join spontaneous group activities.

Group therapy and ward meetings are more structured ways to encourage group participation. Around the hospital, the patients often use the nurse as a focus for group participation and will join a group where she is present. Although she may try not to take too active a part, it is almost impossible for her to remain very inactive, for the patients direct much of the conversation to her or to others by way of her, and constantly look to her for approval and support. Increased ability to participate in groups is a sign of improvement in most of the patients.

Although the general tone of the hospital is permissive, in the time it has been open the staff has found that they cannot be as permissive as they would like to be. Limit-setting, or enforcing the hospital structure as we call it, has been found to be an important part of the milieu. The patients need consistent, reasonable limits; and although they resist being made to follow rules, they respond favorably to them, showing increased movement in therapy and more confidence in the staff. The structure is emphasized to a greater extent with patients who tend to be more disorganized, such as those who have had acute psychotic episodes.

STAFF PROBLEMS

Those who work closely with patients of any kind are aware of the dangers of overidentification. It is not too infrequent for a nurse who spends several hours a day with a patient to become so involved that she is unable to participate objectively in the patient's treatment. She may, for instance, take the patient's side against the doctor for a seeming injustice. The patients are prone to manipulate and will play any and all staff members against each other if they can. Nurses may fall into the trap of helping a patient act out in a neurotic way against authority if they are not alert or if they do not understand the reason for particular restrictions or treatment plans.

Even with such a small hospital and staff, adequate communication is a problem. Consistency is an important aspect of every patient's treatment and this means that each staff member must be aware of all plans and changes in the general structure and in each patient's treatment plan.

Realizing these problems, the staff tries to minimize them by frequent sharing of ideas and problems at team meetings, staff conferences, and informal contacts during the day. The doctors share information freely with the nursing staff and listen to what the nurses have to offer.

We found very little published material about borderline patients and much of what we know about them now has been gained through our own experiences. During the first year, we had to differentiate between problems which came up because the hospital was new and the staff unaccustomed to working together, and those which were related to the milieu and the kind of patient we were treating.

The Mental Health Center of America was set up as a pilot project for the first year. Statistics about admissions and discharges are still too meager to be meaningful, but the hospital has proved its worth to the people involved in it.

40

Freedom for Patients in Mental Hospitals

Josephine T. Lamb*

When the doors of their wards were unlocked and a program of self-government was organized, patients regained hope and the incentive to strive for recovery.

The idea of ground privileges for patients in mental hospitals is not new. But the idea of mental patients governing themselves and enjoying the freedom of unlocked wards *is* new in Texas state hospitals.

In 1954 the superintendent of Terrell State Hospital appointed a committee to study the possibility of instituting an open-door policy and a program of patient self-government. The primary purpose of the new approach was to develop rehabilitation measures which would help patients achieve independence and prepare them for readjustment to society. He hoped also to strengthen the community's understanding of mental illness by setting up a working example—a demonstration project where patients could prove their ability to solve many of their own problems with a minimum amount of supervision. Included on the committee investigating this approach were a psychiatrist, the directors of the hospital's nursing, rehabilitation and social services, a psychologist, and a chaplain.

After careful study, the committee recommended that two wards, one for men and one for women, be used initially for the project; that patients be carefully screened; and that those chosen to take part receive special ther-

---

*From *American Journal of Nursing*, Vol. 58, No. 3 (March, 1958).

Miss Lamb, a graduate of St. Elizabeths in Washington, D.C., and Texas Christian University, did advanced work in psychiatric nursing at the Catholic University of America. Now central director of nursing service in psychiatry, with the Board for Texas State Hospitals and Special Schools, she was previously director of nursing service in Austin (Texas) State Hospital and Terrell State Hospital, at which the program she describes here was originated.

apeutic help and be encouraged in work, play, and resocializing processes. This, the committee pointed out, would help these patients develop a sense of responsibility toward themselves and toward others, and would establish an atmosphere conducive to the organization of a patient-government program.

Recognizing that replacing old ideas with new ones would meet resistance—especially since the old philosophies and their restrictions were so imbedded in both patients and personnel—the committee suggested that this new approach would need to be carefully explained and clearly defined for all concerned.

The superintendent called together the heads of all departments and asked them to serve as team leaders, supporting this plan through their positive attitudes and active participation. He also outlined the plan to the mayor of the town, who agreed with it and asked the support of the Chamber of Commerce in assuring job placement for patients when they were discharged. Through these efforts the entire town was informed of the project and has continuously supported the program.

Obviously, the inauguration of this plan required strong leadership—a person with authority, persistence, and the strength to uproot some of the residual ideas from the past. The unit psychiatrist was appointed to direct the program, assisted by a professional psychiatric nursing supervisor. They made the following recommendations:

1. That the two wards be cleared of all patients and be redecorated.

2. That the employees on these wards be replaced with a carefully selected staff.

3. That the patients selected for these wards be carefully screened according to their behavior, personal habits, physical condition, and treatments they were receiving prior to transfer. Psychotherapy would be continued on the open wards, but patients on insulin or electroshock therapy would not be accepted until their shock series had been completed.

4. That an orientation in self-government be held for all patients transferred to the open wards, and that a special date be announced for the opening of the doors.

5. That a teaching program be started for the ward personnel. (Each unit was to be staffed by one graduate psychiatric nurse technician and four attendants.)

6. That other members of the hospital team, especially the recreational therapist, occupational therapist, chaplain, psychologist, and dietitian, assist with the program when the psychiatrist felt the patient group was ready for their help.

7. That the psychiatrist, professional nurse, and psychiatric nurse technician hold an initial meeting with the patients to describe the patient-government program and point out what they could or could not do.

8. That the patients study these plans and then work out their own program. The ward personnel, on invitation, would meet with the entire group to offer counsel, encouragement, and support.

9. That either the professional nurse or the psychiatric nurse technician attend every meeting and offer suggestions and guidance when needed; that

the professional nurse spend three to four hours on the ward each day, counseling patients and assisting with the initial planning of their self-government program; that the ward psychiatrist spend one to two hours daily, initiating and then directing the program.

THE PLAN IN EFFECT

The patient-government plan was organized as soon as eligible patients were transferred to the wards. They set up their own daily living program under the guidance of the psychiatrist and the professional nurse. An election of officers was planned and handled strictly by the patients themselves. They chose a chairman, vice-chairman, secretary, treasurer, and a vice-secretary and treasurer, a decorating committee, recreation committee, and hosts and hostesses for each ward. The officers were to hold office for one month; this limit was set to prevent establishment of so much individual influence that it might undermine the program and harm the open ward setup. It soon became clear that the patients themselves were the best guardians of their own rights, however, and that they could handle very adequately any attempt at individual administration. Ward routines and assignments were worked out by the officers of the patient government.

Then came the actual unlocking of the ward. The nurse opened the door and asked, "Who will be the first outside?" For a time there was silence, as the patients stood there, unable to realize that they were actually free to go out alone.

As the restrictions were released, some of the older employees expressed their fear that patients who wished to go home would leave immediately. They were reassured, not only by the confidence of the program's supervisors but by the attitude of the patients. This reassurance has been amply justified. There have been no escapes from the open wards.

The patients' reactions to the open ward were interesting. During the day they were happy and secure, but the women's group requested that their doors be locked at sundown, that no patient be allowed to go out at night alone, and that the grills not be removed from the windows. They set up their own fire safety program and requested safety instructions from the fire chief. This was a definite expression of their insecurity at having to reassume some personal responsibility for themselves and each other.

THE PATIENT'S COUNCIL. The patient-government program operates under the guidance of a joint council of 12 to 14 popularly elected patients. The council, whose members represent both the male and female wards, serves as a clearing house for any dissatisfactions that may arise. These are brought to the attention of the ward psychiatrist or the professional nurse. Once a month, two representatives of the council—one from the male and one from the female ward—meet with the superintendent of the hospital, discuss progress and problems, and then bring the superintendent's comments and suggestions back to the council.

The council functions according to its own formally established constitution and bylaws. Its objectives as set forth in its constitution are:

1. To cheerfully carry out the instructions of proper authorities as expressed through our established channels of instruction.

2. To be responsible for the welfare of each individual patient.
3. To be responsible for the conduct and good behavior of each individual.
4. To be responsible for physical maintenance of the ward.
5. To assist one another in solution of personal problems.
6. To provide entertainment and social activities.
7. To promote the closest possible friendly relationship between our ward attendants and patients.
8. To keep the ward clean, friendly, and homelike.
9. To make of ourselves a model ward.
10. To work in close cooperation with other open wards.

From the very beginning, patients began to plan ways to make their wards more livable and homelike. Seeking more attractive dining rooms, they requested table cloths, china, glass and silverware for their tables, and colorful drapes for all the windows. They were permitted to select the colors for their drapes. Gradually, new furniture, some mirrors, a piano, television sets, and other accessories were added.

From the beginning the hospital's Volunteer Services Council has been most enthusiastic about the patient-government plan. They have supported and motivated the open ward group continuously.

The hospital's volunteer garden club helped to beautify the outside of the buildings. The new attitude and enthusiasm were contagious. Soon other volunteer workers were assisting the patient council with projects as they were introduced.

All patients who are physically able are assigned to work in some department of the hospital in which they have indicated interest; they also participate in some specific hobby or recreational activity. The physical operations of the ward are almost entirely in the hands of patients. They also frequently entertain the patients from closed wards at their open house parties, working out the arrangements with the recreation department. There is always a member of the patient council available to assist in other areas of the hospital when requested.

THE NURSING ROLE. In this democratic plan, geared to the patients' freedom of expression and activities, all the nursing principles are based on good common sense. The emphasis in care is on the encouragement of active participation, resocialization, and the rekindling of educational, occupational, and diversional interests. The aims of the nursing personnel are to:

1. Safeguard the patient by providing competent supervision and control without domination. For example, although patients are free to leave the ward to go to other hospital areas, it is important for the nurses to know where they are so that they can be located readily. The patients themselves recognized this and devised a simple check-out system. A large piece of cardbroad with columns of slots labeled with such headings as "In Ward," "Canteen," "Chapel," "Work" and "O.T." was posted on the bulletin board. Each patient's name is printed on a 3 by 5 card which he fits into the appropriate slot whenever he leaves or returns to the ward. The system works extremely well; the patients are very conscientious about reporting in and out.

2. Provide guidance, but without disturbing the challenge of the patient's struggle toward independence. This involves listening to problems, helping the patient to recognize his errors himself, suggesting approaches for overcoming them, and helping him discover and develop his capacity to make decisions.

3. Develop warm interpersonal relationships with patients, providing constructive reassurance, and demonstrating hopefulness and acceptance.

4. Stimulate the patients' active participation in work, hobby, and recreational activities, helping them to choose the type of activity in each category that will give them satisfaction. Encourage patients to take part in the educational programs available to them—home nursing, art, and music classes, for example.

5. Help all patients to feel that they have an important part in the plan and provide them the opportunity to gain status and recognition.

6. Be keenly observant, recognizing physical or mental symptoms that should be brought promptly to the attention of the physician.

7. Recognize patients' physical needs and encourage their concern with personal appearance and personal hygiene.

8. Assist patients in finding ways to meet economic problems, referring them to other sources of help when indicated.

The nurse needs to understand the treatment each patient is receiving and she has to be able to modify situations quickly and skillfully. In order to do this, she keeps in close touch with the patient's therapist and is aware of his progress and his problems. She also works closely with the social worker in her attempts to overcome difficulties in the patient's home or job situation.

The united effort of the nursing team—the understanding, enthusiasm, and sincere attempts to satisfy patients' needs on the part of all categories of nursing personnel—has been a major factor in the success of the open-door policy.

RESULTS OF THE PROGRAM

Perhaps the most tangible indication of the success of the open-door policy and patient-government program is the marked increase in the discharge rate. To help ease the readjustment of patients who have been discharged, or are about to be, "after care clubs" were organized by the hospital chaplain and are now sponsored by local mental health societies throughout the state. At the weekly meetings of these clubs, former patients find a forum where they can air their problems, talk them over with empathic listeners, and share ideas about ways to solve them. Meetings are conducted by a qualified psychiatric leader—either the hospital chaplain, a psychiatrist, or a psychiatric social worker—who is able to discriminate between healthy and unhealthy trends and can offer some professional guidance. This plan also helps in the follow-up of patients, which has often been difficult in the past.

The open-door policy has stimulated initiative and encouraged teamwork throughout the hospital, especially in the nursing program. The positive response of the nursing personnel to their increased responsibilities has been reflected in hopeful attitudes on the part of both patients and personnel.

The volunteer workers have been most helpful, not only in the services they have given but also in furthering community acceptance of mental illness. Many of them have also been instrumental in finding jobs for patients who were able to work part time and live in the hospital during their period of adjustment.

This program of increased freedom for patients has brought certain needs into sharp focus, however—the need for more specially trained therapists, social workers, and psychiatric nurses; inservice education for all hospital personnel; changes in the state commitment law; education of the public about mental illness; greater use of volunteer workers; continuous patient education programs; and sounder methods for screening and utilizing ancillary personnel.

Certainly, the keys to the success of the open-door policy and patient-government program were the coordination of all hospital services and the personnel's acceptance of the philosophy underlying the program.

The outstanding result of the program—and a source of tremendous satisfaction and continued enthusiasm for all those involved in it—was a group of healthier, happier patients, looking into the future with hope and anticipation instead of at the walls of a locked room.

41

What Is
a Therapeutic Community?

Nathaniel H. Siegel*

Some revealing thoughts on what is and is not "good" for patients.

For every psychiatric inpatient there must be many explicit goals and, to the extent that we have a therapeutic environment, we must evidence the wherewithal to implement these goals.

We might also say that *we* have implicit goals in mind and that certain activities make possible their more effective realization. What is usually not done, but is of the greatest importance, is the formalizing of these implicit goals into explicit ones.

Are we, for example, interested in short-term goals or long-term goals, symptom relief, or characterological change? Do we believe that treating people humanely and giving them decent food and housing is good—whether this does or does not relate to a more favorable prognostic status? Is our primary goal to create high staff morale and stability, and, secondly, the effects this will have on the patient population? Often program changes are primarily directed at one goal, but fashion today demands that we twist the primacy of our goal somewhat and call this "a contribution to the therapeutic milieu."

WHAT IS THERAPEUTIC?

A therapeutic community is one in which the staff deliberately employ all relevant physical and interpersonal elements within a given situational

*From *Nursing Outlook*, Vol. 12, No. 5 (May, 1964).

Dr. Siegel (Ph.D., New York University) has had wide experience in teaching, and has written a number of papers for professional journals. He is presently assistant director, Social Science Activities, New York City Department of Health.

sphere to accomplish for their patients the prescribed goals which they know to be beneficial. The premise which underlies the concept of the therapeutic community is that the total environment, of which a patient is a part, is both influenced by the patient and, in turn, contributes to the patient's own behavior and perception. On the basis of available research, we might thus say that given two identical anxious patients in two different treatment settings —one in which there is friction among staff and the other in which there is none—we could predict that in the friction setting, the patient would be more upset and liable to act out. Stanton and Schwartz have shown in this example that because staff are part of the patient's total environment, their own interpersonal problems become entangled in his treatment and his response to it.[1]

In reviewing the literature on the therapeutic community, I find myself responding in certain ways. First, I take as axiomatic that physiological, psychological, and social stimuli all can affect behavior *to some degree* and, therefore, that any stimulus which registers on the individual is going to have some temporal effects on his behavior. Merely to show that all three spheres are interrelated, or that each affects behavior, I think, at this point, provides no great contribution. For example, we know that if people in a cafeteria are seated at 2-person tables, round tables seating 8, and rectangular tables seating 16, they will communicate differently with each other. The same situation is true if one replaces a straight line of chairs in a ward with some grouped pieces of furniture. The sheer physical aspects of the situation make for different possibilities in communication. A finding, then, that changes in patient communication or structure will occur under altered conditions is, I believe, a gratuitous one at present.

In a similar vein, it is no surprise to find that when patients are taken on trips away from a hospital, they talk much more about things outside of the hospital than they would had they not been away. We very often confuse the fact that a particular program may be related to behavioral changes in patients with the idea that these changes are necessarily therapeutic or nontherapeutic. The changes may be important in their own right; they may be therapeutic, *or they may just be changes.*

To return to the example of the cafeteria, if we discover that by changing the seating arrangement, each person speaks with an average of 3.6 rather than 2.4 persons during a given period of time, is this more therapeutic? Without good evidence for doing so, I think many of us too often think and report that the situation per se—in which more persons are spoken with—is preferable for patients. A more valid judgment would involve the question, "What are you trying to accomplish in this situation for this patient?" If a patient seemed to be in need of additional social relationships, one seating arrangement might be preferable; if he were in need of a more limited and possibly deeper relationship, another seating arrangement might be advisable.

HUMANISM

Other changes have been encouraged because they are concordant with humanistic value schemes. These are directed *toward* making the ward an attractive and livable place, and *away from* stripping the individual of his identity by encouraging him to wear street clothes, and keep the watch, eyeglasses, and other personal items which are meaningful to him. While such changes may be generally therapeutic, and in some cases specifically indicated, one might question the wisdom of *generally* identifying a variety of actions commonly conceived to be "nice," "good," "thoughtful," and "considerate" as therapeutic. The therapist is not being "nice" to a patient when he gives him an electroconvulsive treatment—and yet this procedure may best help to lift the patient's depression. Many medical and psychological procedures are not "kind," and yet clinical and scientific evidence would indicate that they serve the best interest of the patient.

We should be aware, then, that seeming humanistic and moral measures are just that and, unless we *know* that they are therapeutic, we should not cloud the picture by calling them therapeutic. I also believe we call things therapeutic without really knowing that they are, and thus give them a status to which they are not really entitled. I would certainly go along with doing humanistic things because they are humanistic. And if they *are* therapeutic, so much the better. But it is quite conceivable that a humanistic action is nontherapeutic—for example, it may contribute to an institutional syndrome. If aspects of humanism prove to be nontherapeutic and our business is therapy, then it is humanistic for the patient that we not indulge in the layman's idea of humanism. In the last 15 years, there has been a very definite swing toward the moral treatment which existed in the early 1800's and while I generally believe that this is a good thing, I think we have to be pretty sophisticated about its present application.[2]

I believe that there is a tremendous amount that psychiatry can learn from the brain washing techniques employed by the Chinese communists, and reported, for example, by Lifton and Schein.[3] These people appear to have developed some rather potent techniques for thought control and re-education. They represent, however, so noxious a force in the ideas of a democratic nation that we tend to reject what they do—along with how they do it. Yet, for example, as a way to encourage the development of a transference relationship, some of their techniques of sensory isolation would seem to be most applicable to our own settings. The classical psychoanalytical setting—in which a patient lies on a couch with the ceiling or walls in view, in a semi-darkened room, in the presence of a relatively noncommunicative therapist—is a situation which employs aspects of a sensory isolation experience for a desired therapeutic outcome. What appears to be antihumanistic in one setting could certainly be humanistic in another, if this proved to help a disturbed population.

Many changes occur within an institutional setting which simply have the status of being *changes*. Yet, they can affect the therapeutic milieu in a positive or negative sense. Most staffs are mobile in some fashion. People enter and leave employment, are promoted or retire. In some settings, patients are moved to new residences as they get better or worse. Major changes can occur in program and staffing as new persons assume positions of authority. These changes are often labeled "therapeutic" because purposeful changes in events which affect the patient's life are supposed to be of a therapeutic nature. When staff alterations occur, we say that patients can form new and different relationships, and that the patient will be seen with "fresh" eyes. While this may be true at times, we do ourselves an injustice by applying this label without really knowing what the behavioral consequences of the action are, and whether it contributes to the change we wish to see occur.

THE INFLUENCE OF COMMUNICATION

As we look at the literature on the "therapeutic community," it is interesting to note that a large portion of it is concerned with communciation—the quality of communication, techniques for promoting communication between staff and staff, staff and patients, and the quantity of communication.

It is not difficult to explain this interest in communication. We know that interpersonal communication can be a potent behavioral influence, both positively and negatively, and that verbal communication is a major psychotherapeutic treatment device.[4] Certainly psychoanalytic literature suggests that we can function more effectively as therapists if we know what and why *we* are communicating to the patient, as well as understanding what *he* is communicating. Since psychotherapists, and certainly psychoanalysts, occupy status positions within the treatment fraternity, I think that we will increasingly find that other members of the club will integrate aspects of these therapists' roles into their own—with a consequently still greater interest in communication.

For example, much remains to be done to make aides more meaningful members of the therapeutic team. The problem is in developing further educational techniques which are appropriate to the group and their general educative and socio-economic level, and in how to help them develop some sense of professional identification with the "team." Awards and rewards to psychiatric aides are only the start of such recognition. The influence of professionalization is an extremely strong force in society today, and, in the next 20 years, we may well see increasing certification of psychiatric aides who will bring to their positions a variety of *formally* derived housekeeping, nursing, and recreational skills.

Central to our interest in communication is the belief that the more that is known and shared about the patient, his behavior, and the events which touch his life, the more effective will be his treatment. To this end, increasing use has been made of the team approach whereby each member of the team contributes to the patient's treatment program and all members are nominally equal. (I say "nominally" equal because the team normally functions under the direction of a psychiatrist who attempts to interrelate the material in the patient's behalf.)

Certainly open communication between staff members is valuable, but we must bear in mind that team meetings often consume time formerly used in giving direct service to patients. Here, it is important to decide what is the optimum mixture of the staff person's time so that the patient may be helped most. I question whether teams, in blurring the barriers to communication, do not often serve to blur professional identification and the rather distinct, if not traditional, roles an individual can play in the treatment process.

It is not necessary to be rigid about this, but to the extent that there is often an interchange of roles within the treatment team, one may well question what a particular person can do—as a nurse or a group worker—that no other person is trained to do. I tend to believe that the blurring of roles, in a negative sense, often distracts from the rather distinctive contribution one can make to the team from the vantage point of one's particular professional allegiance. This is not to suggest that nurses *who are trained to do so* should not do psychotherapy or lead discussion groups but, in general, the question is, "What can one contribute as a nurse doing psychotherapy, versus a physician doing psychotherapy, or as a nurse leading a discussion group, compared with a group worker leading a discussion group?"

When a person is hospitalized as a patient, he is, in a sense, excused from participating in a number of social roles and responsibilities. His major social responsibility is to get well and become a participating member of society. By virtue of his status as a patient, he must be in a dependent relationship (that is, he depends on someone or something to help him). There is much clinical evidence to indicate that the quality of the dependent relationship that is formed does much to foster the patient's *continued* dependence upon the hospital and the manifestation of an institutional syndrome.

HOSPITALIZATION

A good deal of "therapeutic community literature" reports attempts to increase patient participation and responsibility for life within the hospital. In some settings, patients even have a say as to who will remain in the hospital. In most settings, there is an attempt to have patients take increasing responsibility for their living units (beyond mere housekeeping tasks), and to have a voice in the decorating and operation of their wards and recreational areas. In still other settings, psychotherapy is a group affair, with the goal of actively involving as many patients as possible. One major goal underlying these attempts is to allow for conditions under which patients may act more and more autonomously.

We should now study whether patients who are placed in passive relationships, where their dependency needs are met, evidence any different posthospital behavior than patients who are treated in more active relationships, where their dependency needs are somewhat differently met. In both situations, it is quite conceivable that the hospital may gratify the patient, and an institutional syndrome can occur.

While raising these questions about implicitly assuming the therapeutic value of things, we would observe that, generally, treatment settings which most resemble the world outside of the hospital are considered to be most therapeutic. Also inherent in the establishment of the day hospital is the belief that it will, in the nature of things, be a therapeutic community. This is assumed because it permits patients to live at home, engage in social relationships and other such normative pursuits and wear their civilian dress. In a sense they are semi-patients, having one foot in the hospital, and the other outside it. This is considered to be to their advantage, to the extent that these people can continue nonpatient roles. Increasingly, we must know specifically what we want to accomplish, and that we should be able to document the given effects of a particular program—hopefully ones which are therapeutically better for the patient than the given effects of another program.

ENVIRONMENTAL THERAPY

The idea of specific environmental prescriptions is basically an excellent one, and work in this field should be broadened. The "small group" literature, in the social dynamics area, includes tremendous amounts of material on the kind of responses that one can expect from individuals who are imbedded in a variety of social matrices. The Air Force and Navy have spent millions of dollars to learn what one can expect from persons as they become involved in different social situations. How much of this has found its way into mental hospital practices or literature? Practically none! Possibly social psychologists and sociologists fear to contaminate themselves with an applied discipline and yet, truly, this is an area of great potential.

As nurses attempt to broaden their role-participation within the hospital setting, they might do well to become familiar with such social science data. We know, for example, a good deal about the social conditions under which we can either increase or decrease interpersonal dominance and the conditions which block or contribute to the flow of information. For a true therapeutic community, in which all aspects of the interpersonal situation are controlled, this type of data is of vital importance. It is obvious that environmental therapy, a clinical sociology, constitutes a most exciting area to explore—and, potentially, a very fruitful one if we can but keep an open mind about what we are trying to do, and at what cost we accomplish our goals.

REFERENCES

1. Stanton, A. H., and Schwartz, M. S. *Mental Hospital* New York, Basic Books, 1954.
2. Bockoven, J. Moral treatment in American psychiatry. *J. Nerv. Ment. Dis.* 124:- 167-194; 292-321, Aug., Sept. 1956.
3. Group for the Advancement of Psychiatry. *Methods of Forceful Indoctrination.* (Symposium No. 4) New York, 1957, pp. 234-269.
4. Ruesch, Jurgen. *Disturbed Communication.* New York, W. W. Norton Co., 1957.

42

What Makes
a Ward Climate Therapeutic?

Leonard F. Stevens*

Like the weather, the atmosphere of a hospital ward is affected by many forces—some positive, some negative, some poorly understood.

A therapeutic ward climate is an atmosphere that promotes in patients feelings of security and of being accepted. It carries warmth, inspires confidence in patients and motivates their efforts to help themselves. In such a climate, nursing personnel work well together and with others, show sympathetic interest and enthusiastic effort, and make their maximum contributions to their patients' health goals.

Just what makes the social climate of a ward therapeutic? All of us recognize that the environment is affected by color, noise, movement, heat, light, humidity, order, balance, space and other such physical aspects. No one would question the need to assure optimum physical conditions and to reduce physical hazards to an absolute minimum. But are we as well aware of the forces that affect emotional security?

It is unfortunate that we have not been more concerned with emotional security because patients often desperately need support in this area. Moreover, because of our lack of understanding, some of the methods that we have used to provide security have "backfired" on occasion. In many cases, the anxiety engendered by our actions has been more destructive than the physical or psychological threat we were attempting to reduce. For example, any of the following might be frightening to a patient if the situation were

*From *American Journal of Nursing*, Vol. 61, No. 3 (March, 1961).
Mr. Stevens (McLean Hospital School of Nursing; B.S., M.S., Boston University) is chief of the nursing service at the Veterans Administration Hospital in St. Cloud, Minn.

not handled well: "specialing" the patient, moving him to a private room, moving him closer to the nursing station, screening him, having many medical consultations with bedside discussion, or markedly increasing the amount of physical care with little explanation.

It is difficult to identify all of the factors that enter into providing emotional security for a selected patient because they depend so much on his own personal needs. However, we do know that all patients need to feel that they are accepted and that others are genuinely interested in them as individuals. They need to have confidence in those who are caring for them and to see evidence of real teamwork in their own care and that of the other patients around them. They need to have someone spend sufficient time with them so that they will have an opportunity to "talk through" their doubts, worries, fears, and anxieties when they feel a need to do so.

The over-all philosophy of the hospital has a very strong influence on the affective tone of a nursing unit. A hospital philosophy in which the primary consideration is the patient, and in which all treatment programs are aimed at helping him reach his maximum health goal as easily and quickly as possible, contributes appreciably to a therapeutic climate. The attitude of the hospital toward all its personnel directly affects the relationships the personnel have with patients. The philosophy of nursing service is very intimately bound to the patient-personnel relationship. The objective must be the development of a climate within which patients will receive comprehensive nursing care and nursing personnel will want to make maximum efforts to provide it. In so doing, they will attain maximum personal and professional growth.

Many of us have known hospitals or other health agencies with such strong dynamic traditions of service and treatment that just being in the hospital or associated with the institution was a stimulating experience. Patients feel secure just being in such a place. They seem to sense that "here is help," and they respond accordingly. Personnel readily contribute over and beyond the call of duty. Such traditions of service and care contribute much to a therapeutic ward climate.

How do we determine whether a therapeutic ward climate exists? Is it possible to measure?

Completely satisfactory tools for evaluating a ward climate are not available. However, Margaret Schafer has set down criteria by which we may measure, to some degree at least, how the patients and nursing personnel judge the ward climate.[1] She believes that a patient tends to consider that his nursing care is good when the following occurs:

1. He receives courteous, gentle, considerate care.
2. He believes that the nurses and other hospital personnel are interested in him as an individual and not just another patient.
3. His friends, relatives, and belongings receive careful, thoughtful, considerate care.
4. He has a feeling of security because the hospital staff is interested in his recovery, comfort, health, happiness and general well-being.

---

[1]Schafer, Margaret K. These tests help the hospital to measure nursing quality. *Mod. Hosp.* 75:63-65, July 1950.

5. He is kept clean and comfortable.
6. His treatments and medications are administered skillfully, thoughtfully, considerately, and on time.
7. His nourishment—food and drink—is adequate, tasty, attractively served, on time and when he desires it.
8. He has confidence in the skill and ability of the workers.
9. He is aware of a feeling of happiness and job satisfaction among the workers, with no feeling of unrest.
10. His environment is kept clean and attractive and the general sanitation and orderliness of the hospital are good.

Nursing personnel, Miss Schafer believes, tend to feel they are giving good nursing care when the following conditions exist:

1. The primary consideration of the nursing staff is a humanitarian attitude toward its patients.
2. The hospital buildings are free from hazards, and properly equipped to permit comfort and scientific care to patients.
3. The nursing department organization displays the fundamental principles of good management.
4. The nursing department is composed of a sufficient number of nurses with the necessary qualifications to provide safe, adequate nursing care to all patients.
5. The nursing personnel performance satisfies the physical, mental, emotional and health teaching needs of all patients.

FORCES THAT CREATE OR BUILD

A therapeutic ward climate is dependent to a large degree on the personnel who are regularly working on the nursing unit. It is certainly encouraged by nursing personnel who are reasonably secure and who are deriving considerable satisfaction from their jobs; by nursing personnel who have some understanding of their own needs and of the effect of these needs on their day-by-day relationships; by nursing personnel who have considerable understanding of their patients' needs as manifested in their behavior.

A therapeutic climate offers physical security by providing meticulous attention to both safety and comfort measures.

Finally, a therapeutic climate is one in which communications are good. Effective communications must be practiced if a climate of interpersonal understanding is to be achieved.

DESTRUCTIVE FORCES

Conversely, these are forces which could diminish or destroy the therapeutic quality of the ward climate. For example, tensions or anxieties that interfere with the nursing personnel's ability to put maximum effort into providing good care would be destructive forces. These might include practices that give little or no encouragement to initiative, interest, and superior performance; ineffective communication with resulting delays, misinformation, and rumors; inconsistent personnel policies; supervisory or administrative practices that threaten ego structure and diminish status; and poorly defined work roles or factors that keep an employee from fulfilling his proper role.

It is probable that the forces that create tensions in personnel stimulate a reaction that almost immediately initiates a like reaction in the patients they are caring for. This direct transmittal of anxiety emphasizes the need to establish a working climate that reduces such tensions to a minimum.

There are many other avoidable situations that contribute to patients' anxiety. Hospital practices that fail consistently to consider the patient as a person quickly create tensions. The patient has a right to understand activities that directly affect him and he deserves a clear explanation of his treatment and care. To feel secure, he needs to know certain procedures—how to call for a nurse, what happens to him during fire drills, what has happened to his clothing and property, and so on.

Obvious differences in opinions about his treatment program are disturbing to the patient and cause considerable anxiety. This might be a conflict between the administrative personnel and those more directly involved in medical treatment. Such a situation might arise because of a poorly defined organizational plan, or it might be due to ineffective communication practices. Whatever the basis, it would probably be a serious threat to the patient's emotional security.

A failure to establish realistic recognized boundaries for patients is another cause of considerable anxiety. Patients who are uncertain about limits may need to test their environment repeatedly with behavior that is difficult for the other patients, personnel and even the patient himself to tolerate.

The age-old statement that "man does not live by bread alone" may be appropriately recalled when we consider comprehensive care. Specific treatment and care are, of course, important but the atmosphere in which the patient receives that care will markedly influence its effectiveness.